SIGNS AND SYMPTOMS IN
PEDIATRICS

WALTER W. **TUNNESSEN,** JR., M.D.

Associate Professor of Pediatrics
Johns Hopkins University
School of Medicine
Baltimore, Maryland

SIGNS AND SYMPTOMS IN
PEDIATRICS

SECOND EDITION

J. B. LIPPINCOTT **Philadelphia**

London   Mexico City   New York
St. Louis   São Paulo   Sydney

Acquisitions Editor: J. Stuart Freeman
Sponsoring Editor: Sanford Robinson
Manuscript Editor: Marjory I. Fraser
Indexer: Nancy Newman
Design Coordinator: Susan Hess Blaker
Production Manager: Kathleen P. Dunn
Production Coordinator: George V. Gordon
Compositor: Bi-Comp, Inc.
Printer/Binder: R. R. Donnelley & Sons, Company

Second Edition

6   5   4   3   2

Library of Congress Cataloging-in-Publication Data

Tunnessen, Walter W., 1939-
    Signs and symptoms in pediatrics.

    Includes bibliographies and index.
    1. Children—Diseases—Diagnosis. 2. Children—
Medical examinations. I. Title. [DNLM: 1. Diagnosis,
Differential—in infancy & childhood—handbooks.
2. Pediatrics—handbooks.   WS 39 T926s]
RJ50.T86   1988   618.92′0075   87-2898
ISBN 0-397-50863-8

The author and publisher have exerted every effort to ensure
that drug selection and dosage set forth in this text are in accord
with current recommendations and practice at the time of
publication. However, in view of ongoing research, changes in
government regulations, and the constant flow of information
relating to drug therapy and drug reactions, the reader is urged
to check the package insert for each drug for any change in
indications and dosage and for added warnings and precautions.
This is particularly important when the recommended agent is a
new or infrequently employed drug.

To my wife
NANCY and our children WALTER and ANNE for
their support, patience, and understanding.

PREFACE

The flavor of the first edition has been retained in the second edition. Differential diagnoses are listed for various presenting symptoms and physical signs. The primary purpose of this book remains unchanged as a stimulator of recall to assist in formulating an appropriate diagnosis. Obviously, recall of previously learned information is not the only mode of problem solving. We must constantly expand our diagnostic horizons. Many disorders, unusual and uncommon, must be considered in a complete differential diagnosis; thus, the lists may sometimes seem slightly unwieldly. Clinical judgment should allow one to separate out the more likely diagnostic possibilities. The more common diagnostic possibilities are listed first.

Three new chapters have been added to this edition: Chapter 41, Chronic Rhinitis/Nasal Obstruction; Chapter 83, Abnormal Vaginal Bleeding, and Chapter 92, Fragile Bones/Recurrent Fractures. In addition, almost 500 new entries have been incorporated into the lists.

I deeply appreciate the feedback from colleagues at all levels—faculty peers, practitioners, house officers, and medical students. Your suggestions and also your additions are always welcomed.

Walter W. Tunnessen, Jr., M.D.

PREFACE TO FIRST EDITION

Some of us thrive on lists. There is something about a list of diagnostic possibilities that satisfies that quest for thoroughness in our compulsive souls. How this list fetish began is unclear, but the "peripheral brains"—the small pocket notebooks crammed with facts—that all medical students carried around may certainly have helped to create the list habit.

Those notebooks have since become obsolete. They are rarely in evidence today. Mine has been replaced by an office file, which is far more capable of holding ever-increasing amounts of information. Without the file I may as well cross the River Styx. When faced with a diagnostic challenge, the file is my refuge. From the file other tributaries arise, clues to solving the diagnostic problems. The other tributaries may comprise journal articles, textbooks, lecture notes, and articles torn from "throw-aways."

What comprises clinical judgment? How do physicians solve diagnostic problems? According to Elstein and colleagues,* the primary factor involved in clinical judgment is *recall*—the ability to conjure up stored information from the deep recesses of the mind. The amount of information that can be stored in the "cerebral files" is astonishing: The storage capacity of the human mind over a lifetime is far greater than that of any modern computer. It is the retrieval of the information that presents the challenge. This is where lists come in. Many times, review of a list of possible causes for a particular sign or symptom may stimulate the necessary recall. This information can then be combined with probability, other signs, clinical appearance, and so forth to select the most likely cause.

This book is a distillation of lists, designed to help in the retrieval of stored bits of information from the cerebral recesses. For each particular sign or symptom, a list of diagnostic possibilities is offered. The reader may then employ his problem-solving skills to arrive at a tenable diagnosis.

Obviously, there are signs and symptoms other than those presented in this book; only the most common ones, interspersed with some seen less frequently, have been included. (My own experience will undoubtedly be evident in some of the lists as well as in the choice of the signs and symptoms included.) At the end of many chapters, a brief listing of textbooks or journal articles that might be of particular assistance is also included.

---

* Elstein AS, Shulman LS, Sprafka SA: Medical Problem Solving: An Analysis of Clinical Reasoning. Cambridge, Harvard University Press, 1978

This book, then, is intended to act as a catalyst. In combination with information obtained from the history and physical examination, the list of diagnostic possibilities may encourage a release of that stored knowledge that will help the reader arrive at a definitive diagnosis.

Walter W. Tunnessen, Jr., M.D.

ACKNOWLEDGMENTS

Frank A. Oski, M.D., Professor and Chairman of the Department of Pediatrics, Johns Hopkins University School of Medicine, Baltimore, supplied the primary motivation for this endeavor. His continuing support, encouragement, and example are especially appreciated.

I would also like to express my gratitude to Lewis A. Barness, M.D., my pediatric raison d'etre.

CONTENTS

■■■■■■■ SECTION **2** HEAD

■■■■■■■ SECTION **3** EARS

■■■■■■■ SECTION **4** EYES

■■■■■■■ SECTION **5** NOSE

━━━━━━ **SECTION 10** GASTROINTESTINAL SYSTEM

━━━━━━ **SECTION 11** GENITOURINARY TRACT

━━━━━━ **SECTION 12** BACK

━━━━━━ **SECTION 13** EXTREMITIES

■ SECTION **14** NERVOUS SYSTEM

■ SECTION **15** SKIN

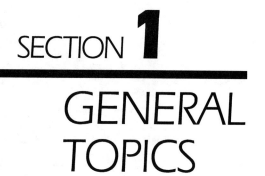

SECTION **1**

GENERAL TOPICS

1

FEVER OF UNDETERMINED ORIGIN

Although fever is a common reason why parents seek medical attention for their children, prolonged fever is a much less frequent complaint. Prolonged fever is generally defined as a temperature of 38.5°C or greater of more than 2 weeks' duration. Fever of undetermined origin (FUO) in this section refers to prolonged fever of undiscernible cause despite careful initial evaluation based on history and physical examination. Some general aspects of FUO are considered first, followed by a list of the most common causes categorized by frequency of occurrence.[1,2]

What temperature is normal? Body temperature depends on many factors, including the time of day, where in the body it is measured, and each person's individual "thermostat setting," and like most other clinical measurements, has a range of normal. With fluctuation associated with the circadian rhythm, body temperature is lowest in early morning and highest in late afternoon. Rectal temperatures are higher than oral temperatures by as much as 0.6°C. Normal rectal temperatures in children may range from 36.2°C (97°F) to 38°C (100.4°F); normal oral temperatures, from 36.0° (96.8°F) to 37.4° (99.3°F). However, although 37.7°C (99.8°F) is quoted as the "normal" rectal temperature, 50% of healthy children may have higher rectal temperatures.

The thermometer is a fairly crude instrument, whose tolerance of error increases at higher temperature levels; nevertheless, it is certainly more accurate than the hand on the forehead. "Low-grade fever," especially as determined by the latter method, occurring in a child every day after school, should be viewed with suspicion: Vigorous physical activity—for example, games such as tag, football, or basketball commonly played on the way home—may temporarily raise body temperature. Temperatures measured too soon after meals may similarly give a false impression of fever. Anxiety can also produce minor temperature elevations. Over-wrapping with clothing may interfere with normal heat escape. Evaluation should rule out these physiologic causes of increased body temperature.

Common causes of prolonged fever in children differ from those in adults. As noted in the study of Pizzo and colleagues,[1] the causes in children over 6 years of age also differ from those in children under 6. Most cases of prolonged fever in children are not due to unusual or esoteric disorders. The majority represent atypical manifestations of common diseases. Similarly, most children with prolonged fever do not have serious diseases or disorders untreatable by ordinary methods.

Differential diagnosis of FUO may be simplified by the following categorization of possible causes.

I. Infectious Causes (40%)

The leading category of causes in FUO in both the report by Pizzo and colleagues[1] and that of McClung[2] was infection. The former attributed infectious causes to 52% of 100 children; the latter, to 29%. A combined list of reported disorders from the two studies, ranking the most common first, follows.

"Viral syndrome"	Osteomyelitis
Urinary tract infection	Septicemia
Pneumonia	Tracheobronchitis
Pharyngitis (chronic)	Pulmonary histoplasmosis
Sinusitis	Brucellosis
Meningitis	Salmonella gastroenteritis
Streptococcosis (chronic)	Malaria
Endocarditis	Peritonsillar abscess
Infectious mononucleosis	Generalized herpes simplex
Tuberculosis	Typhoid fever

II. Collagen–Vascular Disorders (15%)

Rheumatoid arthritis
Systemic lupus erythematosus
Rheumatic fever
Henoch–Schönlein syndrome
Unclassified

III. Neoplastic Disorders (7%)

Leukemia
Reticulum cell sarcoma
Lymphoma
Neuroblastoma

IV. Inflammatory Diseases of Bowel (4%)

Regional enteritis
Ulcerative colitis

V. Undiagnosed (12%)

Three fourths of the cases of FUO in the two studies were assigned to these five categories; the remainder were sprinkled among a mixture of disorders. Noteworthy, however, was a rather large group of 21 patients labeled "no diagnosis established; evidence of resolving disease" as the probable cause of FUO by McClung. Of these patients, 9 were thought to have repeated upper respiratory tract infection (URI). Whether a child has had repeated URI or back-to-back infections of bacterial or viral cause, this possibility must be considered before an extensive investigation for FUO is undertaken. In 3 other patients, recent infectious hepatitis was the probable cause; in another 2, drug fever; and in 4 more, "streptococcal syndromes."

For those readers who desire further diagnostic stimulation, fuel for roundsmanship, or "I once saw a case of . . . ," the following category is included.

VI. Miscellaneous Causes

Factitious (by either child or parents)
Drug fever
Hepatitis, anicteric or chronic active
Central nervous system fever, an "altered thermostat"
Dehydration due to diabetes insipidus or diabetes mellitus
Salicylate toxicity (chronic)
Abscesses, including retroperitoneal, intracranial, subphrenic, hepatic, and perinephric
Ectodermal dysplasia
Ichthyosis
Familial dysautonomia
Congenital sensory neuropathy
Cyclic neutropenia
Familial Mediterranean fever
Hyperthyroidism
Virilizing adrenal hyperplasia
Infantile cortical hyperostosis (Caffey disease)
Allergy
Subdural hematoma
Rat-bite fever
Leptospirosis
Cat-scratch disease
Psittacosis
Sarcoidosis
Diskitis
Dermatomyositis
Periarteritis nodosa
Serum sickness
Other tumors
Acquired immune deficiency syndrome

This list is not complete; however, remember that most causes of FUO are not unusual, although their presentations may be atypical. In the study of Pizzo and colleagues,[1] the history or physical examination suggested or indicated the final diagnoses in 62 of 100 cases. The pattern, height, or duration of the fever did not relate to the final diagnosis or the severity of disease with any significance, nor did symptoms such as anorexia, fatigue, weight loss, toxic appearance, or response to antipyretics.

Careful re-examination, attention to detail, review of historical information, and, of course, time are the most helpful tools in differential diagnosis of FUO.

REFERENCES

1. Pizzo PA, Lovejoy FH, Smith DH: Prolonged fever in children: review of 100 cases. Pediatrics 55:468, 1975
2. McClung HJ: Prolonged fever of unknown origin in children. Am J Dis Child 124:544, 1972

SUGGESTED READINGS

Cone TE Jr: Diagnosis and treatment: children with fevers. Pediatrics 43:290, 1969
Dinarello CA, Wolff SM: Pathogenesis of fever in man. N Engl J Med 298:607, 1978

2

HYPOTHERMIA

Hypothermia refers to the state in which the core body temperature falls below 35°C (95°F). The reduction in temperature reflects a negative balance between heat production and heat loss. The immature infant is especially susceptible to the whims of his environment, but all infants are much more likely to have subnormal body temperatures associated with other insults or derangements ranging from hypoxia and infection to metabolic and endocrinologic problems.

I. Environmental Factors

Hypothermia may occur rather quickly in newborns, especially those delivered in air-conditioned rooms or those exposed to room temperature before amniotic fluids have dried off. Immature or sick infants must be maintained in a thermoneutral environment, a critical factor in their survival.

Older infants, children, and adults may all become hypothermic when exposed to low wind chill factor or immersion with rapid heat loss.

II. Shock

The body temperature may fall dramatically during states of shock. Dehydration, infection, hemorrhage, intestinal obstruction, and trauma may be precipitating causes.

III. Central Nervous System Insults

Hypothermia may reflect severe insult to the central nervous system, particularly when the central temperature-regulating mechanism in the hypothalamic area is involved.

A. Intracranial Hemorrhage or Infarction

B. Trauma (Including Surgical)

C. Severe Birth Asphyxia

D. Tumors
  1. Cranio-
     pharyngioma
                        Hypothalamic disturbances may include hy-
                        perthermia or hypothermia, as well as somno-
                        lence, hypertension or hypotension, obesity,
                        and inappropriate secretion of antidiuretic
                        hormone. The cardinal signs of this tumor are
                        increased intracranial pressure, visual defects,
                        endocrine dysfunction, and the hypothalamic
                        effects.
  2. Astrocytoma
E. Cerebral Malfor-
   mations
  1. Anencephaly
  2. Congenital
     Absence of
     the Corpus
     Callosum
     (Shapiro Syn-
     drome)
                        Children with absence of the corpus callosum
                        may have mild chronic hypothermia or recur-
                        rent attacks of hypothermia associated with
                        mutism or coma. Onset of clinical signs may
                        be delayed until childhood or adolescence.

IV. Infection
Hypothermia is more likely to occur in infants than in older children.
A. Meningitis
B. Encephalitis
C. Sepsis
                        Generalized infection, especially with gram-
                        negative organisms, may significantly lower
                        body temperature.

V. Endocrine–Metabolic Disorders
Subnormal temperatures or impaired temperature regulation may
occasionally occur in these disorders.
A. Addison Disease
B. Hypothyroidism
C. Hypopituitarism
D. Hypoglycemia
                        In infants hypoglycemia may cause hypother-
                        mia, or hypothermia may precipitate hypogly-
                        cemia.
E. Amino/Organic
   Acidurias
                        Occasionally infants with these inborn errors
                        may have hypothermia as part of their tenu-
                        ous metabolic state.

VI. Energy–Protein Undernutrition
In children with kwashiorkor, body temperature may fall below 35°C
despite a high environmental temperature. This risk is highest during
the first week of hospitalization.

VII. Drugs

Heavy sedation from drugs may result in subnormal body temperature.

A. Alcohol
B. Narcotics
C. Barbiturates
D. Phenothiazines
E. Atropine
F. Acetaminophen Overdose

VIII. Miscellaneous Causes

A. Familial Dys-autonomia	This is an autosomal-recessive disorder occurring predominantly in people of Jewish extraction. In addition to altered temperature regulation, features include decreased or absent lacrimation, emotional lability, relative indifference to pain, postural hypotension, and poor muscular coordination.
B. Menkes Kinky-Hair Syndrome	Symptoms usually appear in the first few months of life. Major motor seizures, developmental delay, and the characteristic coarse, short, twisted hair are prominent features.
C. Water Intoxication	Infants fed inappropriately dilute formulas may develop seizures, probably from hyponatremia. Altered sensorium and hypothermia are often present.

3

FAILURE TO THRIVE

The infant or child who is failing to thrive is a common diagnostic challenge to all physicians who care for children. The possible causes encompass malfunction in any of the organ systems of the body as well as nutritional, environmental, social, and psychological factors. Failure to thrive (FTT) is defined as deviation of growth away from previously established channels for weight or height or both, or as weight or height at least two standard deviations below the mean for children of that age.

The index of any textbook of pediatrics may be used as a differential diagnosis of disorders associated with FTT. The lengthy classification below, by no means exhaustive, has been designed to reinforce the concept that the possible causes involve all systems. Obviously the history and physical examination are important, because each may provide evidence that excludes some processes or points to others as causes of this symptom. Growth charts are valuable, particularly if sequential records allow multiple points along the growth curve to be plotted. A sudden deviation from an established growth pattern should focus attention on different disorders from those suggested by a curve that demonstrates a continuing gradual deviation or one that has always been below the third percentile for growth. The prenatal onset of growth retardation should suggest causes other than those for postnatal-onset FTT.

Laboratory methods have been relied on too frequently in the differential diagnosis of FTT. Overuse of blood and radiographic tests should be condemned. The yield from these studies is low, the expense is high, and their performance may interfere with careful consideration of the information already at hand. In a longitudinal study reported by Lacey and Parkin in 1974,[1] 82% of children with growth retardation had no evidence of an organic disease. Of 23 children with organic disease, only in 3 was the disease asymptomatic; 1 had probable growth-hormone deficiency, 1 had early chronic renal failure, and 1 a chromosomal abnormality. The history and physical examination deliver the most useful information. Other studies have reported up to a 50% incidence of organic disease in children with the symptom of FTT. The source of the study populations, however, must be considered: In a referral center, for example, it is more likely that organic causes of FTT will constitute a larger percentage. In a primary-care setting most children will have nonorganic causes of FTT.

The nonorganic causes of FTT are normal variants and nutritional deprivation. However, children who fall below the third percentile for height because of genetic endowment may be inappropriately labeled as having FTT. Evaluation should include determination of parental and grandparental stature. In these children, the bone age is equivalent to chronologic age. The superb study by Smith and colleagues clearly demonstrates that the deceleration in growth seen after the first 3 to 6 months of life in many infants may reflect the genetic growth factors passed on by their parents.[2] A new growth channel is achieved at a mean age of 13 months. In older children, delayed adolescence (constitutional delay) may be responsible for the shift in growth channels. A history of similar pubertal delay in one of the parents may occasionally be reported. With delayed adolescence, the bone age is appropriate for the height age (the age at which the child's measured height is at the 50th percentile on standard growth curves), but both are less than the chronologic age of the child.

Nutritional deprivation as a nonorganic cause of FTT represents a variety of diagnoses, but all have in common a lack of adequate caloric intake for one reason or another. Worldwide, caloric deprivation on an economic basis is the most common cause of FTT. More common in this country, however, are psychosocial factors accounting for deficient caloric intake. An excellent general outline of psychosocial FTT was written by Barbero and Shaheen in 1967.[3] Their diagnostic criteria for "environmental FTT" included the following:

- Weight below the third percentile with accelerated gain during appropriate nurturing. (The height is generally less affected than weight.)
- Developmental retardation with subsequent acceleration of development following appropriate stimulation and feeding.
- No evidence of systemic disease or abnormality. Laboratory investigation is also unrevealing.
- Clinical signs of deprivation that improve in a more nurturing environment. Signs include poor hygiene, cradle cap, diaper rash, and impetigo.
- Significant environmental psychosocial disruption in the family, such as alcoholism, unwanted pregnancies, or marital discord. It is often difficult to extract this kind of information on first contact with the parents.

In addition to these five diagnostic criteria, Barbero and Shaheen described four clinical patterns of "environmental FTT"[3]: Group I has signs of FTT without obvious symptoms or signs of systemic disease, but with the presence of family discord. Group II has FTT with various clinical manifestations such as vomiting, diarrhea, neuromuscular disorders, or recurrent infections, but these symptoms do not account for the FTT. Group III has FTT associated with signs of abuse; Group IV demonstrates FTT with underlying primary systemic disease that does not account for the growth disturbance. Examples of Group IV include the infant with a poor start such as a premature infant separated from the mother, or the infant with a cleft lip or congenital heart disease. With adequate nurturing, in a hospital setting perhaps, the infant begins to thrive. Too frequently, the infant with FTT admitted for evaluation is subjected to a multitude of tests that can interfere with adequate nurturing. The infant who undergoes successive radiologic examinations and blood tests during hospitalization may continue to lose weight. Observation, tender care, and stimulation by a team of health professionals (nurses, aides, and social workers) are critical. A difficult task in cases of "environmental FTT" is finding appropriate support systems for the family.

Psychosocial deprivation, like any other disorder, has a spectrum of clinical presentations. The most severe and bizarre form is labeled "deprivation dwarfism." Reversible growth-hormone insufficiency may be associated with its macabre symptoms and behavior.[4,5]

The reason for the emphasis here on normal variants and nutritional deprivation should be obvious to all who have cared for children in a primary-care setting. These two categories account for most children with FTT, perhaps as many as 90%. The myriad of other causes make up a small proportion of the total group. In addition, the organic causes usually have signs and symptoms that direct attention to them. Few of these causes are truly hidden. Nevertheless, the etiologic classification follows.

I. Normal Variants

A. Familial (Genetic) Factors — Height and weight are proportionately below the third percentile and follow the growth curves, though below it. The history and physical examinations do not suggest organic disease. Short stature is usually uncovered in the family history. The bone age equals the chronologic age.

B. Constitutional Factors

1. Early-Onset Growth Retardation — Length and weight are within the normal range at birth, but deviation away from previously established growth curves begins at 3 to 6 months of age. An acceptable growth pattern resumes before 2 years of age. The head circumference is normal, and the history and physical examination are unrevealing, except for occasional similar patterns in other family members. The bone age may be slightly retarded.

2. Delayed Adolescence — Children in this group fail to demonstrate the normal pubertal growth spurt until much later in adolescence. History and physical examina-

tion are unrevealing except for signs of delayed puberty and perhaps a similar pattern of growth in relatives. The bone age equals the height age, demonstrating potential for future growth.

II. Nutritional Deprivation (Inadequate Intake)

A. Caloric Deprivation	Signs of insufficient or inappropriate intake may be obvious or subtle. A careful feeding history must be obtained.
B. Psychosocial Factors	
1. "Environmental FTT"	This is an important, common cause of FTT, especially in children under 3 years of age. Factors include maternal depression and family disruption. The child's weight is affected before length.
2. "Deprivation Dwarfism"	This striking syndrome of FTT is associated with unusual behavior of the child, significant family psychosocial disruption, and endocrinologic aberrations.

III. Renal Disease

A. Urinary Tract Infection	Even when systemic symptoms are absent, a urine culture should be part of the evaluation in all children with FTT. Vomiting and diarrhea are common presenting symptoms in young infants and children.
B. Renal Tubular Acidosis	Several different types of renal tubular acidosis (RTA) have been described. Proximal RTA may present only with FTT clinically, with hyperchloremic acidosis apparent on laboratory studies. In distal RTA, polyuria, polydipsia, and recurrent episodes of dehydration may also be noted. Hyperchloremic acidosis with a urinary pH that fails to drop below 7.0 is typical.
C. Chronic Renal Insufficiency	
1. Congenital Obstructive Uropathy	Obstructive uropathy may go unnoticed until growth failure becomes evident. Patients with posterior urethral valves may have few symptoms until renal failure occurs.

2. Primary Hyperoxaluria (Oxalosis)

Renal failure, nephrolithiasis, and hematuria occur with deposition and excretion of calcium oxalate.

D. Malformations or Cystic Disease

Enlarged kidneys or an abdominal mass may be palpable.

E. Diabetes Insipidus

Polyuria and a low urinary specific gravity despite dehydration are important clues. There may be episodes of unexplained fever.

IV. Cardiorespiratory Disease

A. Upper Airway Obstruction

Chronic partial obstruction of the upper airway from enlarged tonsils and adenoids may lead to chronic hypoxemia, with resulting pulmonary hypertension and eventually cor pulmonale.

B. Congenital Heart Disease

Chronic hypoxemia or congestive heart failure may interfere with growth.

C. Myocardiopathy

D. Acquired Heart Disease
   1. Endocarditis
   2. Myocarditis

E. Mulibrey Nanism

This is an unusual syndrome that features short stature, a characteristic facies, and hepatomegaly secondary to constrictive pericarditis.

F. Chronic Lung Disease
   1. Asthma

Severe asthma in young children may interfere with growth for several reasons; however, this condition may obscure psychosocial causes of FTT.

   2. Bronchiectasis

Bronchiectasis may follow pneumonia or aspiration and occurs in immunocompromised patients.

   3. Bronchopulmonary Dysplasia

The neonatal history is essential for diagnosis.

   4. Cystic Fibrosis

In young infants respiratory or gastrointestinal symptoms may be subtle. Cystic fibrosis must always be considered in an infant who is failing to thrive despite a voracious appetite.

V. Gastrointestinal Factors

A. Upper Tract
   Disorders

   1. Cleft Palate
      or Lip

      The severity of the anomaly may interfere occasionally with adequate nutritional intake. Parental reaction to the clefting may also be a factor in FTT. The possibility of other associated defects should be considered.

   2. Esophageal
      Compression

   3. Gastroesophageal Reflux

      A variety of presentations with or without vomiting may occur in gastroesophageal reflux (GER). Recurrent wheezing, coughing or pneumonitis, "colic," apneic episodes, and anemia are but a few.

   4. Hiatal Hernia

      The patient may have symptoms such as those in GER. Torsion spasms of the neck (Sandifer syndrome) may be a clue.

B. Pyloric Stenosis

   Projectile vomiting with epigastric distension usually makes the diagnosis obvious.

C. Enzymatic Deficiencies

   Patients with lactase, fructase, maltase–isomaltase, and other enzyme deficiencies generally present with chronic diarrhea.

D. Cystic Fibrosis

   Examination of the stool for steatorrhea is indicated in suspected cases.

E. Celiac Disease

   Chronic diarrhea, FTT, and irritability with abdominal distension suggest celiac disease in the differential diagnosis. However, up to 30% of patients have no diarrhea. Flattened villi are found on intestinal biopsy.

F. Pancreatic Disorders

   Chronic pancreatitis from infection or trauma or, more rarely, pancreatic insufficiency with neutropenia (Schwachman syndrome) may produce FTT.

G. Food Sensitivity
   or Intolerance

   Expressions include diarrhea, vomiting, and abdominal pain and distension.

H. Hepatic Disorders

   1. Hepatitis

      Congenital as well as acquired infections, metabolic disorders, and certain drugs may produce chronic hepatic inflammation.

   2. Cirrhosis

      A variety of disorders, both acquired and inherited, may result in cirrhosis.

I. Biliary Disorders

    1. Biliary Atresia — Prolonged and increasing jaundice suggests biliary atresia.

    2. Choledochal Cyst

J. Inflammatory Bowel Disease

    1. Regional Enteritis — Symptoms other than weight loss, such as diarrhea, fever, abdominal pain, and an abdominal mass, may not be evident.

    2. Ulcerative Colitis — Diarrhea, often bloody, with tenesmus is characteristic.

K. Hirschsprung Disease — The chronic constipation may be obscured by intermittent loose stools.

VI. Endocrine Disorders

A. Thyroid Disorders — Hyperthyroidism and hypothyroidism may both produce FTT.

B. Pituitary Disorders — Hypopituitarism may not be noticeable until late in the first year of life when the child's growth rate drops off. Hypoglycemic episodes and micropenis may be early clues.

C. Adrenal Disorders

    1. Adrenal Insufficiency — Lethargy, fatigue, and increased pigmentation with hyperkalemia and hyponatremia suggest this diagnosis.

    2. Adrenocortical Excess (Cushing Syndrome) — Cushing syndrome may result from exogenous steroid therapy, a primary adrenal tumor, or a central nervous system problem. The child's growth velocity falls off, but truncal obesity is prominent.

D. Diabetes Mellitus — Juvenile-onset diabetes is usually rapid in development. Glucosuria is easily detected with urine dipsticks.

E. Parathyroid Disorders — Tetany and seizures secondary to hypocalcemia are common presenting symptoms.

F. Sexual Precocity — Early closure of epiphyses leads to ultimate short stature.

G. Hyperaldosteronism — Muscle weakness, hypertension, and low serum potassium levels suggest hyperaldosteronism.

VII. Central Nervous System Disorders
  A. Chronic Sub-
      dural Hema-
      toma
  B. Cerebral Insults
      1. Anoxia
      2. Trauma
      3. Vascular
          Bleed or
          Thrombosis
      4. Infection
  C. Degenerative   Neurologic abnormalities overshadow the FTT.
      Disorders
  D. Diencephalic   This striking disorder is usually caused by a
      Syndrome   tumor in the area of the third ventrical and
                         results in severe weight loss with euphoria,
                         vertical nystagmus, and papilledema. "Hand-
                         edness" in an infant prior to 18 months of age
                         may be an early sign of a central nervous sys-
                         tem tumor.

VIII. Skeletal Disorders
  A. Chondrodystro-   Various disorders have been described but are
      phies   generally associated with short stature rather
                         than FTT.
  B. Rickets
      1. Vitamin-D
          Deficiency
      2. Vitamin D-
          Resistant
  C. Osteopetrosis   In osteopetrosis marble bones, pallor, and
                         splenomegaly may be early findings.

IX. Chronic Infections or Infestation
  A. Tuberculosis
  B. Parasites
  C. Recurrent Infec-   Infants with school-age siblings may be sub-
      tions   jected to recurrent infections.

X. Intoxications
  A. Lead
  B. Mercury   Poisoning is uncommon, but signs are dra-
                         matic, including irritability, hypotonia, photo-
                         phobia, and a macular eruption.

C. Hypervitamin- osis	Vitamin A excess may cause irritability, in- creased intracranial pressure, and bone pain.
D. Fetal Exposure	
1. Anticonvul- sants	The fetal hydantoin syndrome may include impressive FTT with other phenotypic abnor- malities.
2. Alcohol	Features of the fetal alcohol syndrome may not be striking. Prenatal onset of growth defi- ciency, microcephaly, and short palpebral fis- sures are best recognized.

XI. Metabolic Disorders

A. Galactosemia	The combined symptoms of vomiting, diar- rhea, jaundice, and FTT mandate urine exami- nation to detect reducing substance.
B. Hypercalcemia	
C. Amino-Acid and Organic-Acid Disorders	Recurrent episodes of lethargy, poor appetite, vomiting, seizures, or stupor suggest amino- acid or organic-acid disorders.
D. Storage Disease	Phenotypic and physical abnormalities suggest the possibility of a storage disorder.
1. Mucopolysac- charidoses	
2. Lipidoses	
3. Glycogenoses	
E. Acrodermatitis Enteropathica	Diarrhea, hair loss, and acral, perianal, and perioral rashes are commonly found.
F. Dietary Chloride Deficiency	This deficiency has been described in formula errors as well as one case of inadequate chlo- ride in breast milk. Additional features include anorexia, hypotonia, metabolic alkalosis, and low serum electrolytes.

XII. Chronic Anemias

A. Iron Deficiency Anemia	
B. Thalassemia Major	Hepatosplenomegaly is an early and progres- sive finding.
C. Sickle Cell Ane- mia	

XIII. Primordial Dwarfism

The onset of growth failure may be *in utero* or shortly after birth secondary to genetic, infectious, or undetermined insults.

  A. Placental Insuffi-
    ciency

B. Chromosomal Disorders

C. Congenital Infection

D. Dysmorphogenetic Syndromes — All children with FTT should be examined closely for phenotypic abnormalities that may suggest described syndromes of malformation.

XIV. Miscellaneous Disorders

A. Malignancies — Patients with occult tumors occasionally present with FTT before associated symptoms surface.

    1. Vasoactive Intestinal Peptidase-Secreting Tumors — Infants with these tumors present with growth failure, intermittent diarrhea, soiling, and, occasionally, flushing, sweating, and hypertension. The tumors are generally ganglioneuromas and ganglioneuroblastomas.

B. Reticuloendothelioses — Skin rashes, adenopathy, and bony lesions suggest disorders in this category.

C. Immune Deficiency Disorders — Recurrent infections, often with unusual organisms that are difficult to control, are common.

D. Collagen–Vascular Disorders — Chronic inflammation may lead to FTT.

    1. Juvenile Rheumatoid Arthritis

    2. Systemic Lupus Erythematosus

    3. Dermatomyositis

    4. Periarteritis Nodosa

E. Muscular Dystrophy — Failure to thrive may be an early sign of Duchenne muscular dystrophy.

F. Acquired Immune Deficiency Syndrome — Opportunistic infections, diffuse lymphadenopathy, and hepatosplenomegaly are common findings.

The list of causes could go on, but enlargement would serve no useful purpose. Remember that categories I and II account for perhaps 80% to 90% of causes of FTT in a primary-care setting. Extensive laboratory testing should be avoided. The most effective diagnostic tools are a careful history and physical examination, sequential growth records, determination of parental stature, and evaluation for psychosocial problems.

REFERENCES

1. Lacey KA, Parkin JM: Causes of short stature; a community study of children in Newcastle-upon-Tyne. Lancet 1:42, 1974
2. Smith DW, Truog, W, Rogers JE et al: Shifting linear growth during infancy: Illustration of genetic factors in growth from fetal life through infancy. J Pediatr 89:225, 1976
3. Barbero GJ, Shaheen E: Environmental failure to thrive: A clinical view. J Pediatr 71:639, 1967
4. Silver HK, Finkelstein M: Deprivation dwarfism. J Pediatr 70:317, 1967
5. Powell GF, Brasel JA, Blizzard RM: Emotional deprivation and growth retardation simulating idiopathic hypopituitarism. N Engl J Med 276:1272, 1967

SUGGESTED READING

Cupoli JM, Hallock JA, Barness LA: Failure to thrive. Curr Prob Pediatr X, No 11, Sept 1980

4

TALL STATURE AND ACCELERATED GROWTH

Accelerated linear growth and tall stature are much less frequent complaints than is short stature. Most children who grow more rapidly than their peers do so because of their genetic potential. A careful analysis of family growth patterns is usually rewarding. A careful physical examination should be performed to look for signs of precocious sexual development. An assessment of skeletal maturation by means of roentgenograms of the hand and wrist should be made.

I. Physiologic Causes

Constitutional Factors	Most children who grow rapidly and attain what is perceived as excessive stature usually do so because of genetic predisposition. There is no underlying organic abnormality. The problems that arise are psychological ones: Tall men are accepted readily in society; therefore, tall boys are not usually seen for medical evaluation. Parents, however, are often concerned if their daughters seem to be growing at excessive rates.

II. Endocrinologic Causes

A. Precocious Puberty	Children with early onset of puberty grow more rapidly than do their peers, but their ultimate height is not excessive. (For causes, see Chap. 80, Precocious Puberty.)
B. Congenital Adrenal Hyperplasia	This inherited disorder should be suspected in any child with excessive linear growth and signs of virilization or ambiguous genitalia. Muscle mass is usually increased and skeletal maturation advanced. If the disorder is not treated, the ultimate adult height is diminished because of early closure of epiphyses.

C. Hyperthyroidism | There is usually an initial growth spurt in children with untreated hyperthyroidism. Most patients present with tachycardia, systolic hypertension, restlessness, weight loss, heat intolerance, tremors, and frequent stools.

D. Gigantism and Acromegaly | Gigantism occurs if there is excessive secretion of growth hormone before epiphyseal closure. In both gigantism and acromegaly, an anterior pituitary tumor is usually responsible; significant enlargement of the hands and feet occurs with coarsening of facial features. The bone age is not advanced. The jaw becomes markedly prominent in acromegaly but less so in gigantism.

III. Chromosomal Abnormalities

A. Klinefelter Syndrome | This syndrome should be considered in males who are relatively tall and slim and have hypogonadism. The limbs tend to be long, and the penis and testes small. Gynecomastia occurs in 40% of the cases during adolescence. The karyotype is XXY.

B. XYY Karyotype | There are no diagnostic phenotypic features except for tall stature. Severe personality disorders seem to be common.

IV. Miscellaneous Causes

A. Marfan Syndrome | Children with this autosomal-dominant disorder have a tendency toward tall stature. Long limbs, joint laxity, pectus deformities, subluxation of the lenses, scoliosis, and aortic dilation are characteristic features.

B. Homocystinuria | The clinical picture in this disorder inherited as an autosomal-recessive trait resembles that in Marfan syndrome. Arachnodactyly, pectus deformities, subluxation of lenses, and aortic degeneration are common. The hair tends to be sparse, dry, and light in color. A malar flush is often present; arterial and venous thromboses are common. Over half of affected individuals have mental deficiency.

C. Beckwith–Wiedemann Syndrome | Infants with this syndrome tend to be large at birth or grow rapidly after the neonatal period. Omphalocele or umbilical hernia and macroglossia are often present. Hypoglycemia is common in the neonatal period. The skeletal age is advanced. Renal or adrenal tumors occur in significant numbers.

D. Cerebral Gigantism
Children with cerebral gigantism have marked acceleration of growth in infancy and acromegalic features; macrocephaly and developmental and mental retardation are common. The palate is high and arched, and the face is long with frontal bossing, hypertelorism, and an antimongoloid slant to the eyes. The bone age is advanced.

E. Lipodystrophy
Children with generalized lipodystrophy have accelerated growth with enlargement of the hands and feet. The loss of subcutaneous tissue creates a muscular appearance. Hepatomegaly with abdominal distension is common.

F. Marshall Syndrome
The few cases reported have had accelerated linear growth with failure to gain weight. The bone age is advanced prenatally. The facial appearance is unusual, featuring a prominent forehead, elongated skull, shallow ocular orbits, upturned nose, and bluish sclerae.

G. Weaver Syndrome
This rare syndrome is associated with accelerated growth and prenatal advancement of skeletal maturation. The infants described have an unusual appearance characterized by large ears, ocular hypertelorism, mild micrognathia, broad thumbs, and broad forehead. Limited knee and elbow extension and mild hypertonia, with signs of delayed development, are other features.

H. Proteus Syndrome
A rare disorder in which affected children have asymmetric growth. An unusual thickening of the skin and subcutaneous tissue leads to gyriform convolutions, especially of the feet.

5

ANOREXIA

A brief loss of appetite commonly occurs during acute infections. Prolonged anorexia, accompanied by weight loss or poor weight gain, usually denotes a serious underlying organic or psychological disorder.

The hypothalamus is thought to be the center of appetite control, but the stimuli that influence this control are poorly understood. Nevertheless, the differential diagnosis of anorexia may be simplified by the following categorization into ten groups, including infection, psychosocial factors, and specific disease.

I. Infection

A. Acute Infection	Acute infection, whether bacterial, viral, or of other types, is the most common cause of anorexia in children. Generally, the diminished appetite is short-lived and coincident with the illness.
B. Chronic Infection	Chronic infections may be associated with anorexia over prolonged periods of time, with resulting poor weight gain or weight loss. Pyelonephritis, hidden abscesses, chronic lung infections, tuberculosis, amebiasis, and many other subacute or occult infections may be responsible.

II. Psychosocial Factors

A. Parental Expectations	The parents may have unrealistic expectations about food consumption by the child, especially the toddler, whose caloric requirements diminish with the deceleration in growth rate normally seen in this age group. The small but normal child may be perceived as anorectic by the parents, who want him to grow beyond his genetic capacity.
B. Parental Pressures	Children may respond to parental overconcern about eating by refusing to eat.
C. Response to Stress	Fear, anger, depression, and mania may result in diminished food intake. Family discord,

meal-time disruption, and unpleasantness may also affect the appetite.

D. Anorexia Nervosa
This striking disorder occurs much more frequently in adolescent girls than boys. Hallmarks in girls include amenorrhea, weight loss, and the maintenance of or an increase in physical activity. Onset often follows a change in the child's life such as during trips, separations from the family, or school changes, or an awareness of parental discord. Bradycardia, low blood pressure, and constipation are common. Plasma cortisol levels are usually increased in this disorder, whereas they are decreased in adrenal insufficiency.

E. Pregnancy
Anorexia and morning sickness may be present in the early months of pregnancy.

F. Psychiatric Disturbances
Anorexia may be present in various forms of mental illness including major depressive disorders, schizophrenia, and paranoid disorders.

III. Metabolic and Endocrine Disorders

A. Liver Failure
Disorders associated with significant acute or chronic insult to the liver may be associated with anorexia.

B. Renal Failure

C. Adrenocortical Insufficiency (Addison Disease)
Adrenocortical insufficiency may be associated with anorexia, fatigue, muscle weakness, postural hypotension, and increased skin pigmentation. The heart rate is generally increased rather than decreased as in anorexia nervosa.

D. Hypothyroidism
The general demeanor of hypothyroid patients is one of sluggishness, including diminished appetite.

E. Diabetes Insipidus
Although affected patients have polydipsia, anorexia is usually present.

F. Adrenogenital Syndrome
In the salt-losing form in infants, early presenting symptoms are vomiting, weight loss, anorexia, and dehydration.

G. Lead Poisoning
Chronic plumbism features anorexia with abdominal pain, irritability, and anemia.

H. Hypercalcemia
1. Williams Syndrome
The cause may be excessive intake of vitamin D by the mother during pregnancy. Infants may have hypercalcemia, failure to thrive,

	irritability, anorexia, abnormal facies, and heart defects.
2. Hyperpara-thyroidism	Symptoms may include nausea, vomiting, abdominal pain, muscle weakness, and poly-uria.
3. Immobili-zation	Children in traction, casts, or otherwise immo-bilized may develop hypercalcemia with its attendant problems.
I. Renal Tubular Acidosis	Growth retardation, excessive vomiting and constipation are additional clues.
J. Inborn Errors	A number of amino and organic acidurias may have episodes of poor feeding as prominent symptoms.
K. Pseudohypo-aldosteronism	The cause of this unusual disorder is un-known. Biochemically, it is characterized by increased plasma renin and aldosterone and renal salt wasting associated with hyponatre-mia, hyperkalemia, and acidosis. Failure to thrive and lethargy are found in young chil-dren.
L. Hypervitamin-osis A	Irritability, pain in the legs and forearms, ano-rexia, and hepatomegaly are clinical findings.
M. Dietary Chlo-ride Deficiency	
N. Panhypopitui-tarism	
O. Polycystic Ovary Syn-drome	

IV. Gastrointestinal Disorders

A. Obstruction	Distension of the bowel from obstruction or stenosis may result in anorexia.
B. Diarrhea	Disorders associated with diarrhea may pro-duce anorexia when the child decreases oral intake to prevent the diarrhea.
C. Constipation	The child with chronic constipation tends to eat less to prevent discomfort elicited by peris-taltic activity following meals.
D. Inflammatory Bowel Disease	
1. Ulcerative Colitis	The presenting symptoms are usually bloody diarrhea with pus and mucus and crampy abdominal pain. Anorexia, nausea, and vomit-ing are later symptoms.

2. Regional Ileitis (Crohn Disease)	Chronic inflammation of the bowel and cramps brought on by eating lead to a diminished appetite.
E. Superior Mesenteric Artery Syndrome	With significant weight reduction following illness or a prolonged fast, omental fat may be lost, with resulting compression of the duodenum by the artery. The first symptom is often early satiety, and, later, vomiting. Patients may be misdiagnosed as having anorexia nervosa. Roentgenographic findings include delayed emptying of the stomach and dilatation of the duodenum up to the position of the superior mesenteric artery.
F. Appendicitis	Anorexia is an important early symptom.
G. Pancreatitis	
H. Achalasia	

V. Malignancy
Anorexia may be an early sign of an occult malignancy.

VI. Cardiopulmonary Disease

A. Congestive Heart Failure	
B. Chronic Hypoxemia	Cyanotic congenital heart disease and chronic lung disorders may be associated with anorexia.
C. Polycythemia	Neonates may present as poor feeders with lethargy and cyanosis.

VII. Inflammatory Disorders
A. Juvenile Rheumatoid Arthritis
B. Systemic Lupus Erythematosus
C. Acute Rheumatic Fever
D. Sarcoidosis

VIII. Nutritional Deficiencies

A. Iron Deficiency	Anorexia and irritability may be the only symptoms.
B. Zinc Deficiency	Decreased sensation of taste and smell may lead to anorexia.
C. Kwashiorkor	

IX. Neurologic Disorders

A. Increased Intra-
cranial Pressure

B. Diencephalic
Syndrome

A tumor in or near the third ventricle is the usual cause. Patients become emaciated and are anorectic; despite their appearance they have a disproportionately happy affect. A vertical nystagmus is often present.

C. Degenerative
Diseases

D. Neuromuscular
Disorders with
Defective Swal-
lowing

X. Drugs

A large number of drugs may cause anorexia. The more commonly used drugs include antihistamines, digitalis, antimetabolites, morphine, aminophylline, methylphenidate, amphetamines, diphenylhydantoin, and ephedrine.

SUGGESTED READING

Ulshen MH In Hoekelman RA (ed): Principles of Pediatrics, 2nd ed, Chap 114, pp 867–868. New York, McGraw-Hill, 1987

6

WEIGHT LOSS

Growth rates below average for both height and weight are common and are related to intrinsic and extrinsic factors, such as genetic potential and an inadequate nurturing environment. Actual loss of weight, unless transient in the course of an acute illness, is a worrisome symptom requiring careful evaluation.

Some of the many disorders that may cause weight loss have been covered in other chapters (see Chaps. 3 and 5); this chapter deals primarily with causes of weight loss in children beyond infancy, especially diseases that may be subtle in presentation.

I. Infection

Acute or chronic infections are the most common causes of weight loss. In acute infections the weight loss is transient, and once the infection clears, the child generally regains the lost weight. Signs and symptoms of acute infections are usually present and recognizable. In chronic infections there may be no obvious signs of illness; a careful evaluation based on history and physical examination may reveal subtle signs and symptoms.

The following chronic infections may be more difficult to detect.

A. Urinary Tract Infection

B. Pulmonary Infection   Tuberculosis is less common today.

C. Abdominal Abscess

D. Osteomyelitis

II. Gastrointestinal Disorders

Vomiting and diarrhea are obvious symptoms of disturbance that may lead to weight loss. Some disorders, however, may not be associated with blatantly obvious features.

A. Inflammatory Bowel Disease   Although many children present with diarrhea, abdominal pain, or rectal bleeding, unexplained weight loss may be the only overt symptom in some. The diarrhea or abdominal cramping may go unnoticed. Anorexia may be a prominent symptom producing the weight loss.

B. Hepatitis — Chronic hepatitis—low-grade smoldering inflammation—may produce anorexia and a general sense of ill health.

C. Pancreatitis — Recurrent episodes of pancreatic inflammation may pass relatively unnoticed. The location of abdominal pain, usually part of the picture, may vary.

D. Celiac Disease — This disorder is usually apparent by 3 years of age, when the classic triad of steatorrhea, abdominal enlargement, and malnutrition may be noted. Stool examination for fat absorption is essential in suspected cases.

E. Cystic Fibrosis — The abdominal and pulmonary symptoms may not be obvious. A sweat test should be performed if steatorrhea is found.

F. Constipation — Chronic constipation can affect the appetite and result in decreased appetite with weight loss.

G. Intestinal Parasites — Giardiasis is a typical parasitic infestation that may produce weight loss with a minimum of other symptoms.

H. Superior Mesenteric Artery Syndrome — Intentional weight loss by dieting or immobilization in a body cast may lead to diminished omental fat, with resultant compression of the duodenum by the superior mesenteric artery. The compression creates a sense of early satiety with resultant decreased appetite and weight loss.

I. Malabsorption — In addition to fats, carbohydrates and proteins may be poorly absorbed, leading to weight loss.

III. Physiologic Causes

A. Dieting — Older children may embark on "fad" diets without their parents' knowledge.

B. Increased Physical Activity — Otherwise healthy-appearing youngsters may lose considerable weight when they are involved in supervised or unsupervised athletic activities. Despite eating their usual or even increased amounts of food at home, weight loss may follow. Despite the weight loss, other symptoms are lacking and they keep up with peers.

IV. Emotional Factors

A. Depression	Weight loss, loss of interest in activities, and insomnia are warning signals of depression.
B. Anorexia Nervosa	This disorder is more frequent in adolescent girls. Despite the loss of weight they remain active and are superficially interested in food, but not in eating it.

V. Metabolic and Endocrine Disorders

A. Diabetes Mellitus	Polyphagia, polydipsia, and polyuria are usually present.
B. Diabetes Insipidus	Anorexia may accompany the polyuria.
C. Hypercalcemia	In addition to anorexia, there may be nausea, vomiting, abdominal pain, muscle weakness, and polyuria.
D. Addison Disease	Hypoadrenocorticism may mimic anorexia nervosa, but lethargy is a key feature. Skin pigmentation may increase.
E. Thyrotoxicosis	The hypermetabolic state may result in weight loss. There may be other signs and symptoms such as tachycardia, tremors, and increased sweating.
F. Hypopituitarism	Onset may be later in childhood following encephalitis or as the result of destruction of the hypothalamus by a tumor. The clinical picture may falsely suggest anorexia nervosa.
G. Renal Failure	Uremia may be subtle.

VI. Cardiopulmonary Disease

A. Asthma
B. Chronic Congestive Heart Failure
C. Constrictive Pericarditis
D. Infective endocarditis

VII. Malignancy

Occult tumors are often the primary concern of parents whose children are losing weight.

VIII. Nutritional Deficiencies

A. Iron Deficiency	Anorexia may be a subtle symptom leading to weight loss. Other unusual signs include pa-

gophagia (craving for ice), geophagia (craving for dirt), and the abnormal ingestion of cornstarch.

B. Zinc Deficiency — Anorexia results from an altered sensation of taste and smell.

IX. Neurologic Causes

A. Increased Intra-cranial Pressure — Usually present with other symptoms, especially headache. Pseudotumor cerebri, of various causes, may be subtle and produce anorexia with weight loss.

B. Degenerative Disorders — Various inherited disorders, such as Wilson disease and Friedreich ataxia, may be associated with weight loss, but neurologic symptoms predominate.

C. Diencephalic Syndrome — A tumor in or near the third ventricle is the cause. Despite an emaciated appearance, patients have a happy affect. A vertical nystagmus is often present.

X. Miscellaneous Causes

A. Chronic Inflammatory Disease — Patients with connective-tissue disorders such as juvenile rheumatoid arthritis and systemic lupus erythematosus may have weight loss as a prominent complaint.

B. Drugs — Amphetamines and methylphenidate among other drugs may affect appetite.

C. Poisonings — Chronic lead and mercury poisonings may cause anorexia and weight loss.

D. Sarcoidosis

7

OBESITY

Obesity is the most common form of malnutrition in the United States. Various studies have found that approximately 10% of prepubertal and 15% of adolescent age groups are obese. Obesity has been defined as a 20% excess of the calculated ideal weight for age, sex, and height. More recently, in the past decade, triceps skin-fold measurements have been recommended as the best single method for defining the problem.

Most children (and adults) who are obese have exogenous obesity. In the not-too-distant past, exogenous obesity meant that one simply ate too much. The problem of exogenous obesity is, however, much more complex. Physical activity and genetic influences must be taken into account. The review by Weil is recommended if your appetite has been whetted.[1]

Perhaps less commonly today than in the past, "glandular" problems are blamed as the cause of obesity. Endocrine causes of obesity are distinctly uncommon and, more importantly, usually can be readily differentiated from exogenous obesity by a simple physical examination and an assessment of linear growth. Children with exogenous obesity tend to have an accelerated linear growth, whereas children with endocrine, metabolic, or malformation syndromes are usually short.

I. Exogenous Causes

Most obese children are classified as having exogenous obesity, but there is a great deal of controversy regarding the actual mechanism or mechanisms involved. Implicated in exogenous obesity are the following factors.

A. Excessive Intake — Overeating was previously considered to be the primary cause of obesity, but some investigators think that an excessive intake beyond caloric requirements is operative only in a few cases.

B. Diminished Activity — Failure to utilize the calories taken in results in a gradual increase in fat stores. Forced inactivity, such as after surgery or orthopedic procedures, without a concomitant reduction in calorie intake will generate weight gain.

C. Genetic Factors — The mechanisms involved remain poorly understood, but a familial tendency toward excessive weight is well recognized. In families with obese members, the effects of environment versus those of heredity are still controversial.

II. Endocrine Disorders

A. Hypothyroidism
This condition is often blamed as the cause of obesity, but seldom is. Evidence of delayed growth with a bone age of less than normal separates children with hypothyroidism from those with exogenous obesity.

B. Hyperadrenocorticism (Cushing Syndrome)
Although most frequently the result of exogenous steroid therapy, hyperadrenocorticism may occur in patients with adrenal tumors or disorders of the hypothalamic-pituitary axis that result in overproduction of adrenocorticotropic hormone. Growth usually decelerates or stops. Truncal obesity, acne, hirsutism, purplish striae, and hypertension are prominent diagnostic clues.

C. Pancreatic Tumors
Insulinomas may produce hypoglycemia with resultant hyperphagia and secondary obesity.

D. Growth-Hormone Deficiency
Fat accumulation, if it occurs, involves the trunk and buttocks.

E. Hypothalamic Lesions
A number of lesions affecting the hypothalamus may result in hyperphagia and obesity. Injury to the hypothalamus may occur following encephalitis and with craniopharyngiomas, optic gliomas, histiocytosis X, and pituitary tumors.

F. Central Nervous System Disorders
Hydrocephalus, pinealomas, porencephalic cysts, meningeal leukemia, and trauma have all been implicated as causes of obesity.

G. Fröhlich Syndrome (Adiposogenital Dystrophy)
This rare disorder is caused by a hypothalamic tumor, resulting in polyphagia, dwarfism, hypogonadism, and optic atrophy.

H. Stein–Leventhal Syndrome
Girls with this syndrome have polycystic ovaries and are overweight; hirsutism occurs in 50% of the cases. Some girls may show signs of virilization.

I. Pseudohypoparathyroidism
This disorder, also known as Albright's hereditary osteodystrophy, is characterized by short stature, moderate obesity, mental deficiency,

short fourth and fifth metacarpal bones, and variable hypocalcemia and hyperphosphatemia.

III. Chromosomal Abnormalities

A. Klinefelter Syndrome (XXY Karyotype)

Boys with this abnormality have a tendency toward long limbs and are tall and slim. Without testosterone therapy they become obese as adults. The testes remain small.

B. Turner Syndrome (XO Karyotype)

Some girls with the XO karyotype may be short and overweight.

C. Down Syndrome

D. XXXXY Karyotype

This abnormality may occasionally be associated with obesity. Wide-set eyes, mental deficiency, a low nasal bridge, small penis, hypoplastic scrotum, and limited elbow movement are prominent features.

IV. Congenital or Inherited Disorders Associated with Obesity

A. Prader–Willi Syndrome

Hypotonia, bizarre eating habits, hypogonadism, mental deficiency, small hands and feet, and obesity are characteristic.

B. Laurence–Moon–Biedl Syndrome

Prominent features include obesity, mental retardation, polydactyly and syndactyly, hypogonadism, and retinitis pigmentosa. Height is less than average.

C. Beckwith–Wiedemann Syndrome

Infants and children with this inherited disorder generally grow excessively and may appear obese. Macroglossia, visceromegaly, an omphalocele or umbilical abnormality, and neonatal hypoglycemia are common.

D. Carpenter Syndrome

Findings include obesity, mental deficiency, brachydactyly, preaxial polydactyly, and syndactyly. The shape of the skull is usually abnormal.

E. Cohen Syndrome

In this rare syndrome, obesity becomes apparent in mid-childhood. Hypotonia, weakness, mental deficiency, a high nasal bridge, narrow hands and feet, and prominent central incisors are present.

F. Grebe Syndrome

Children with this rare, inherited syndrome have obese and very short limbs, very short fingers, and hypoplastic bones of the arms and legs.

G. Alstrom Syn-   Characteristics include obesity from infancy,
   drome   progressive loss of vision, and, later, progres-
                         sive neurosensory hearing loss.

V. Miscellaneous Disorders

A. Glycogen Storage   Children with von Gierke disease may appear
   Disease, Type I   obese. The abdomen is protuberant because of
   (von Gierke Dis-   massive hepatomegaly.
   ease)
B. Mucopolysac-   Children with Hurler or Hunter syndrome
   charidoses   may appear obese, but the striking features of
                         these disorders should make the diagnosis
                         obvious.

REFERENCE

1. Weil WB: Current controversies in childhood obesity. J Pediatr 91:175–187, 1977

SUGGESTED READINGS

Dietz WH Jr: Childhood obesity: Susceptibility, cause, and management. J Pediatr 103:676–686, 1983
Garn SM: Continuities and changes in fatness, from infancy through adulthood. Curr Prob Pediatr 25(2), 1985
Golden MP: An approach to the management of obesity in childhood. Pediatr Clin North Am 26:187–197, 1979

8
FATIGUE

Fatigue is characterized by a general state of decreased endurance for or interest in activities and is usually associated with tiredness, irritability, and sleepiness. Physiologic causes (such as lack of sleep, excessive exercise, or inadequate caloric intake) or infections are frequently blamed for this symptom. Depression as a cause of fatigue frequently goes unrecognized, especially in adolescents.

The following classification is not a comprehensive one, but it is intended to suggest several general categories for consideration in the differential diagnosis.

I. Physiologic Causes

A. Lack of Rest	
B. Excessive Exercise	
C. Insufficient Caloric Intake	Kwashiorkor is the end stage in the spectrum of nutritional deficiency.
D. Obesity	Overweight children are likely to fatigue more rapidly than children whose weight is appropriate for body build and age. Rarely, markedly obese children may have excessive and dangerous periods of somnolence with elevated $PaCO_2$ levels (the Pickwickian syndrome).
E. Anemia	A significant reduction in oxygen-carrying capacity of the blood will result in fatigue. The onset may be insidious.
F. Polycythemia	Neonates with polycythemia are frequently lethargic with cyanosis and feeding problems.

II. Infectious Causes

Any bacterial, viral, or other infection may be associated with fatigue. The following infections, both acute and chronic, are particularly noteworthy.

A. Meningitis
B. Encephalitis
C. Bacteremia

D. Infectious Mononucleosis	This is probably the most commonly suspected cause of fatigue in adolescents. In young children, results of the slide agglutination test may be negative despite the presence of infection.
E. Chronic Epstein–Barr Virus Infection	Recurrent episodes of fever, pharyngitis, malaise, and adenopathy occur in the presence of persistently elevated anti-early antigen. A second syndrome occurs primarily in teenagers who are chronically exhausted. Malignancy is frequently mistaken for this syndrome.
F. Hepatitis	A variety of disorders may cause disruption of liver function. Infectious hepatitis and serum hepatitis are both relatively common causes. Fatigue may be the initial and most prominent symptom.
G. Tuberculosis	Signs and symptoms other than fatigue may be minimal.
H. Histoplasmosis	
I. Cytomegalic Inclusion Disease	The acquired form must be considered as a cause of seronegative mononucleosis.
J. Toxoplasmosis	
K. Brucellosis	Weight loss, low-grade fever, and back pain are among the subtle symptoms of chronic brucellosis.
L. Intestinal Parasites	Fatigue may result from interference with a variety of body functions, such as food digestion and absorption or blood loss.

III. Psychological Factors

Fatigue is a common presenting symptom of depression, although in many cases other signs and symptoms have been ignored.

IV. Allergy

Allergic individuals commonly seem fatigued. Clinical signs of allergy may be mistaken for other disorders: rhinorrhea and cough for infections, and allergic "shiners" (dark circles under the eyes) for lack of sleep.

A. Tension–Fatigue Syndrome	Intolerance to certain foods has been suggested to cause a variety of symptoms including recurrent abdominal pain, headaches, and "growing pains."

B. Asthma — Chronic, low-grade bronchospasm may be responsible for fatigue. Wheezing may not be clinically evident.

V. Endocrine Disorders
A. Hypothyroidism
B. Hyperthyroidism — Initial overactivity soon leads to fatigue. Tachycardia, increased sweating, tremor, and systolic hypertension are important clues.
C. Adrenocortical Insufficiency — Progressive weakness and hyperpigmentation are usually present.
D. Cushing Syndrome — Adrenocortical excess leads to metabolic changes and fatigue. Obesity and growth retardation are prominent features.
E. Primary Aldosteronism — Potassium loss results in muscle weakness and fatigue.

VI. Drugs
Many kinds of drugs may produce fatigue. Important groups to consider include antihistamines, anticonvulsants, tranquilizers, and opiates.

VII. Metabolic Disorders
A. Hypoglycemia — Fatigue, irrational behavior, irritability, headaches, and seizures may be symptoms of hypoglycemia.
B. Diabetes Mellitus — Poorly controlled disease results in insufficient fuel for energy and excessive water and mineral losses.
C. Inborn Errors of Metabolism — Fatigue is rarely recognized because of the generally early age at onset and the presence of more dramatic symptoms such as vomiting, lethargy, convulsions, and coma.

VIII. Gastrointestinal Disorders
A. Inflammatory Bowel Disease — Both regional enteritis and ulcerative colitis are frequently associated with impressive fatigue before the onset of other symptoms.
B. Liver Disease — Fatigue may be an early finding in infections or metabolic or physiologic disorders that interfere with liver function.
C. Intussusception — In addition to intermittent episodes of abdominal pain, diarrhea (that may become bloody late in the course), and vomiting, other frequently prominent symptoms are lethargy and fatigue.

IX. Collagen–Vascular Diseases

A. Juvenile Rheumatoid Arthritis — Fatigue in children with this disease is frequently more severe than expected with the degree of involvement.

B. Systemic Lupus Erythematosus

C. Dermatomyositis — Muscle weakness, pain, and fatigue are early symptoms.

D. Progressive Systemic Sclerosis

X. Cardiovascular Disorders

A. Congestive Heart Failure — Easy fatigability, tachypnea, tachycardia, and dyspnea on exertion are prominent signs.

B. Pericarditis — Fatigue and dyspnea may precede other physical signs including the friction rub.

C. Cyanotic Congenital Heart Disease

D. Primary Pulmonary Hypertension — Fatigue and dyspnea are the prominent symptoms.

XI. Renal Disease

A. Uremia — Anorexia, nausea, vomiting, and fatigue are common symptoms

B. Renal Tubular Acidosis — In both early-onset and late-onset forms, fatigue and weakness are common. Growth retardation, anorexia, polyuria, and rickets eventually appear.

XII. Miscellaneous Causes

A. Pulmonary Disease — Any lung disorder interfering with gas exchange or resulting in chronic inflammation may be associated with fatigue. Children with cystic fibrosis commonly are fatigued, but cough, diarrhea, and other symptoms are more prominent.

B. Malignancy — Children with leukemia, lymphoma, central nervous system and other solid tumors may manifest fatigability as an early symptom of their disease.

C. Myasthenia Gravis — Muscle weakness and fatigue are prominent features.

D. Tonsillar–Adenoidal Hypertrophy

The mass of posterior pharyngeal lymphoid tissue may be large enough to compromise air exchange, particularly during sleep. Snoring and retractions during inspiration are usually impressive. Fatigue and lethargy often characterize the waking state.

E. Familial Periodic Paralysis

Episodic attacks of flaccid paralysis and areflexia, occurring most commonly at night, are characteristic. Although the attacks may only last a few hours, fatigue may follow the episodes.

F. Sarcoidosis

9

IRRITABILITY

All children, as well as adults, have episodes of irritability at various times for various reasons. Stressful situations, infections, trauma, and bodily dysfunctions are only a few of the causes. This chapter focuses on causes of irritability that are relatively long-lasting; "irritable" here refers to those children who are unable to be soothed.

The tension produced by an unconsolable child often leads to a great deal of family discord and may result in child abuse if the symptom is prolonged. Although psychosocial disruption is a relatively common cause of irritability, particularly in infants, the disruption may also be produced by the persistent crying of the child; this relationship should be considered in the evaluation. Clues of bodily as well as psychological dysfunction must be sought in the differential diagnosis of irritability.

I. Behavioral and Psychosocial Factors

A. Altered Parent–Child Interaction   The child may be vulnerable to a number of familial disruptions resulting in irritability from a loss of security.

    1. Mismatch of Temperaments   The irritable child may not fit into the family structure and personalities.

    2. Marital Discord

    3. Battered Child

    4. Unwanted Child

B. Attention Deficit Disorder   This term is a rather nebulous catch-all for various disorders. Hyperactivity and learning disabilities may create frustrations for the child as well as the parents.

C. Infantile Autism   Autistic children are resistant to changes and fail to respond to human contact, even from their parents.

II. Infections

Any infectious process may result in irritability. Generally the onset is rather acute and the irritability coincident with the duration of the infectious process. A few noteworthy examples are meningitis, encephalitis, otitis media, urinary tract infection, osteomyelitis, acute cerebellar ataxia, measles, and the staphylococcal "scalded-skin" syndrome.

III. Skeletal Disorders

A. Fractures	Inapparent fractures, especially the "toddler fracture" (a spiral fracture of the lower leg often inapparent on roentgenograms for 1 week to 10 days), may produce irritability.
B. Infantile Cortical Hyperostosis (Caffey Disease)	Onset of symptoms in this bizarre disorder is before 6 months of age and is characterized by bony swelling, most commonly of the jaw and thorax, but which may affect any part of the skeleton. Soft tissues over the involved bone are usually swollen. The child is often febrile and usually irritable.

IV. Metabolic Disorders

A. Hypoglycemia	Symptoms of hypoglycemia may include restlessness and irritability as well as lethargy, pallor, and seizures.
B. Hypocalcemia	
C. Hypercalcemia	
D. Hyponatremia	Water intoxication, for various reasons, is a relatively common cause of hyponatremia.
E. Hypernatremia	
F. Gluten-Induced Enteropathy (Celiac Disease)	The classic picture is one of irritability with failure to thrive; stools are greasy, foul-smelling, and bulky. The onset ranges from late infancy to early childhood. A small percentage of children may have constipation. Irritability may be a primary feature.
G. Hypervitaminosis A	Ingestion of high doses of vitamin A may result in irritability, bone pain, and increased intracranial pressure.
H. Acrodermatitis Enteropathica	Prominent features include skin lesions ranging from bullae to verrucous plaques, especially on the distal limbs, perioral region, and perineum, and hair loss and diarrhea. Irritability and emotional disturbances are common along with photophobia, stomatitis, and paronychiae. The average age of onset is 9 months.

I. Scurvy	Irritability is the result of bone pain from periosteal bleeding.
J. Phenylketonuria	A quick screening test may be performed by adding a few drops of ferric chloride to an aliquot of urine. Irritability may be seen in infancy.
K. Gaucher Disease	The juvenile form features gradually increasing dementia during middle or late childhood, often with behavioral changes and irritability, seizures, and extrapyramidal signs. Organomegaly is mild.
L. Acute intermittent Porphyria	Symptoms include attacks of neurologic dysfunction, abdominal pain, constipation, sweating, labile hypertension, back or limb pain, and irritability.
M. Hypophosphatasia	The hypoplastic fragile bones are easily broken, resulting in irritability.
N. Pompe Disease (Glycogen Storage Disease, Type II)	The heart becomes massively enlarged, and affected children usually die by 1 year of age.
O. Pheochromocytoma	During intermittent release of epinephrine and norepinephrine by the tumor, children may be irritable, pale, and sweaty and may vomit and complain of headache along with their hypertension.
P. Vitamin B$_6$ Dependency (Pyridoxine)	Symptoms usually develop in the perinatal period and include convulsions, hyperirritability, hyperacusis, and feeding difficulties.
Q. Tryptophan Malabsorption	A bluish discoloration of the diapers may be noted in infancy. Other features include failure to thrive, unexplained fevers, infections, constipation, and irritability.
R. Hyperammonemia	Vomiting, lethargy, and coma are associated with increased ammonia levels following protein ingestion. Other findings are mental retardation, agitation, and seizures.
S. Hyperglycinemia, Nonketotic	Lethargy usually appears in the first few days of life, with convulsions shortly thereafter. The few children described were microcephalic, severely retarded, and irritable.
T. Argininemia	Periodic lethargy and irritability have been described in most patients. The onset may be delayed until 2 or 3 years of age or may be within the first 6 months.

U. Tyrosinemia | The onset is usually between 2 and 7 months of age with fever, irritability, lethargy, failure to thrive, hepatomegaly, vomiting, edema, and ascites. Death usually occurs before 1 year of age.

V. Pyruvate Carboxylase Deficiency with Lactic Acidemia | Infants are normal at birth, but development is slow. By 1 year of age, failure to thrive, vomiting, irritability, apathy, hypotonia, areflexia, spasticity, and seizures become apparent.

W. Biotin Deficiency | In addition to irritability, findings include periorificial dermatitis, conjunctivitis, alopecia, and hypotonia.

X. Argininosuccinic Lyase Deficiency | The subacute form presents a Reye syndrome–like picture with vomiting, lethargy, and irritability progressing to coma. Infants have marked hepatomegaly.

V. Drugs, Poisoning, and Toxins

A. Narcotic Withdrawal | Neonates may demonstrate symptoms of withdrawal from drugs taken by the mother during pregnancy. Irritability, tremors, diarrhea, and a shrill cry are common.

B. Phencyclidine Poisoning | Lethargy, ataxia, miosis, a trance-like stare, increased salivation, and hypertension are symptoms in addition to irritability.

C. Lead Poisoning

D. Drugs | Commonly used drugs that may produce irritability include phenobarbital, theophylline, amphetamines, antihistamines, ephedrine, imipramine, phenothiazines, and salicylates.

E. Mercury Poisoning (Acrodynia) | Prominent symptoms include irritability, restlessness alternating with apathy, insomnia, hypotonia, anorexia, hypertension, and excessive sweating. A pink macular rash may be seen.

F. Scorpion Bite | Restlessness and extreme agitation are common.

G. Chinese Restaurant Syndrome | Monosodium glutamate is the causative agent. Dizziness, sweating, flushing, headaches, and palpitations are prominent symptoms.

H. Carbon Monoxide Poisoning

I. Fetal Alcohol Syndrome

VI. Neurologic Disorders

A. Increased Intracranial Pressure

B. Subdural Hematoma or Effusion

C. Cerebral Contusions — Infants who are shaken usually show no cutaneous evidence of trauma. Retinal hemorrhages are an important clue.

D. Neurologic Impairment — Children who are neurologically impaired, for various reasons, may be excessively irritable.

E. Degenerative Diseases — Deterioration of cerebral function may be associated with irritability in several disorders.

F. Migraine — Diagnosis is especially difficult in infants and young children.

G. Convulsions

H. Brain Stem Tumors — Even before increased intracranial pressure is evident, irritability may be noted.

VII. Hematologic Disorders

A. Iron Deficiency — Children with iron deficiency may be more irritable than children whose stores of iron are sufficient.

B. Sickle Cell Anemia — Vaso-occlusive crises produce extreme irritability. Dactylitis with the hand–foot syndrome is a relatively common presentation.

C. Leukemia

D. Hemolytic–Uremic Syndrome — A hemolytic anemia with thrombocytopenia, hypertension, convulsions, and renal failure may follow a diarrheal illness.

VIII. Cardiac Disease

A. Congestive Heart Failure

B. Paroxysmal Atrial Tachycardia — During attacks young children may be fretful.

C. Endocardial Fibroelastosis — Irritability may precede cardiac symptoms.

D. Tetralogy of Fallot — During hypoxic attacks, children are anxious and irritable.

E. Myocardial Infarction — In infancy sweating, circumoral pallor and irritability may be subtle signs. Older children have chest pain as a helpful clue.

IX. Miscellaneous Conditions

A. Infantile Colic — Colic is a much-invoked but poorly understood condition characterized by episodes of uncontrollable crying with drawing up of the legs. The cause is uncertain and probably of multiple origin.

B. Hidden Food Allergy — Allergic symptoms may be obvious or at times covert, including unexplained irritability. Allergy is difficult to prove except by elimination of and re-exposure to various food products. Cow milk has been implicated as a cause of "colic."

C. Atopic Dermatitis — Pruritus, characteristic of this disorder, makes the child irritable but also elicits the scratching that results in the rash. It is an "itch that rashes." Any chronic pruritic condition may result in irritability.

D. Corneal Abrasions — Particularly in infants, the discomfort may manifest as irritability.

E. Glaucoma — Infants and children with glaucoma are irritable and have photophobia, tearing, and an enlarged, steamy cornea.

F. Deafness — Young children who are deaf may become frustrated and irritable.

G. Urticaria Pigmentosa — The release of histamine from the mast cells may produce cutaneous flushing and diarrhea accompanied by irritability.

H. Strangulated Hernias

I. Familial Dysautonomia — Suggestive findings include absent lacrimation, absent filiform papillae on the tongue, recurrent aspiration, unexplained fevers, and postural hypotension.

J. Lipogranulomatosis — The cardinal feature is discrete, lumpy masses over the wrists and ankles. Hoarseness occurs early; later findings include noisy respirations, restricted joint movement, delayed development, irritability, and recurrent pulmonary infections leading to death.

K. Smith–Lemli–Opitz Syndrome — Important features include anteverted nares, ptosis, hypospadias and cryptorchidism, syndactyly of second and third toes, microcephaly, and mental retardation.

L. De Lange Syndrome — Striking phenotypic features are anteverted nares, hirsutism, downturned corners of the mouth, a mottled skin, growling cry, and limb abnormalities.

M. Testicular Torsion

N. Anal Fissure

Irritability may be associated with defecation in infants. Bright red blood is often present on the stool.

O. SGA (Small-for-Gestational-Age) Infants

Beginning at a few weeks after birth, SGA infants often seem irritable and cry excessively for hours on end. The irritability may last as long as 9 months.

P. Respiratory Failure

Increasing agitation may indicate impending respiratory failure.

Q. Water Intoxication

R. Kwashiorkor

10

LYMPHADENOPATHY

Lymph nodes are easily palpated in children, particularly because nodal response to a variety of stimuli is rapid and often prolific in this age group compared to that in adults. The peak of lymphoid tissue development is between the ages of 8 and 12 years.

Infections are the most common cause of enlarged lymph nodes. Viral infections are more likely to cause generalized enlargement than any other type of infection. To many parents, however, lymphadenopathy suggests a malignant disorder, and they should be carefully reassured when the cause is merely infectious.

In this chapter lymphadenopathy has been divided into two principal categories, generalized and regional. All infectious causes have not been enumerated. In addition, it would be unnecessarily repetitious to include localized infectious and inflammatory disorders under each regional sub-section.

I. Generalized Lymphadenopathy

A. Benign Lymphoid Hypertrophy	This is probably the most common cause of lymphadenopathy in children. The enlarged nodes represent a benign response to minor infections, particularly upper respiratory infections.
B. Systemic Infections	Generalized lymphadenopathy commonly occurs in a variety of systemic infections. In some cases regional adenopathy may be more prominent.
1. Bacterial Infection	Sepsis, salmonellosis, scarlet fever, brucellosis, syphilis, leptospirosis, typhoid fever, and plague may all cause lymph node enlargement.
a. Streptococcosis	Chronic streptococcal infection in young children may feature excoriative rhinorrhea, prolonged fever, weight loss, and generalized adenopathy.
2. Viral Infection	Rubella, rubeola, infectious mononucleosis, infectious hepatitis, cytomegalovirus, and enteroviruses are common causes.
3. Other Infections	Mycoplasma, tuberculosis, toxoplasmosis, histoplasmosis, malaria, trypanosomiasis,

	schistosomiasis, and rickettsial diseases may produce nodal enlargement.
C. Skin Disorders	Chronic irritation of the skin will lead to adenopathy in lymph drainage areas. Children with atopic dermatitis tend to have generalized adenopathy, more prominent with subtle secondary infections.
D. Drug Reactions	Various drugs may produce generalized lymphadenopathy.
1. Diphenylhydantoin	
2. Other Drugs	Aspirin, barbiturates, penicillin, tetracycline, iodides, sulfonamides, and mesantoin are a few that have been reported to cause nodal enlargement.
E. Collagen–Vascular Diseases	
1. Juvenile Rheumatoid Arthritis	The adenopathy is more prominent during the acute phase of the illness.
2. Systemic Lupus Erythematosus	
F. Malignancies	
1. Acute Stem-Cell Leukemias	
2. Neuroblastoma	Occasionally, adenopathy is the first physical abnormality.
3. Histiocytosis X	
G. Immunologic Disorders	
1. Chronic Granulomatous Disease	Children with this disorder have multiple, chronically enlarged nodes that frequently suppurate owing to infection with pyogenic organisms.
2. Serum Sickness	Arthralgias, arthritis, fever, and an urticarial rash occur after sensitization to foreign proteins, often drugs.
3. Autoimmune Hemolytic Anemia	During episodes of hemolysis the lymph nodes may become greatly enlarged but are not tender.
4. Immunoblastic Lymphadenopathy	This disorder occurs mainly in adults; features resemble those of Hodgkin disease. Fever, sweats, weight loss, and hepatosplenomegaly are common; there may be a hemolytic anemia as well as hyperglobulinemia.

5. Acquired Immune Deficiency Syndrome (AIDS)

Prominent features include recurrent, opportunistic infections, failure to thrive, and hepatosplenomegaly.

H. Storage Diseases

1. Gaucher Disease

Hepatosplenomegaly is also present.

2. Niemann–Pick Disease

Patients have prominent hepatosplenomegaly.

3. Tangier Disease

Hepatosplenomegaly, large yellowish gray or orange-colored tonsils, and peripheral neuropathy are also found.

I. Endocrine Disorders

1. Hyperthyroidism

2. Adrenal Insufficiency

J. Miscellaneous Causes

1. Gianotti Crosti Syndrome

Papulonodular lesions on the extremities, adenopathy, and hepatomegaly are common findings. Hepatitis B virus has been suggested as the pathogenic organism, particularly in Europe and Japan but other infectious agents are responsible in North America.

2. Sarcoidosis

3. Chédiak–Higashi Syndrome

In this autosomal recessive disorder there is an increased susceptibility to pyogenic infections. Partial albinism with related ocular signs and progressive hepatosplenomegaly are also found.

4. Sinus Histiocytosis

This benign disorder is characterized by massively enlarged lymph nodes that appear over a few weeks' time; the cause is poorly understood. Children under 10 years of age are affected most often. Laboratory findings include anemia, neutrophilia, an increased sedimentation rate, and elevated serum concentration of IgG.

5. Angiofollicular Lymph Node Hyperplasia

A rare, benign tumor of unknown origin. The plasma cell type can be associated with systemic signs and symptoms: fever, malaise, anemia, hyperglobulinemia, and increased sedimentation rate.

II. Regional Adenopathy
A. Cervical Region

1. Viral Infections of the Upper Respiratory Tract	These are the most common causes of cervical adenopathy. The nodes are usually soft and slightly tender.
2. Other Viral Infections	Patients with infectious mononucleosis, cytomegalovirus infection, rubella, rubeola, or varicella frequently have prominent cervical nodes.
3. Bacterial Infections	The nodes are usually tender; erythema of the overlying skin is frequently seen. Pharyngeal infections, particularly with streptococci, commonly produce cervical adenitis. Staphylococci are often recovered from involved nodes. Patients with diphtheria may present with a "bull-neck" appearance.
4. Parasitic Infections	Toxoplasmosis may mimic infectious mononucleosis. Sore throat is not prominent.
5. Mycobacterial Infections	
a. Tuberculosis	The incidence of scrofula has decreased in recent years. Bilateral nodal enlargement is common.
b. Atypical Forms	Nodal enlargement is usually unilateral.
6. Fungal Infections	Aspergillosis, cryptococcosis, histoplasmosis, and coccidioidomycosis have been implicated.
7. Cat-Scratch Fever	The involved nodes are often red and tender and frequently suppurate. Fever, malaise, and headache follow a kitten scratch by days to weeks.
8. Mucocutaneous Lymph Node Syndrome	Fever, rash, conjunctival injection, fissured lips, and, later, peeling of the finger tips are prominent features. The cervical adenopathy is nonsuppurative and often unilateral.
9. Malignancies	
a. Lymphoma and Leukemia	Adenopathy tends to be bilateral. Nodes are painless and firm.
b. Hodgkin Disease	Unilateral involvement is typical.
c. Carcinoma of Thyroid	

d. Hand–Schüller–Christian Disease	Cervical node involvement and skull lesions are found.
10. Sarcoidosis	Adenopathy is generalized, but cervical involvement is most prominent.
11. Benign Sinus Histiocytosis	
12. Following Immunization	Diphtheria–pertussis–tetanus (DPT) vaccine given in the deltoid muscle may be followed by painless cervical node enlargement.
13. Suppurative Thyroiditis	

B. Occipital Region
  1. Seborrheic Dermatitis
  2. Tinea Capitis
  3. Pediculosis
  4. Folliculitis of Scalp
  5. External Otitis Media
  6. Rubella
  7. Tick Bites
  8. Roseola
C. Preauricular Region

1. Chronic Eye Infections	Nodal enlargement is seen especially with chlamydia.
2. Tularemia	Eye infection is associated with a suppurative preauricular adenitis.
3. Adenovirus Infections	
a. Type 3	Symptoms include pharyngitis, conjunctivitis, fever, and enlarged nodes.
b. Type 8	Epidemic keratoconjunctivitis is associated with a follicular conjunctivitis.
4. Cat-Scratch Fever	Suppurative preauricular adenopathy may occur if the scratch is near the eye.
5. Styes or Chalazion	
6. Ear Infections	Infections of the auricle and ear canal may cause preauricular adenopathy.

D. Submaxillary and
Submental Regions
1. Gingivitis
2. Dental Infec-
tions
3. Glossitis
4. Herpetic
Gingivostoma-
titis
5. Cystic Fibrosis

E. Axillary Region
1. Infection — Bacterial, viral, fungal, or other infection of an upper extremity, lateral chest wall, or breast is the most common cause of tender adenopathy.

2. Inflammation — Chronic irritation of an extremity, involving either skin or joints, may result in axillary adenopathy. Juvenile rheumatoid arthritis and atopic dermatitis are examples.

3. Vaccination — BCG vaccine or smallpox or other immunizations administered in the upper arm may cause axillary node enlargement.

F. Inguinal Region
1. Infection — The inguinal nodes drain the lower extremities, genitalia, perineum and buttocks, and lower abdominal wall. Bacterial, viral, fungal, and other infections in any of these areas may cause inguinal node enlargement.

   a. Lympho-
   granuloma
   Venereum — Large, matted nodes often suppurate.

   b. Chancroid — A ragged-edged, shallow ulcer on the genitalia precedes the adenopathy.

   c. Rickettsial
   Infections — Arthropod bites of the lower extremities are a common cause.

   d. Blastomyco-
   sis — Violaceous papules occur at the inoculation site, followed by lymphangitis and lymphadenopathy.

   e. Filiariasis — Repeated infection in this tropical disorder leads to lymphadema and elephantiasis.

2. Inflammation — Irritation of skin or inflammation of joints may cause nodal enlargement. Diaper dermatitis, mosquito or flea bites, and contact dermatitis may be overlooked in the differential diagnosis.

G. Supraclavicular
Region

  1. Left   Nodal enlargement in this area suggests malignant disease arising in the abdomen.

  2. Right   Nodes in this area drain the superior parts of the lungs and the mediastinum; therefore, thoracic disorders are usually responsible for the adenopathy.

SUGGESTED READINGS

Barton LL, Feigin RD: Childhood cervical lymphadenitis: A reappraisal. J Pediatr 84:846–852, 1974

Lake AM, Oski FA: Peripheral lymphadenopathy in childhood. Am J Dis Child 132:357–359, 1978

Zuelzer WW, Kaplan J: The child with lymphadenopathy. Semin Hematol 12:323–334, 1975

11

EDEMA

Four major pathogenetic mechanisms are responsible for edema, or the accumulation of fluid in body tissues: (1) increased capillary permeability; (2) decreased oncotic pressure; (3) increased hydrostatic pressure; and (4) impaired lymphatic drainage. The responsible mechanism should be determined in each case. Other diagnostic considerations include whether the edema is generalized or localized; whether it is acute or chronic; whether inflammation is associated with the swelling; whether there are systemic signs or symptoms of other diseases; and whether there is a familial history of edema.

In this chapter the causes of edema have been broken down into four groups based on the pathogenetic mechanism involved. The distinction, however, is not always clear-cut: In some instances, more than one mechanism may be involved, and in a number of disorders the exact mechanism is unknown.

Of the numerous causes of edema—some common, others rare—most have associated signs or symptoms that should make the diagnosis clear. Other chapters that cover specific areas of edema, such as Chapter 32, Periorbital Edema, may be helpful, as well as Chapter 63, Ascites.

I. Increased Capillary Permeability

A. Hereditary Angioneurotic Edema
Intermittent brawny swelling of the extremities is more common than facial or subglottic swelling. The edema is often precipitated by trauma. Recurrent, crampy abdominal pain is common. The edema usually lasts 24 to 72 hours. Laboratory findings include decreased serum levels of C4 and of C1 esterase inhibitor.

B. Infections
1. Bacterial Infections
a. Scarlet Fever
Pharyngitis and a fine, papular, sandpaper-like rash suggest this possibility.
b. Diphtheria
A mousey odor, serosanguineous nasal discharge, cervical adenopathy, and stridor may be present.
c. Pertussis
Periorbital edema may occur.

2. Viral Infections

   a. Mumps — Parotid swelling is the classic sign, but marked presternal edema may be seen.

   b. Epstein–Barr Virus Infection — Periorbital edema is common in mononucleosis.

   c. Roseola — Periorbital edema may be marked. The rash appears after defervescence on the third to fourth day.

3. Other Infections

   a. Rocky Mountain Spotted Fever — Generalized, non-pitting edema occurs to some degree in all patients. The rash, at first macular, then papular and petechial, appears on the fourth day of illness, at first distally and then centrally. Headache, anorexia, photophobia, and periorbital edema are characteristic features.

C. Allergic Reactions

   1. Insect Bites — Tissue edema commonly occurs after insect bites, particularly those of Hymenoptera. A papule is present at the site of the bite.

   2. Contact Dermatitis — A rash is usually present; scaling, often weeping or with linear vesicles, occurs especially in poison ivy.

   3. Ingestants — The swelling is often accompanied by urticaria. Drugs may produce a serum-sickness reaction with arthralgias or arthritis. Certain foods, especially shellfish, may produce an allergic reaction.

   4. Inhalants — Angioneurotic edema may occur upon exposure.

D. Collagen–Vascular Diseases

   1. Serum Sickness — Fever, urticaria, edema, and arthralgias or arthritis may occur secondary to infections, injections, or drug ingestion.

   2. Henoch–Schönlein Purpura — A petechial or purpuric rash, and abdominal pain, arthritis, or nephritis suggest this disorder. Striking areas of edema are commonly found.

   3. Allergic Vasculitis — Palpable purpura is often found with edema.

   4. Rheumatoid Arthritis — Periarticular swelling may obscure the arthritis.

5. Systemic Lupus Erythematosus	Various signs and symptoms may be present including rashes and arthritis.
6. Polyarteritis Nodosa	Extremity edema may be present with nephritis, hypertension, and arthralgias.
7. Mucocutaneous Lymph Node Syndrome	Brawny edema of the hands and feet, peeling of the fingers, conjunctival injection, cracked and bleeding lips, rashes, and fever lasting longer than 5 to 7 days are characteristic.
8. Dermatomyositis	Facial edema is common. Key features include muscle weakness with erythematous, scaly papules over the elbows and knees and erythematous lesions over the knuckles.
9. Progressive Systemic Sclerosis	The skin becomes increasingly tight. Raynaud phenomenon is a common finding.
10. Thrombotic Thrombocytopenic Purpura	Edema may be prominent with purpuric lesions.
11. Stevens–Johnson Syndrome	Facial and generalized edema may be marked. Mucous membrane involvement is often severe, along with the erythema multiforme.

E. Miscellaneous Causes

1. Scurvy	Easy bruising and bleeding gums are early signs.
2. Beriberi	Thiamine deficiency is rare in the United States. Peripheral neuritis and cardiac failure may be present.
3. Vitamin E Deficiency	Premature infants not given vitamin E supplements may develop edema.
4. Hyperthyroidism	Pretibial myxedema is rare in children. Tachycardia, weight loss, and nervousness suggest this diagnosis.
5. Hypothyroidism	Children may have a generalized puffy appearance, particularly around the eyes.
6. Mucopolysaccharidoses	The skin appears coarse and thickened in several types. Phenotypic characteristics suggest the diagnosis.
7. Pancreatitis	Abdominal (epigastric) pain is generally present. Ascites and extremity swelling may occur.
8. Sickle Cell Anemia	The hand–foot syndrome produces symmetrical, tender swelling of the hands or feet. Children are often febrile.

9. Eosinophilic Cellulitis	Resembles bacterial cellulitis and usually affects the extremities or trunk. Marked edema and moderate erythema with minimal tenderness and lack of warmth is found. Recurrent episodes are typical. A peripheral eosinophilia of the blood is found.
10. Episodic Angioneurotic Edema and Hypereosinophilia	An unusual disorder of unknown etiology with recurrent attacks of edema and hypereosinophilia. Pruritic papules and fever may be present.

II. Decreased Oncotic Pressure (Hypoproteinemia)

A. Hereditary Causes	
1. Analbuminemia	Patients are usually asymptomatic; mild pretibial edema may be seen.
2. Trypsinogen Deficiency	Diarrhea and marked hypoalbuminemia are characteristic findings.
B. Renal Disorders	
1. Nephrosis	
a. Nil Disease	Generalized edema, with proteinuria, hypoproteinemia, and hypercholesterolemia, is characteristic.
b. Nephrotic Syndrome	A wide variety of disorders may be responsible. See references.
2. Nephritis	Hematuria and casts are generally found with proteinuria.
a. Hereditary	Hereditary forms may become symptomatic during infections.
b. Infectious	The infection may be viral or bacterial.
c. Drug-Induced	Commonly used drugs include methicillin, sulfonamides, and mercurial diuretics.
d. Immune-Complex Disease	Prototypes are post-streptococcal acute glomerulonephritis and subacute bacterial endocarditis.
C. Liver Disease	
1. Cirrhosis	
2. Galactosemia	Jaundice, vomiting, diarrhea, and the presence of a reducing substance in the urine strongly suggest this disorder.
3. Malnutrition	
a. Kwashiorkor	Deficient protein intake may be associated with edema.

b. Marasmus	Edema may accompany severe caloric deficiency.
4. Hepatocellular Failure	Elevated levels of liver enzymes are present.
5. Hypervitaminosis A	In chronic overdosage a cirrhotic picture may develop. Bone pain, headache, and a scaly dermatitis are more prominent findings.

D. Gastrointestinal Disorders

1. Cystic Fibrosis	Edema is more likely to occur in breast-fed or soy-fed infants. Despite a usually voracious appetite, the infant fails to thrive.
2. Exudative Enteropathy	
a. Chronic Allergic Gastroenteropathy	Intermittent diarrhea, abdominal pain, or vomiting occurs after ingestion of certain foods, particularly milk.
b. Ulcerative Colitis	Bloody diarrhea with mucus is suggestive.
c. Protein-Losing Enteropathy	Conditions associated with intestinal protein loss include regional enteritis, constrictive pericarditis, lymphoma, and congenital ileal stenosis.
d. Transient Protein-Losing Enteropathy	This occurs most often in children less than 3 years of age. It may follow a viral infection and is acute in onset. Edema resolves spontaneously within weeks to months. Presenting symptoms are anorexia, emesis, or abdominal pain, followed soon by generalized edema.
e. Neuroblastoma	A protein-losing enteropathy has been described with this tumor.
f. Intestinal Lymphangiectasia	This may be part of a generalized congenital abnormality of the lymphatic system. Steatorrhea and diarrhea with enteric loss of protein are usually present.
g. Congenital Megacolon	Hyperplastic mucosal changes in the colon resemble pseudopolyposis of ulcerative colitis.
h. Polypoid Adenomatosis	Involvement of the entire intestinal tract with protein loss is rare. Blood is present in the stool.
i. Trypsinogen Deficiency	Other pancreatic proteolytic enzymes are deficient because of trypsinogen deficiency. Protein malabsorption is present. Onset is early and anemia is present.

3. Malabsorption

   a. Gluten-Induced Enteropathy — Chronic diarrhea, weight loss, abdominal distension, and wasting of the buttocks are classic findings.

   b. Infections and Infestations — Chronic infections or infestations (*e.g.*, with *Giardia*) may lead to malabsorption.

4. Bezoar — Gastrointestinal protein loss may occur.

E. Miscellaneous Causes

   1. Pancreatic Pseudocyst — In addition to edema, ascites and abdominal pain may be present.

   2. Severe Anemia — Children with severe iron deficiency anemia may appear edematous.

   3. Zinc Deficiency — Low-birth-weight infants may present at 1 to 2 months of age with edema secondary to hypoproteinemia.

III. Increased Hydrostatic Pressure

A. Venous Hypertension

   1. Cardiac Failure — Tachycardia, tachypnea, hepatomegaly, and cardiomegaly characterize heart failure. Periorbital edema generally is noted before peripheral edema.

   2. Arteriovenous Fistula — A large fistula may produce high-output cardiac failure and edema. Bruits, especially cranial or hepatic, may be heard.

   3. Venous Thrombosis — Edema may occur distal to the obstruction.

   4. Failure of Venous Valves — Varicosities are uncommon in children, unless proximal obstruction is also present.

   5. Orthostatic Hypertension

      a. Casts — Children in casts may have edema of dependent parts.

      b. Causalgia — Decreased vascular tone secondary to neurogenic injury may lead to venous pooling and edema of affected parts.

      c. Paralysis — Paralyzed extremities may appear edematous.

   6. Obstruction from Tumors

   7. Constrictive Pericarditis — Hepatomegaly and neck vein distension are characteristic findings.

8. Superior Vena Cava Syndrome	Swelling of the face, neck, and upper torso may cause a cyanotic or plethoric appearance.
9. Primary Hypertriglyceridemia	Recurrent episodes of leg swelling, often bluish in color, have been described in patients with marked elevations in chylomicrons.

B. Increased Vascular Fluid

1. Inappropriate Antidiuretic Hormone Secretion	This problem is associated with various illnesses including central nervous system and pulmonary disorders. Decreased urine output, hyponatremia, and seizures may follow.
2. Salt-Retaining Steroids	
3. Excessive Intravenous Fluid	
4. Androgen Therapy	
5. Hyperaldosteronism	Edema is unusual. Muscle weakness and hypertension are prominent findings.
6. Hydrops Fetalis	Various disorders may produce hydroptic infants (see Chap. 63, Ascites).

IV. Impaired Lymphatic Drainage

A. Hereditary Disorders

1. Milroy Disease	Lymphedema is present at or shortly after birth. The inheritance pattern is autosomal dominant.
2. Meigs Syndrome	The onset of lymphedema occurs at about the time of puberty. The inheritance pattern is autosomal dominant.
3. Recurrent Lymphangitis	Recurrent infection or inflammation of lymph vessels results in edema. The onset is in childhood or teenage years and the inheritance pattern is autosomal dominant.
4. Yellow Nail Syndrome	The edema may begin at any age. Dystrophic yellow nails are characteristic; the inheritance pattern is autosomal dominant. Recurrent pleural effusions, bronchiectasis, and sinusitis may occur.
5. Edema with Distichiasis	The edema develops at any time from late childhood on. An extra row of eyelashes is the

key to diagnosis. Inheritance is autosomal dominant.

6. Edema with Recurrent Cholestasis

Onset is usually in the neonatal period with prolonged jaundice. Cirrhosis often develops later. The inheritance pattern is autosomal recessive.

7. Edema with Lymphangiectasis

Edema develops in infancy with diarrhea, vomiting, hypoproteinemia, chylous effusions, and failure to thrive. The inheritance pattern is autosomal dominant.

8. Edema with Cerebral Arteriovenous Anomaly

Edema develops in late childhood or early teens. Pulmonary hypertension is common. The inheritance pattern is autosomal dominant.

B. Congenital Disorders

1. Lymphedema Praecox

Onset may be at any age, with no family history. Aplasia or hypoplasia of the lymphatics is found on lymphangiogram.

2. Turner Syndrome

The classic presentation is lymphedema of the hands and feet in the neonate. The edema may recur later. Other stigmata may be associated with the XO genotype.

3. Noonan Syndrome

The phenotypic appearance is similar to that in Turner syndrome, but there is no chromosomal abnormality and it affects both boys and girls. The lymphedema of the hands and feet is similar to that in Turner syndrome.

4. Idiopathic Chylous Ascites

Abdominal ascites is present with the edema.

5. Constriction from Amniotic Bands

The extremity is edematous below the level of tissue constriction.

6. Chylothorax

Pleural effusions are obvious clinically and radiologically.

7. Edema with Capillary Hemangiomas

8. Congenital Absence of Nails

9. Xanthomatosis and Chylous Reflux

10. Thrombocyto-
penia with
Aplasia of the
Radius (TAR)
Syndrome

Dorsal pedal edema may be seen in children
with this syndrome.

C. Infections
  1. Protozoal In-
     fection
     a. Filiarisis

Elephantiasis, occurring mainly in tropical
regions, is caused by disruption of lymphatic
drainage.

     b. Trichinosis

Periorbital and pretibial edema with muscle
pain and eosinophilia are characteristic findings.

  2. Cat-Scratch
     Fever

A history of chills, fever, and adenopathy
proximal to the involved extremity is usually
obtained.

D. Trauma
  1. Tissue Injury
  2. Burns
  3. Surgical
     Trauma
  4. Extrinsic Pres-
     sure

E. Tumors
  1. Primary Tu-
     mors

Obstruction of lymphatics by the tumor results
in edema distal to the block.

  2. Metastatic Tu-
     mors
  3. Carcinoid

This uncommon gastrointestinal tumor is associated with recurrent diarrhea and cutaneous
flushes.

  4. Retroperitoneal
     Fibrosis

Various drugs and disorders may result in
fibrosis and lymphatic obstruction.

V. Mimics of Edema

A. Scleredema

A rare connective tissue disorder of unknown
cause sometimes follows streptococcal infections. Firm, nonpitting edema typically begins
in the nape of the neck and spreads to involve
the face, shoulders, and trunk. The lower extremities, hands and feet, and genitalia are
rarely involved. The face may become mask-
like.

B. Scleroderma	The skin appears thickened and often becomes shiny with decreased or increased pigmentation at the borders. Raynaud phenomenon and systemic symptoms are usually present.
C. Dermatomyositis	The skin may feel indurated. Erythematous papules over the knuckles, elbows, and knees are characteristic.
D. Myxedema	
E. Eosinophilic Fasciitis	An unusual disorder characterized by the rapid onset of scleroderma-like thickening of the skin, pain and swelling of the distal extremities, and the rapid development of contractures. Peripheral eosinophilia is common. The relationship to progressive systemic sclerosis is blurred.

SUGGESTED READINGS

Burke, MJ, Seguin J, Bove KE: Scleredema: An unusual presentation with edema limited to scalp, upper face, and orbits. J Pediatr 101:960–962, 1982

Fisher DA: Obscure and unusual edema. Pediatrics 37:506–528, 1966

Holmes LB, Fields JP, Zabriskie JB: Hereditary late-onset lymphedema. Pediatrics 61:575–579, 1978

Kent LT, Cramer SF, Moskowitz RW: Eosinophilic fasciitis. Arthritis Rheum 24:677–683, 1981

Lewis JM, Wald ER: Lymphedema praecox. J Pediatr 104:641–648, 1984

Oliver WJ, Kelsch RC: Nephrotic syndrome due to primary nephropathies. Pediatr Rev 2:311–317, 1981

Smeltzer DM, Stickler GB, Schirger A: Primary lymphedema in children and adolescents: A follow-up study and review. Pediatrics 76:206–218, 1985

12

PALLOR

The pale child is usually brought to medical attention because of parental concern about anemia. Although the various causes of anemia are important considerations, constitutional factors are by far the most common causes of pallor. Pale skin is more likely to be the result of a familial trait or lack of sun exposure, or part of the atopic diathesis, than of a pathologic process.

Pallor has been divided into chronic and acute classifications in this chapter.

I. Chronic Pallor

A. Constitutional Factors

1. Hereditary (familial) Traits — Heredity is probably the most common cause. Pallor frequently accompanies light hair coloration.

2. Lack of Sun Exposure — Children who live in northern climates during the winter months may have pale skin.

3. Atopic Individuals — Children with a predisposition to allergies or atopic dermatitis often have a striking pallor. Other clinical signs and symptoms of allergy are usually present such as allergic "shiners," Dennies lines, and the allergic salute.

B. Anemia — Pallor is usually attributed to anemia by most laymen, but the various causes of anemia are not the most common cause of this sign. In early infancy pallor may be the presenting sign of erythroblastemia.

C. Inflammatory Diseases — Chronic inflammatory diseases are often associated with pallor. The pallor may be due in part to lack of sun exposure, depending on the severity of the illness, and may be associated with the anemia of chronic disease. Pallor is a common finding in juvenile rheumatoid arthritis, inflammatory bowel disease, and systemic lupus erythematosus.

D. Edema	Disorders that result in edema, such as idiopathic nephrosis, frequently have associated pallor.
E. Cystic Fibrosis	Children with cystic fibrosis commonly demonstrate pallor, unrelated to the severity of the disease.
F. Juvenile Diabetes Mellitus	Many diabetics appear pale, irrespective of disease control.
G. Uremia	Children with uremia as a result of chronic renal disease have a pallor related partly to their associated anemia. Lethargy, fatigue, anorexia, and weight loss are commonly associated complaints.
H. Hypothyroidism	Part of the pallor may be related to edema.
I. Celiac Syndrome	Diarrhea is a more prominent symptom than pallor.
J. Lead Poisoning	Pallor may be due in part to anemia.

II. Acute Pallor

A. Infection	
1. Bacteremia	Some infections, particularly those in which bacteremia is a finding, are likely to be associated with a pallid appearance. Bacteremia seems more frequent in infections by gram-negative organisms.
2. Pyelonephritis	
3. Subacute Bacterial Endocarditis	
B. Shock	Peripheral vasoconstriction produces a striking pallor in any of the various causes of shock. Poor peripheral perfusion, such as that found in paroxysmal atrial tachycardia, produces a pronounced pallor.
C. Neurologic Disorders	
1. Closed Head Injury	Vomiting, pallor, and irritability are common. There may be a history of loss of consciousness.
2. Cerebral Hemorrhage	
D. Paroxysmal Disorders	
1. Migraine	Headache and visual disturbances are usual in

	older children. Young children may only have pallor, nausea, and vomiting.
2. Breath-Holding Spells	Most episodes are associated with cyanosis as the breath is held, but a pallid form has been described in which, after the precipitating event, the child does not cry but suddenly becomes pale and faints.
3. Psychomotor Seizures	Onset is rarely before 10 years of age. Auras, such as anxiety, visceral sensations, olfactory hallucinations, and déjà vu, precede the seizure. Following the aura the child may suddenly stop all activity, stand still, stare, and turn pale and then perform some minor motor acts. There is complete amnesia for these events.
4. Benign Paroxysmal Vertigo	Recurrent attacks of vertigo are associated with pallor, nystagmus, vomiting, and sweating. There is no loss of consciousness.
5. Infantile Spasms	Sudden muscular contractions with the head flexed, arms extended, and legs drawn up are characteristic. The infant may become pale, appear flushed, or turn cyanotic during these attacks.
E. Syncope	Pallor is pronounced just prior to the loss of consciousness.
F. Hypoglycemia	During episodes of hypoglycemia the child is often pale, sweaty, and nauseated and frequently demonstrates altered behavior.
G. Intussusception	During the paroxysms of abdominal pain the child often appears pale as if in shock.
H. Pheochromocytoma	Common symptoms include episodes of headache, sweating, pallor, and palpitations. Hypertension may be chronic or associated with the episodic attacks during release of catecholamines.
I. Henoch-Schönlein Purpura	Petechiae and ecchymoses, particularly over the lower extremities, are almost invariably present.
J. Hemolytic-Uremic Syndrome	A major cause of the pallor is the development of anemia.
K. Infantile Cortical Hyperostosis (Caffey Disease)	Onset is usually before 6 months of age. Irritability, fever, and soft-tissue swelling over the bony swellings are common findings.
L. Heavy Sedation	

13

CYANOSIS

Cyanosis, the bluish color imparted to the skin by unsaturated hemoglobin in capillaries, is often difficult to quantify clinically. At least 5 grams of reduced hemoglobin must be present before cyanosis is apparent. Clinical assessment is affected by several factors including skin pigmentation and light source. It may be difficult to decide if the bluish color is peripheral, most commonly from vasoconstriction, or central, a result of true unsaturation of hemoglobin.

Cardiac, pulmonary, and central nervous system disorders usually first come to mind in the differential diagnosis of cyanosis. It is important to ascertain that the bluish discoloration is not just "skin deep": Blue dye imparted to the skin from fabric, especially that of blue jeans, may initially be mistaken for a potentially serious problem.

I. Cardiac Abnormalities
   A. Cyanotic Congenital Heart Disease
      1. Tetralogy of Fallot
      2. Transposition of the Great Vessels
      3. Tricuspid Atresia
      4. Truncus Arteriosus
      5. Total Anomalous Pulmonary Venous Return
      6. Pulmonary Atresia or Severe Stenosis with a Ventricular Septal Defect

7. Severe Aortic Stenosis or Atresia

8. Ebstein Anomaly

9. Eisenmenger Complex   A large left-to-right shunt through a ventricular septal defect results eventually in increased obstruction to pulmonary flow, producing a right-to-left shunt.

10. Atrioventricular Canal

11. Hypoplastic Left Heart

12. Preductal Coarctation of the Aorta

13. Pulmonary Stenosis with a Patent Foramen Ovale

B. Failure of the Heart as a Pump

1. Congestive Heart Failure

   a. Congenital Heart Defects   Left-to-right shunts such as in ventricular septal defect, postductal coarctation of the aorta, and severe aortic stenosis may cause cyanosis.

   b. Dysrhythmias   Paroxysmal atrial tachycardia in particular may cause cyanosis.

   c. Myocarditis   Myocarditis may be of viral origin or associated with inflammatory diseases.

   d. Endocardial Fibroelastosis

2. Constrictive Pericarditis   Venous pressure is increased, leading to increased deoxygenation of hemoglobin in the capillaries during stasis.

3. Heart Block   Severe bradycardia may affect blood flow enough to cause cyanosis.

4. Atrial Myxoma   Symptoms include the sudden onset of dyspnea, fainting spells, or cyanosis when the tumor obstructs the mitral valve.

II. Disorders Affecting the Pulmonary System

A. Airway Compromise

  1. Upper Airway

a. Nasal Obstruction	In infants who are obligate nose breathers, or those with choanal atresia or even obstruction by mucus, cyanosis may be present. Similarly, rebound mucosal swelling from the use of sympathomimetic nose-drop preparations may result in symptoms of airway compromise.
b. Glossoptosis	The tongue may fall back and obstruct the airway in infants with micrognathia or poor neuromuscular control.
c. Foreign Body	
d. Croup Syndrome	Laryngotracheitis, acute and spasmodic, may result in severe subglottic narrowing. Various other disorders may mimic croup and cause narrowing of the airway (see Chap. 58, Respiratory System: Stridor).
e. Pharyngeal Infections	Retropharyngeal abscesses, epiglottitis, pharyngeal diphtheria with pseudomembrane formation, and peritonsillar abscesses may compromise airflow.
f. Vocal Cord Paralysis	
g. Laryngeal Webs or Cysts	
h. Angioedema	
i. Tumors	Hemangiomas, papillomas, and lymphangiomas have been implicated.
j. Congenital Goiter	
k. Tonsillar-Adenoidal Hypertrophy	Snoring, noisy respirations, and disturbed sleep are the more prominent symptoms.

  2. Lower Airway

    a. Foreign Body

    b. Aspiration   Inhalation of food or drink or of gastric contents and near-drowning are examples.

    c. Mucous Plugs

    d. Mediastinal Masses

    e. Tracheo-esophageal Fistula

    f. Vascular Rings

    g. Broncho-stenosis

B. Interference with Lung Expansion

    1. Pneumothorax and Pneumomediastinum

    2. Pleural Effusions

    3. Abnormalities of the Thoracic Cage   Severe pectus excavatum, flail chest following rib fractures, thoracic asphyxiant dystrophies, and the hypophosphatasia syndrome are examples.

    4. Severe Scoliosis

    5. Diaphragmatic Hernia

    6. Hypoplastic Lung

    7. Lobar Emphysema

    8. Pulmonary Sequestration

    9. Cystic Adenomatoid Malformation

    10. Severe Abdominal Distension   Lung expansion may be blocked by ascites or abdominal masses; patients with peritoneal irritation may hypoventilate.

    11. Obesity   Profound obesity may compromise pulmonary function (Pickwickian syndrome).

C. Disorders Affect-
ing the Lung
1. Atelectasis
2. Pneumonia
3. Bronchial
Asthma
4. Cystic Fibro-
sis
5. Bronchiolitis
6. Pulmonary
Edema
7. Hypersensi-
tivity Pneu-
monitis
8. Broncho-   Chemicals or noxious gases may produce
spasm   spasm.
9. Hyaline
Membrane
Disease
10. Pulmonary
Hemor-
rhage
11. Idiopathic
Pulmonary
Hemosider-
osis
12. Bronchopul-
monary Dys-
plasia
13. Pulmonary
Fibrosis
14. Alveolar
Proteinosis
D. Pulmonary Vas-
cular Disorders
1. Pulmonary
Emboli
2. Pulmonary
Thromboses
3. Persistent
Fetal Circula-
tion
4. Oxygen Toxic-
ity

III. Neurologic and Muscular Disorders

A. Central Nervous
   System Insults
   1. Intracerebral
      Hemorrhage
   2. Subarachnoid
      and Subdural
      Hemorrhages
   3. Cerebral
      Edema
   4. Meningitis or
      Encephalitis
   5. Seizures

B. Drugs   Various drugs may cause central nervous sys-
                         tem depression or affect the muscles involved
                         in respiration. Narcotics, tranquilizers, muscle
                         relaxants, and anesthetics are but a few.

C. Disorders Affect-
   ing the Muscles
   of Respiration
   1. Botulism
   2. Muscular Dys-   Pulmonary function may be affected in ad-
      trophy   vanced disease.
   3. Myasthenia
      Gravis
   4. Werdnig–
      Hoffman Dis-
      ease
   5. Poliomyelitis
   6. Diaphragmatic
      Paralysis

IV. Disorders Affecting the Oxygen-Carrying Capacity of Blood

A. Polycythemia   Cyanosis may be a finding in disorders in
                         which hemoglobin is increased, because the
                         amount of unsaturated hemoglobin is also
                         increased to as much as 5 grams.

B. Methemoglo-
   binemia
   1. Congenital   Deficiency of hemoglobin reductase
   2. Acquired   Various chemicals including nitrites, nitrates,
                          benzocaine, sulfonamides, and aniline dyes
                          may be responsible.

C. M Hemoglobins — Five hemoglobin variants, with an autosomal-dominant inheritance pattern, have been described. All produce clinical cyanosis. Hemoglobin M can be detected electrophoretically. The cyanosis either is present at birth or appears within 3 to 6 months of age.

D. Hemoglobins with Low Oxygen Affinity — Six variants have been described, the most common of which is hemoglobin Kansas. Patients have a hemoglobin oxygen saturation of 60% in arterial blood despite a PaO_2 of 100 torr.[1]

V. Shock and Sepsis
A. Blood Loss
B. Septic Shock
C. Septicemia
D. Adrenal Insufficiency — The defect may be congenital or acquired, particularly after withdrawal from exogenous steroid therapy.

VI. Peripheral Cyanosis
A. Vasoconstriction — The most common cause of cyanosis is vasoconstriction in response to cold exposure. Vasoconstriction may also occur in response to drugs and in some autonomic nervous system disturbances (see also Chap. 101, Raynaud Phenomenon and Acrocyanosis).

B. Deficient Blood Supply — Arterial compromise caused by a thrombus, vasculitis, or disseminated intravascular coagulation or venous stasis from interference with blood return results in cyanosis. Occasionally after trauma a limb may be cool, cyanotic, and slightly edematous (reflex sympathetic dystrophy).

VII. Miscellaneous Causes
A. Breath-Holding — Cyanosis may be marked during breath-holding episodes in infants and young children.

B. Crying — The mechanism of cyanosis apparent during crying is thought to be increased venous pressure resulting in stasis of blood in the capillaries and an increased extraction of oxygen.

C. Hypoglycemia — Cyanosis is most likely to occur in hypoglycemic infants, perhaps because of right-to-left shunting through a patent foramen ovale and hypoventilation.

D. Familial Dys-
   autonomia

Infants and children with this disorder have an abnormal response to hypoxia and a decreased sensitivity to hypercapnia.

E. Superior Vena
   Cava Syndrome

Swelling of the face, neck, and upper torso may take on a cyanotic or plethoric appearance.

REFERENCE

1. Vichinsky EP, Lubin BH: Unstable hemoglobins, hemoglobins with altered oxygen affinity, and M-hemoglobins. Pediatr Clin North Am 27:421–428, 1980

SUGGESTED READING

Lees MH: Cyanosis of the newborn infant. J Pediatr 77:484–498, 1970

14

JAUNDICE

Jaundice, a yellow discoloration of the skin, is the result of the presence of excess bile pigment and reflects a disturbance in the mechanisms for formation or elimination of this pigment. The causes are many, but evaluation should include a blood test to determine whether the bilirubin is of the conjugated or unconjugated form. The presence of large amounts of unconjugated bilirubin in the blood reflects excessive pigment formation from hemolysis or disturbances of the hepatic conjugating mechanisms. Hyperbilirubinemia with the conjugated form is an indication of difficulties in pigment elimination caused by liver parenchymal disease or obstruction of intrahepatic or extrahepatic bile ducts.

In this chapter, causes of jaundice are considered under the two types of hyperbilirubinemia, in which either unconjugated or conjugated bilirubin is present. A category of causes of yellow skin unrelated to jaundice is also included.

I. Hyperbilirubinemia with Unconjugated Bilirubin

A. Transient Neonatal Jaundice

1. Physiologic Jaundice

This mild form, common in newborns, has been defined as a total bilirubin serum level of not more than 12 mg/dl and conjugated bilirubin serum level of not more than 1.5 mg/dl. Any of several mechanisms may be involved: A transient deficiency of liver glucuronide transferase; low hepatic levels of the binding protein γ resulting in impaired hepatic uptake of unconjugated bilirubin; decreased intestinal elimination of bilirubin due to lack of intestinal flora necessary to reduce conjugated bilirubin to urobilinogen; and regeneration of free bilirubin from its conjugated form with resorption owing to the presence of glucuronidase in the intestinal epithelium (increased enterohepatic circulation).

77

2. Breast Milk Jaundice	Some mothers' milk contains a hormone that inhibits bilirubin conjugation. In most cases the inhibition is thought to be caused by a high concentration of saturated free fatty acids or lipoprotein lipase activity in the milk. The jaundice usually does not appear before 4 to 5 days of age. Discontinuation of breast feeding results in a rapid reduction of serum bilirubin levels in 24 to 48 hours.
3. Intestinal Obstruction	Especially in infancy, intestinal obstruction may result in an increased enterohepatic circulation. Various causes are intestinal atresia, annular pancreas, Hirschsprung disease, meconium plug syndrome, pyloric stenosis, and cystic fibrosis.
4. Lucey–Driscoll Syndrome	The mother's serum contains an inhibitor of bilirubin conjugation; thus, all of the mother's offspring are affected.

B. Increased Bilirubin Production
  1. Hemolytic Disorders

a. Maternal-Fetal Blood Group Incompatibilities	Most commonly affected are the Rh and ABO systems.
b. Red-Blood-Cell Enzyme Deficiencies	An increasing number of enzyme deficiencies, including glucose-6-phosphate dehydrogenase, fructokinase, pyruvate kinase, and glutathione peroxidase, are being reported.
c. Congenital Disorders	
1. Spherocytosis	Onset of symptoms may be in infancy or later in life, with pallor, abdominal pain, splenomegaly, and occasionally an aplastic crisis.
2. Thalassemia Major	Jaundice is rare, but pallor and hepatosplenomegaly become prominent at a few months of age.
3. Sickle-Cell Anemia	
4. Vitamin-E Deficiency	Jaundice related to vitamin-E deficiency is most likely to occur in premature infants, especially if acidotic.

d. Acquired Disorders

1. Drug-related Jaundice — Hemolysis may follow the ingestion of various drugs or toxins.

2. Autoimmune Disease — Various diseases may cause hemolytic processes, in which results of Coombs' test may be positive. Viral infections and systemic lupus erythematosus are best known.

3. Infantile Pyknocytosis — Pallor, jaundice, hepatosplenomegaly, and the presence of burr cells on peripheral smear are characteristic.

2. Resorption of Extravascular Blood — In infants increased bilirubin production may be the result of absorption of blood from hematomas (*e.g.,* cephalohematomas, subdural hematoma) or even ingestion of maternal blood during birth.

3. Polycythemia — Delayed clamping or stripping of the cord or maternal-fetal transfusion may produce polycythemia.

C. Mixed or Undefined Causes

1. Sepsis — Infection may cause hemolysis as well as cholestasis.

2. Hypothyroidism — Prolonged jaundice may be the only early clue.

3. Hyperthyroidism

4. Infant of Diabetic Mother

5. Dehydration

6. Hypoxia

7. Acidosis

8. Hypoalbuminemia — Premature infants are especially predisposed.

9. Drugs — Sulfonamides, acetylsalicylic acid, and other drugs may interfere with bilirubin transport.

D. Hereditary Causes of Defective Conjugation

1. Crigler–Najjar Syndrome — The hepatic enzyme glucuronide transferase is deficient. Type I, the autosomal-recessive form, is associated with death in infancy. In type II, the autosomal-dominant form, sur-

vival into adulthood is the rule, and phenobarbital therapy is effective.

2. Gilbert Syn-   Onset of symptoms is usually in late child-
drome   hood, with mild jaundice, vague abdominal
                       pain, and nausea. Jaundice is responsive to
                       phenobarbital therapy.

II. Hyperbilirubinemia with Conjugated Bilirubin

A. Neonatal Hepati-   Manifestations of neonatal hepatitis may ap-
tis Syndrome   pear at any time after birth. In addition to
                       elevated serum levels of conjugated bilirubin,
                       poor appetite, failure to thrive, and irritability
                       may be seen. Although identifiable causes of
                       neonatal hepatitis have been split away from
                       this group, this syndrome still accounts for a
                       considerable number of cases of neonatal con-
                       jugated hyperbilirubinemia and should remain
                       a diagnosis of exclusion.

B. Biliary Obstruc-
tion (Idiopathic
Ductal Cholestatic
Jaundice)

1. Biliary Atresia   Despite recent advances in diagnosis and
                       treatment 90% of the cases remain uncorrect-
                       able.

2. Biliary Hypo-
plasia

3. Paucity of In-
trahepatic Bile
Ducts

4. Choledochal   The classic triad of findings includes upper-
Cyst   abdominal pain, jaundice, and an abdominal
                       tumor, the result of cystic dilatation of the
                       common bile duct.

5. Inspissated Bile   This syndrome is a rare cause of jaundice to-
Syndrome   day but was more prevalent when severe Rh
                       isoimmunization reactions were more com-
                       mon. Plugging of bile ducts has been sug-
                       gested as the mechanism; hepatic injury was
                       found in some cases following severe hemo-
                       lytic disease.

6. Fibrosing Pan-   Most patients also have abdominal pain,
creatitis   weight loss, steatorrhea, and glucose intoler-
                       ance.

7. Primary Sclerosing Cholangitis — A rare disorder, occasionally associated with ulcerative colitis. Hepatomegaly, progressive liver failure, weight loss, and steatorrhea are other features.

C. Acquired Cholestatic Jaundice

1. Bacterial Infections — Jaundice may be the presenting symptom or a common finding in sepsis, pyelonephritis, and other bacterial infections, including liver abscesses and cholangitis.

2. Viral Infections
   a. Viral Hepatitis — Infectious hepatitis (caused by virus A), serum hepatitis (caused by virus B), and other forms must be considered.
   b. Coxsackie Virus Infections
   c. Infectious Mononucleosis — Jaundice occurs in 5% to 10% of cases.

3. TORCH Infection — Neonatal hepatitis may follow intrauterine infection with any of a complex of diseases referred to as TORCH—toxoplasmosis, rubella, cytomegalovirus infection, and herpes simplex—as well as syphilis.

4. Fungal Infection — Systemic histoplasmosis may involve the liver.

5. Parasitic Infestation — Visceral larva migrans caused by *Toxocara canis* or *T. cati* may produce inflammation of the liver with jaundice, hepatomegaly, and a marked eosinophilia.

6. Chemical Injury — Carbon tetrachloride exposure may result in hepatic necrosis.

7. Drugs — Potential hepatotoxins include acetylsalicylic acid, acetaminophen, iron, isoniazid, and vitamin A. Other drugs that appear to cause allergic hepatocellular damage are erythromycin, sulfonamide, oxacillin, rifampin, halothane, and isoniazid. Ethanol, steroids, tetracycline, and methotrexate may all cause jaundice.

8. Reye Syndrome — Jaundice may occur during the fatty infiltration of the liver.

9. Chronic Active Hepatitis — This form, more common in adolescent girls, may present as an apparent viral hepatitis, but

the jaundice does not resolve when expected. Malaise, fever, weight loss, and other systemic complaints may be present.

D. Metabolic Disorders

1. Alpha$_1$-Antitrypsin Deficiency — Onset of symptoms including jaundice and hepatomegaly may be at any age including the neonatal period. The diagnosis may be made by serum–protein electrophoresis.

2. Cystic Fibrosis — Liver involvement includes plugging of periportal canaliculi.

3. Galactosemia — The urine of jaundiced infants should always be tested for reducing substance, before vomiting, diarrhea, failure to thrive, and cataracts develop.

4. Galactokinase Deficiency — Hyperbilirubinemia and cataracts are the only manifestations. Signs develop later than in galactosemia.

5. Wilson Disease (Hepatolenticular Degeneration) — Liver dysfunction may occur at any age after infancy. Ceruloplasmin serum levels should be determined in any child with unexplained liver disease.

6. Hereditary Tyrosinemia — Other features include vomiting, diarrhea, failure to thrive, rickets, renal tubular defects, and hypoglycemia.

7. Hereditary Fructose Intolerance — Vomiting, diarrhea, and weight loss appear with the introduction of fructose into the diet.

8. Niemann–Pick Disease — Hepatosplenomegaly, failure to thrive, neurologic deterioration, and the presence of cherry red spots on funduscopic examination are characteristic.

9. Wolman Disease — In infancy, diarrhea and failure to thrive are followed by rapid demise. Adrenal calcification is present on roentgenograms.

10. Glycogen Storage Disease

a. Type IV — The cause is a defect in the brancher enzyme. Failure to thrive, jaundice, and hepatomegaly appear in the first 2 months of life, followed by progressive deterioration.

b. Type III — This form, caused by a defect in the debrancher enzyme, is more benign than type IV.

	Jaundice and increased serum levels of transaminase may be present.
11. Zellweger (Hepatocerebrorenal) Syndrome	In the neonatal period the physical appearance is striking; features include high forehead and epicanthal folds. Severe hypotonia, hepatomegaly, and poor appetite are other findings.
E. Familial Cholestasis Syndromes	
1. Benign Recurrent Cholestasis	Recurrent attacks of jaundice with severe pruritis began in early childhood.
2. Recurrent Cholestasis with Lymphedema	Infants with this syndrome may have prolonged jaundice, often followed by cirrhosis. Pedal edema develops in childhood.
3. Byler Disease	Loose, fatty stools appear in the first month of life. Jaundice and then hepatosplenomegaly develop, followed by cirrhosis and death in childhood.
4. Syndrome with Growth and Mental Retardation	In addition to findings of hepatosplenomegaly and jaundice, the toes and fingers are short and the skin thick.
F. Inherited Noncholestatic Syndromes	
1. Dubin–Johnson Syndrome	Jaundice may be noted at birth. A family history of jaundice is often present. The serum bilirubin usually does not exceed 6 mg/dl, of which one third to three fourths is the conjugated form. Constitutional symptoms may include weakness, fatigue, anorexia, nausea, and vomiting. On liver biopsy the hepatic cells are pigmented.
2. Rotor Syndrome	Findings are identical to those in Dubin–Johnson syndrome, but on liver biopsy there is no pigment in hepatic cells.
G. Miscellaneous Disorders	
1. Hyperthermia	
2. Chromosomal Defects	Infants with Turner syndrome or the trisomy 18 syndrome are predisposed to hyperbilirubinemia.
3. Hyperalimentation	

III. Mimics of Jaundice

A. Carotenoderma	A yellow-orange discoloration of the skin may be caused by pigments absorbed from yellow, orange, or red vegetables and fruits. The sclerae of the eyes are not involved.
B. Lycopenoderma	A yellowish skin discoloration may also occur following prolonged ingestion of excessive amounts of red pigment in foods, especially tomatoes.
C. Drugs	Antimalarials such as Quinacrine, in particular, may produce a yellow cast.

SUGGESTED READINGS

Kaye R. In Kaye R, Oski FA, Barness LA (eds): Core Textbook of Pediatrics, pp 109–126. Philadelphia, JB Lippincott, 1982

Mathis RK, Andres JM, Walker WA: Liver disease in infants. J Pediatr 90:864–880, 1976

15

RECURRENT INFECTIONS

Fortunately most children with recurrent infections are normal, without inherent problems in handling infections; recurrence is a simple matter of re-exposure. However, a large group of children have recurrent infections of certain organ systems because of anatomic or physical problems, especially those causing obstruction or poor circulation. Bronchial asthma, for instance, may be the most common cause of recurrent "pneumonia."

Immunodeficiencies and disorders of phagocytosis are relatively uncommon, but the nature of recurrent infections may suggest the presence of one of these disorders. The following pathogens in particular have been implicated: bacteria of high virulence, especially staphylococci and *Hemophilus influenzae;* bacteria of low virulence, such as *Serratia marcescens;* and fungal organisms, especially *Candida albicans.* A history of unusual reactions to vaccines, recurrent diarrhea, and failure to thrive may also be important clues, as is a history of recurrent severe infections in other family members.

Children with B-cell immunodeficiencies tend to have recurrent bacterial infections, especially pneumonia or otitis media. Those with T-cell disorders or with defects in cell-mediated immunity are predisposed to viral, fungal, or protozoal infections. Children with phagocytic defects commonly have recurrent pyodermas and systemic infections caused by organisms of usually low virulence; those with disorders in which complement activity is decreased have recurrent pyogenic infections, sometimes with lupus erythematosus–like syndromes.

I. Physiologic Causes

By far most common cause of recurrent infections is repeated exposure to infectious agents of an otherwise healthy child. The average child has 6 to 8 respiratory infections per year. This number may increase in the child attending school or the preschool child or toddler who attends nursery school or is enrolled in a day-care center. Older siblings may also bring home the infections. An extensive laboratory evaluation is not indicated in these cases, unless the infections are unusual, severe, or prolonged.

85

II. Anatomic and Physical Problems

A. Pulmonary Disorders

1. Bronchial Asthma — Asthma is the most common cause of recurrent "pneumonia." Decreased bronchial lumen and mucus plugs may predispose to repeated infections.

2. Cystic Fibrosis — Repeated respiratory infections may be prominent before gastrointestinal symptoms and signs appear.

3. Foreign Body

4. Recurrent Aspiration

   a. Gastroesophageal Reflux

   b. Hiatal Hernia

   c. Neuromuscular Disorders — Central nervous system damage causing difficulty in handling secretions or a poor cough reflex should be considered.

   d. Familial Dysautonomia

   e. Tracheoesophageal Fistula

   f. Vascular Ring

5. Congenital Heart Disease — Conditions causing pulmonary congestion may predispose to infection.

6. Tracheal Bronchus — An accessory or aberrant bronchus may lead to recurrent pneumonia and stridor. May be associated with Down syndrome.

B. Urinary Tract Obstruction — Repeated infections may be caused by various obstructive diseases such as ureteral stenosis, stones, and ureteral reflux, as well as compression of the urinary system by extrinsic causes such as chronic constipation.

C. Central Nervous System Disorders

1. Ventricular Shunts

    2. Skull Frac-   Basilar fractures in particular may be associ-
       tures   ated with infections.
    3. Midline Sinus
       Tracts
  D. Metabolic Dis-
    eases
    1. Diabetes Mel-   Part of the cause of repeated infections may be
       litus   poor circulation, but probably more important
           is impaired leukocyte chemotactic activity.
    2. Galactosemia   Young infants are particularly prone to gram-
           negative infections.
  E. Hematologic
    Disturbances
    1. Sickle Cell   Functional asplenia develops following re-
       Disease   peated infarctions. Defective opsonic function
           is the likely cause.
    2. Leukemia   Several factors may be involved including a
       and Lympho-   decreased number of leukocytes and defective
       mas   phagocytosis.
    3. Neoplasms   Neoplasms may cause obstructive problems as
           well as defective leukocyte function.
  F. Skin Defects
    1. Atopic Der-   Repeated skin infections are common.
       matitis
    2. Burns

III. Disorders of Phagocytic Function

  A. Chemotaxis
    1. "Lazy Leuko-   Recurrent upper respiratory infections, sto-
       cyte" Syn-   matitis, gingivitis, otitis media, abscesses, and
       drome   staphylococcal furuncles are common. Periph-
           eral neutropenia with depressed migration of
           neutrophils is present, but normal mature
           neutrophils are found in the bone marrow.
    2. Familial Neu-   Recurrent, severe infections are characteristic.
       tropenia   The neutropenia may be cyclic.
    3. Autoimmune   Infants may develop an absolute neutrophil
       Neutropenia   count of 0–500/ul, usually associated with
       of Infancy   monocytosis and eosinophilia. Recurrent fe-
           vers and infections are typical. Circulating
           antibodies to neutrophils are present.
    4. Job Syn-   Severe eczema of early onset and almost con-
       drome   stant staphylococcal infections are characteris-
           tic. Affected children have a coarse facies with

a broad nasal bridge. Serum IgE levels are markedly increased.

5. Chédiak–Higashi Syndrome

This uncommon inherited disorder is associated with partial oculocutaneous albinism and peripheral neutropenia. The white cells have abnormal granules and inclusions.

6. Kartagener Syndrome

Chronic or recurrent sinopulmonary and middle ear infections are characteristic. Situs inversus is a finding in about one half of the cases. Cilia of respiratory tract appear to be immotile. Decreased chemotaxis is also present.

B. Ingestion
  1. Neutropenia

Neutropenia may be inherited or may be caused by certain drugs or overwhelming infections.

  2. Defective Opsonization

This defect occurs after splenectomy and in sickle-cell disease. Newborns are deficient in the ability to opsonize coliform bacteria.

C. Phagocyte Killing
  1. Chronic Granulomatous Disease

Most patients are boys who have recurrent suppurative and granulomatous lesions, colonized usually by staphylococci, *E. coli, Pseudomonas,* and *Klebsiella.* Adolescents usually have severe and antibiotic-resistant acneiform lesions and seborrheic dermatitis as well. The onset in most cases is by 1 year of age. Hepatosplenomegaly, pneumonitis, and osteomyelitis are also common.

  2. Myeloperoxidase Deficiency

Chronic moniliasis is common.

  3. Leukocyte Glucose-6-Phosphate Dehydrogenase Deficiency

Findings are similar to those in chronic granulomatous disease, but infections are less severe.

IV. Disorders of the Complement System
  A. C1q Deficiency

This form has been found in association with severe immunologic deficiency states, especially T-cell disorders. Clinical findings include severe wasting, chronic debilitation, chronic candidiasis, and diarrhea. Persistent infections may be caused by various organisms.

B. C2 Deficiency — In the United States this is the most frequently described homozygous deficiency of a complement component. In addition to recurrent severe pyogenic infections, affected individuals, both homozygous and heterozygous, are at increased risk of rheumatoid and other autoimmune diseases.

C. C3 and C5 Deficiencies — Children with deficiencies of these components have had recurrent severe infections such as pneumococcal pneumonia and meningococcal meningitis.

D. C5 Dysfunction (Leiner Disease) — A generalized seborrhea-like dermatitis, recurrent infections (especially by gram-negative organisms), diarrhea, and failure to thrive are important features.

E. C6, C7, and C8 Deficiencies — Meningococcal and gonococcal bacteremias may be recurrent in families with these deficiencies.

V. Disorders of Antibody Production

A. Transient Hypogammaglobulinemia — The production of immunoglobulins may be delayed in some infants until 18 to 30 months of age. Recurrent respiratory infections and unexplained fevers are common.

B. X-Linked Hypogammaglobulinemia — All classes of immunoglobulins are deficient. Lymphoid tissue, including the tonsils, is hypoplastic. Recurrent severe, life-threatening infections are common after 6 months of age. A rheumatoid arthritis-like picture develops in some patients.

C. X-Linked Hypogammaglobulinemia with Normal or Increased Serum IgM — Infections are similar to those in the form described above, but lymphoid tissue may be enlarged. Neutropenia, thrombocytopenia, hemolytic anemia, and lymphomas are relatively common.

D. Transcobalamin II Deficiency and Hypogammaglobulinemia — Megaloblastic anemia, granulocytopenia, and thrombocytopenia with absent antibody production are other findings in this rare disease. Large doses of vitamin B_{12} may correct these abnormalities.

E. Common Variable Immuno-Deficiency — Recurrent infections may not begin until late childhood or adulthood. Malabsorption and autoimmune disorders are also common.

F. Selective IgA Deficiency — This is the most common primary immunodeficiency, but many affected children are asymptomatic. Recurrent respiratory infections of both upper and lower airways, intractable asthma, chronic diarrhea, autoimmune disorders, and malignancies are common.

G. Selective IgM Deficiency — Recurrent bacteremias, meningitis, and gastrointestinal problems are common.

H. Secondary Immunodeficiencies — These may occur in malnutrition, during immunosuppressive therapy, in protein-losing enteropathies and uremia, after splenectomy, and with lymphomas.

I. Ataxia Telangiectasia — Recurrent sinopulmonary infections with bronchiectasis are most common. The ataxia is progressive, leading to eventual complete debility. Telangiectasiae develop gradually, first on the conjunctivae and ears. IgA and IgE deficiencies are common.

J. Wiskott–Aldrich Syndrome — This is an X-linked recessive disorder characterized by recurrent infections, eczema, and thrombocytopenia. Serum IgM is decreased, but serum IgA and IgE levels are elevated.

K. Acquired Immune Deficiency — Increasing numbers of cases of AIDS are being reported in children as a result of blood transfusions or are acquired *in utero.* Symptoms include failure to thrive, chronic diarrhea, recurrent pneumonia, candidiasis, otitis media, and so forth.

VI. Disorders of Cellular Immunity

A. DiGeorge Syndrome — The thymus and parathyroid glands fail to develop. Congenital heart disease, an abnormal facies (hypertelorism, micrognathia, low-set abnormally shaped ears, antimongoloid slant to the eyes), and tetany from hypocalcemia are found.

B. Chronic Mucocutaneous Candidiasis — Chronic candidal infections of the skin, nails, and mucous membranes may be associated with endocrinopathies (especially hypoparathyroidism).

C. Severe Combined Immunodeficiency	Combined T-cell and B-cell deficiencies result in early severe recurrent infections, usually before 6 months of age. Diarrhea and pneumonia with failure to thrive are present; inheritance is autosomal recessive or X-linked recessive.
D. Adenosine Deaminase Deficiency	Both B-cell and T-cell deficiencies are also present; the clinical picture may be that of a severe combined immunodeficiency. Another enzyme deficiency, that of nucleoside phosphorylase, has similar findings, but onset of infections may be later (at 6 to 12 months of age).
E. Nezelof Syndrome	In this cellular immunodeficiency there is a variable degree of normal immunoglobulin synthesis. The cases are sporadic in occurrence. The age at onset of recurrent infections is variable. Eczema, chronic otitis media, and sinusitis are common.
F. Immunodeficiency with Short-Limbed Dwarfism	Several forms have been described: one with severe combined immunodeficiency; another with cellular immunodeficiency; and a third with humoral immunodeficiency. Redundant skin folds are found around the neck and large joints.

VII. Drug-Related Causes

A. Corticosteroids	Recurrent infections may be a problem in children taking corticosteroids.
B. Antineoplastics	
C. Antibiotics	Resistant bacterial infections may develop in some children on chronic antibiotic therapy.

VIII. Chronic Infections

A. Chronic Epstein–Barr Virus	An unusual disorder characterized by recurrent episodes of pharyngitis with fever, cervical lymphadenopathy, and malaise. Edema of the eyelids and fingers, arthralgias, and myalgias are often present. Anti-EBV antibody pattern is typical in this syndrome is a persistently elevated anti-early antigen or absent anti-EB nuclear antigen.
B. Other	Other infectious agents associated with this syndrome include cytomegalovirus, Coxsackie B virus, toxoplasmosis, and mycoplasma.

SUGGESTED READINGS

Ammann AJ: T cell and T-B cell immunodeficiency disorders. Pediatr Clin North Am 24:293–312, 1977

Gallin JI, Wright DG, Malech HL et al: Disorders of phagocyte chemotaxis. Ann Int Med 92:520–538, 1980

Goldman AS, Goldblum RM: Primary deficiencies in humoral immunity. Pediatr Clin North Am 24:277–292, 1977

Jones JF, Ray CG, Minnich LL et al: Evidence for active Epstein–Barr virus infections in patients with persistent unexplained illnesses: Elevated anti-early antigen antibodies. Ann Intern Med 102:1–7, 1985

Lalezari P, Khorshidi M, Petrosova M: Autoimmune neutropenia of infancy. J Pediatr 109:764–769, 1986

Miller ME: Cutaneous infections and disorders of inflammation. J Am Acad Dermatol 2:1–22, 1980

16

UNUSUAL ODORS AS CLUES TO DIAGNOSIS

With increasing reliance on laboratory findings for diagnosis, the art of clinical diagnosis using the physical senses may be neglected. In particular, the physician's sense of smell may not be used to full advantage.

Certain disorders may produce characteristic odors of body, sweat, urine, or breath. Many of these disorders are rare, but a quick and accurate diagnosis based on odor will make the physician "smell like a bed of roses."

I. Unusual Body or Urine Odor

A. Foreign Body	Nasal foreign bodies are perhaps the best-known cause of a pervasive foul body odor that may even permeate the clothing. A unilateral nasal discharge should always suggest a nasal foreign body. Vaginal foreign bodies and, much more rarely, foreign bodies in the external ear canal may also produce a generalized odor.
B. Urinary Tract Infection	An ammoniacal odor may be prominent in infection by urea-splitting bacteria.
C. Foods	Asparagus and garlic are examples of foods that may impart their distinctive odors.
D. Drugs	Various drugs may produce strong "medicinal" odors of the urine and occasionally of the skin. The odors from ampicillin and its derivatives are most pungent and are found frequently in children.
E. Phenylketonuria	The odor is often described as mousey, musty, or horse-like. If neonatal screening for this disorder were omitted, diagnosis may be based on the clinical features of developmental delay, fair complexion, microcephaly, eczema, and seizures.

F. Maple Syrup Urine Disease

Infants present in the first week or two of life with decreased appetite, vomiting, acidosis, seizures, coma, and the characteristic urine odor. The disorder is caused by a defect in amino acid metabolism.

G. Isovaleric Acidemia (Sweaty Sock Syndrome)

Isovalericacidemia, resulting from a defect in leucine catabolism, is characterized by recurrent vomiting, acidosis, and coma. (Another enzyme defect, green acyl dehydrogenase, has been reported in some cases to produce the same odor. The infants, who had poor appetite, vomiting, seizures, and severe acidosis, died within a few months of age.)

H. Oasthouse Urine Disease

A yeast-like odor is produced in this rare defect in methionine absorption. The two patients described had white hair, convulsions, and attacks of hyperpnea.

I. Hypermethioninemia

Three siblings between the ages of 2 and 8 weeks developed a fishy smell along with lethargy and irritability. All died of infection within a few months.

J. Beta-Methylcrotonyl CoA Carboxylase Deficiency

Only two cases of this disorder, associated with the smell of cat urine, have been described. Poor appetite and lethargy are findings in early infancy.

K. Stale Fish Syndrome

One patient with the stigmata of Turner syndrome has been described. The fishy odor was due to large amounts of trimethylamine in the urine.

L. Rancid Butter Syndrome

Hypermethionemia and hypertyrosinemia were found in three siblings who developed poor appetite, irritability, seizures, and coma in the first few months of life along with the offensive odor.

M. Schizophrenia

A pungent body odor has been described in patients with schizophrenia, apparently caused by the presence of trans-3-methyl-2-hexanoic acid in the sweat.[1]

N. Scurvy

The sweat is said to smell putrid.

O. Typhoid Fever

An odor of freshly baked bread is said to be emitted by patients with this disease.

P. Skin Disturbances

Disorders of the skin, such as some forms of ichthyosis, keratosis follicularis (Darier disease), or any disorder resulting in marked thickening and fissuring, may be associated with an unusual body odor. Ulcers or other necrotic skin lesions or tumors may also produce a generalized foul odor.

Q. Gout — Although a medical rarity in children, gout is said to produce a characteristic odor.

II. Unusual Breath Odors

A. Diabetic Ketoacidosis — A fruity breath odor is found in ketoacidosis, whether produced by diabetes, salicylates, or other causes.

B. Hepatic Failure — The fetor hepaticus of liver failure resembles musty fish or raw liver.

C. Gingivitis — Infection of the gingiva produces a pungent breath odor. Decaying food particles between the teeth are a common cause of bad breath.

D. Tonsillitis — Infection of tonsils and adenoids with any infectious agent may produce an abnormal odor.

E. Lung Abscess — Anaerobic organisms produce a foul breath odor.

F. Uremia — An ammoniacal smell is often noticeable on the breath of patients with uremia.

REFERENCE

1. Mace JW, Goodman SI, Centerwall WR et al: The child with an unusual odor. Clin Pediatr 15:57–62, 1976

SUGGESTED READINGS

Hayden GF: Olfactory diagnosis in medicine. Postgrad Med 67:110–118, 1980
Liddell K: Smell as a diagnostic marker. Postgrad Med J 52:136–138, 1976

17

EXCESSIVE SWEATING

Children who sweat excessively do so most frequently in response to exercise, in reaction to stress, and with fever. The classification below enumerates both common and uncommon causes of excessive perspiration.

I. Physiologic Causes
A. Exercise
B. Increased Environmental Temperature
C. Fever
D. Emotional Stimuli   The increased perspiration may be generalized or localized, especially in the axillae or on the perineum, forehead, and palms of the hands and soles of the feet.
E. Gustatory Stimuli   The forehead, upper lip, and cheeks may show an increase in perspiration accompanying the ingestion of certain foods, especially spicy and hot ones.

II. Sweating with Infection
A. During Defervescence   Excessive sweating is most likely to occur as the body temperature falls toward normal, during infections or inflammatory diseases.
B. Chronic Illnesses
  1. Pulmonary Tuberculosis   Night sweats are a classic sign of active pulmonary tuberculosis, but this is an uncommon cause of excessive sweating in children.
  2. Brucellosis   Although in acute infection the symptoms are variable, constitutional symptoms include fatigue, vague muscle aches, headaches, fever, and hyperhidrosis.
  3. Malaria

III. Endocrine and Metabolic Disorders

A. Hypoglycemia — In the newborn, symptoms include tremors, sweating, cyanosis, poor appetite, and apneic episodes. In older infants and children, pallor, staring episodes, and abnormal behavior, as well as sweating and tachycardia, may be findings.

B. Hyperthyroidism — Tremor, fatigue, tachycardia, elevated systolic blood pressure, and hyperhidrosis are common signs.

C. Pituitary Gigantism or Acromegaly — Increased perspiration is common, probably secondary to hypermetabolism.

D. Pheochromocytoma — Episodic elevations of the blood pressure are a classic sign, but headaches, sweating, pallor, and palpitations are the most common symptoms.

E. Phenylketonuria — Infants and children with untreated phenylketonuria are reported to sweat excessively.

F. Citrullinemia

IV. Drugs and Toxins

A. Salicylate Intoxication — Fever, sweating, vomiting, and hyperpnea are common.

B. Narcotic Withdrawal — This possibility must be considered in infants with tremors, irritability, increased appetite, and sweating.

C. Organophosphate Poisoning — Symptoms depend on the severity of the exposure. Excessive salivation, lacrimation, and sweating are common. Muscle cramping, anxiety, vomiting, diarrhea, and bronchospasm may also be seen.

D. Acrodynia — In mercury poisoning, the gradual onset of irritability, anorexia, and low-grade fever is followed by generalized erythema, or a miliarial-like rash, profuse sweating, photophobia, and hypotonia, and painful, peeling fingers.

E. Emetics — Ipecac may cause sweating as well as its desired effect.

F. Insulin Overdose

G. Carbon Monoxide Poisoning

V. Cardiovascular Disorders

A. Congestive Heart Failure — More prominent signs include tachycardia, tachypnea, hepatomegaly, and dyspnea. Sweating is most common about the head and neck.

B. Syncope — Pallor, sweating, and restlessness may precede syncopal episodes.

C. Raynaud Phenomenon — Sweating of the involved hands and feet commonly accompanies the color change.

D. Cluster Headaches — Thought to be a form of migraine, the headaches are severe and often short-lived but recur frequently during attacks. Conjunctival injection, tearing, nasal stuffiness, facial flushing, and sweating accompany the attacks.

E. Myocardial Infarction — Although infarctions are rare, disorders such as Kawasaki syndrome may produce coronary occlusion. Chest pain, syncope, hypotension, and tachycardia are other features.

VI. Neurologic Disorders

A. Spinal Cord Lesions — Following cord disruption, stimulation of the affected limbs causes a mass reaction with spasm and sweating.

B. Benign Paroxysmal Vertigo — The recurrent attacks of vertigo are short-lived and associated with pallor, nystagmus, and often marked sweating.

C. Diencephalic Syndrome — Infants with tumors in the diencephalon (usually optic gliomas) sweat excessively; failure to thrive, nystagmus, and a happy affect are other features.

D. Subacute Sclerosing Panencephalitis — In the terminal stages, profuse sweating may occur.

E. Auriculotemporal Syndrome — A unilateral facial flush and sweating may accompany food intake as a result of disruption of the auriculotemporal nerve.

VII. Miscellaneous Causes

A. Lymphoma — Occult tumors, especially lymphomas, may be associated with excessive sweating.

B. Atopic Disposition — Children with atopic dermatitis and allergic conditions may sweat excessively.

C. Familial Dysautonomia — In this rare autosomal-recessive disorder, there may be many unusual responses such as difficulty in swallowing, repeated aspiration and infection, absent lacrimation, blotchy skin, temperature swings, emotional lability, relative indifference to pain, and excessive sweating.

D. Familial Periodic Paralysis

Episodic attacks of flaccid paralysis and areflexia occur most commonly at night. The attacks last a few hours and then subside. Increased thirst and perspiration may precede the attacks.

E. Carcinoid Syndrome

The malignant carcinoid syndrome is rare in children. The classic features include right-sided valvular heart disease, sudden flushing of the skin, frequent watery stools, and asthmatic attacks.

F. Chédiak–Higashi Syndrome

Prominent features of this rare inherited disorder include areas of depigmented skin, photophobia accompanying ocular albinism, decreased lacrimation, hepatosplenomegaly, increased susceptibility to infection, and progressive granulocytopenia. Large inclusions are seen in the cytoplasm of white blood cells. Children with this syndrome have been noted to have increased sweating.

G. Thrombocytopenia with Aplasia of the Radius (TAR) Syndrome

H. Respiratory Failure

Increased sweating is a clinical index of the degree of failure.

I. Juvenile Rheumatoid Arthritis (JRA)

Children with JRA are frequently noted to perspire excessively, even without fever.

J. Pyridoxine Deficiency

Sweating, especially of the head, has been reported in this rare vitamin deficiency.

K. Vasoactive Intestinal Peptide Secreting Tumor

Infants usually present with growth failure, intermittent diarrhea and, occasionally, flushing, sweating, and hypertension. Tumors are usually ganglioneuromas and ganglioneuroblastomas.

18

POLYDIPSIA

Polydipsia, or excessive thirst, is a rather uncommon symptom in childhood. The underlying causes that come first to mind include diabetes mellitus and diabetes insipidus. Diabetes mellitus is probably the most common cause of polydipsia; however, other symptoms, particularly weight loss and polyuria, outweigh the increased thirst as the primary complaint. Psychogenic polydipsia (also called hysterical or primary polydipsia or compulsive water drinking) is probably underrated in frequency, especially after one considers the disorders listed below.

I. Psychogenic Polydipsia

Affected children are compulsive water drinkers and may have other neurotic traits such as immature behavior. Social history is important. Water deprivation usually increases urine osmolality, but diagnosis is difficult to confirm.[1,2]

II. Metabolic–Endocrine Causes

A. Diabetes Mellitus — Polydipsia is usually fairly abrupt in onset, with progression to weight loss and acidosis. In suspected cases the urine can be quickly checked for glucose.

B. Hypercalcemia — Several disorders including vitamin D intoxication and malignancies may produce hypercalcemia with resultant hyposthenuria and polydipsia. Anorexia, constipation, lethargy, failure to thrive, and renal stones may be present. In hyperparathyroidism, repeated bone fractures or deformities may also be findings.

C. Hypokalemia

D. Bartter Syndrome — Growth failure, polydipsia and polyuria, constipation, and episodes of fever and dehydration may be seen as early as 2 months of age. Symptoms are secondary to severe hypokalemia caused by excessive aldosterone secretion.

E. Pheochromocytoma — All patients have hypertension at some time although usually paroxysmal. During attacks of hypertension, symptoms of headache, palpitations, sweating, vomiting, and pallor may be present.

F. Neuroblastoma and Ganglioneuroblastoma
Catecholamines may be secreted by these tumors, resulting in hypertension, flush, pallor, polydipsia and polyuria, and diarrhea.

G. Cystinosis
Onset of symptoms is in the first year of life, with irritability, slow growth, anorexia, polydipsia and polyuria, constipation, and heat intolerance. Photophobia, cherubic facies, and decreased pigment of hair and skin are other findings, as well as glucosuria with hyperglucosemia.

H. Diabetes Insipidus
Antidiuretic hormone production is deficient owing to destruction of the neurohypophysis or hypothalamic lesions from various causes including histiocytosis, trauma, infection, cysts, tumors, leukemia and sarcoidosis. Water deprivation fails to increase urine osmolality. This form responds to Vasopressin therapy.

III. Renal Causes

A. Nephrogenic Diabetes Insipidus
This form is seen principally in boys; inheritance is probably X-linked, although girls may be affected. This possibility must be considered in a child with hypertonic dehydration who continues to excrete urine of low specific gravity. Failure to thrive, repeated bouts of dehydration, and fever are common manifestations. Vasopressin therapy is ineffective.

B. Sickle-Cell Anemia
Hyposthenuria is thought to be secondary to sludging of sickle cells in the renal medulla. Polydipsia follows the resultant water loss from the kidneys.

C. Interstitial Nephritis
Renal parenchymal inflammation may occur for no apparent reason. In these cases, onset of polyuria and dipsia is at 3 to 4 years of age, but most cases are diagnosed in the teens with the development of hypertension.[3] Known causes of interstitial nephritis include analgesic abuse, mercury poisoning, methicillin reaction, diphenylhydantoin, and sulfonamides.

D. Renal Tubular Acidosis
This clinical syndrome has several causes and should be considered in children with dehydration and constipation with polyuria. In

infants, vomiting, failure to thrive, anorexia, and lethargy are common. Laboratory findings include hyperchloremic acidosis, hypokalemia, and an alkaline urine with low specific gravity.

E. Medullary Cystic Disease of Kidney (Nephronophthisis)

There may be a history of polyuria and polydipsia beginning at 2 to 6 years of age. Growth failure and rickets may be present; renal failure occurs later. Inheritance is autosomal recessive.

IV. Miscellaneous Causes

A. Congestive Heart Failure

B. Hypertension

Renin-induced hypertension and secondary Angiotension II production may cause polydipsia.

C. Increased Salt Intake

REFERENCES

1. Kohn B, Norman ME, Feldman H et al: Hysterical polydipsia (compulsive water drinking) in children. Am J Dis Child 130:210–212, 1976
2. Stevko RM, Balsley M, Segar WE: Primary polydipsia—compulsive water drinking. J Pediatr 73:845–851, 1968
3. Stickler GB, Kelalis PP, Burke EC et al: Primary interstitial nephritis with reflux. Am J Dis Child 122:144–148, 1971

19
SLEEP DISTURBANCES

Interference with normal sleep patterns is relatively common in children. Fortunately, most of these disturbances are benign and are commonly precipitated by changes in the child's routine. Nightmares, difficulty in falling asleep, and even night terrors may follow daytime stresses, activities, and excitement. Genuine serious psychological problems manifesting as sleep disturbances are much less common in children than in adults.

I. Disturbances Causing Wakening

A. Nightmares	This is a common sleep disturbance during which the child usually awakes in terror from a dream. The disturbing incident is remembered, and the child is oriented after the event. Nightmares often occur following disturbances in routines during the day.
B. Night Terrors (Pavor Nocturnus)	In this uncommon disorder most prevalent in mid-childhood, an intense anxiety reaction, with physical signs such as screaming, agitation, hallucinations, sweating, and tachycardia, occurs. The child appears awake but does not recognize surroundings. The episode lasts a few minutes; the child falls back to sleep and does not remember the event.
C. Sleepwalking (Somnambulism)	Sleepwalking may occur in up to 5% of children. The eyes are open, but the child seems not to recognize the environment. Motor skills are clumsy. The duration is usually only a few minutes, and the child has amnesia for the event, which often follows a stressful event during the preceding day. The incidence increases in families where there is a history of this disorder.
D. Sleep-talking (Somniloquy)	Usually the child does not wake but may awaken others with the talking, which often accompanies sleepwalking.

E. Pinworms	In infected young girls, the pinworm may crawl out of the anus during the night and migrate forward onto the hymenal ring. The associated irritation may awaken the child.
F. Bronchial Asthma	In some children, the onset of attacks during sleep causes repeated wakening accompanied by anxiety.
G. Nocturnal Seizures	Tonic-clonic motor activity may waken others in the household. Other clues include incontinence or injuries to the tongue from biting.
H. Milk Allergy	Chronic sleeplessness has been described in milk-sensitive infants. All infants had atopic dermatitis. Daytime fussiness is present as well.
I. Airway Obstruction	Frequent episodes of wakening and sleeplessness are common in upper-airway obstruction.
J. Gastroesophageal Reflux	

II. Disturbances Causing Excessive Sleepiness

A. Depression	Depressed individuals, including children, are often lethargic and sleep excessively although restlessly.
B. Migraine	Prolonged episodes of sleep may occur with episodic attacks of migraine.
C. Narcolepsy	This disorder is uncommon in childhood; attacks usually begin after age 15. The characteristic feature is an uncontrollable, episodic change in consciousness, usually of short duration (less than 15 minutes), commonly associated with a sudden loss of muscle tone (cataplexy), sleep paralysis, and, much less commonly, states of auditory or visual hallucinations.
D. Head Trauma	
E. Postencephalitic Disturbances	
F. Drugs	Various drugs may cause excessive sleepiness including antihistamines, anticonvulsants, analgesics, and opiates.
G. Increased Intracranial Pressure	
H. Hypoglycemia	
I. Hypothyroidism	

J. Airway Obstruction	Some children with enlarged tonsils and adenoids or those who have a falling back of the tongue (glossoptosis) during the pharyngeal muscular relaxation of sleep may have excessive lethargy, snoring, and episodic periods of apnea.
K. Pickwickian Syndrome	Excessively obese individuals may experience hypercapnia and excessive sleepiness owing to respiratory insufficiency.
L. Kleine–Levin Syndrome	This rare disorder has been described in boys over 10 years of age, who have episodes of excessive sleep lasting for days to weeks. They may awake intermittently and eat excessively.

III. Difficulty Falling Asleep

A. Anxiety	Children may have difficulty sleeping because of fears or emotional stimulation or following parental discipline, or, particularly in older infants and toddlers, because of fear of separation from parents.
B. Depression	
C. Overstimulation	Young children need a period of relaxation prior to bedtime.
D. Curiosity	Activity in the environment may make it difficult to sleep.
E. Hyperthyroidism	This condition is a rare cause of insomnia.

IV. Other Disturbances

A. Sleep Myoclonus	Sudden, single, generalized jerks as the child is falling to sleep are common and benign.
B. Sleep Apnea	Short periods of apnea (less than 10 seconds) are common in infants. Children with narcolepsy and upper-airway obstructive disorders may also have apneic episodes. Prolonged episodes of sleep apnea may be a cause of sudden infant death syndrome.

SUGGESTED READINGS

Anders TF, Weinstein P: Sleep and its disorders in infants and children: A review. Pediatrics 50:312–324, 1972

Kahn A, Mozin MJ, Casimir G et al: Insomnia and cow's milk allergy in infants. Pediatrics 76:880–884, 1985

Kales A, Kales JD: Sleep disorders: Recent findings in the diagnosis and treatment of disturbed sleep. N Engl J Med 290:487–499, 1974

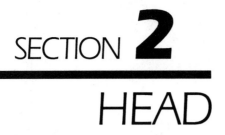

SECTION 2

HEAD

20

HEADACHE

Headache is a common complaint in children. In most children, episodes are short-lived and infrequent, so that medical advice is not sought; children with persistent or recurrent headaches are the ones usually brought for evaluation. Headaches come in all shapes and sizes. However, certain features of headache, especially patterns, can often be related to a specific cause.

Overall, the most frequent cause of headaches is infection, in which the associated fever results in vasodilatation of the intracranial vessels, producing the pain. In the evaluation of recurrent or persistent headache in children, the history is especially important and should include information about location, severity, associated symptoms, duration, and usual time of onset. A family history of migraine may be obtained, but headaches may also be the learned somatic expression of anxiety or stress in the family.

In the differential diagnosis of headache, it is important to discover patterns if they exist. Unfortunately, not all causes of headaches have a typical pattern, and specific characteristics of headache may be associated with several disorders. The atypical presentation in particular poses a greater diagnostic challenge.

Many parents consider that a brain tumor is the most likely cause of their child's headache, although they are usually reluctant to voice this fear. Fortunately, brain tumors are uncommon. Anticipation and dismissal of this concern after a thorough examination can be an important therapeutic intervention.

I. Vascular Causes

A. Fever — Generalized dilatation of cranial arteries is the most common cause of headaches, particularly in acute infectious diseases. Fever associated with chronic systemic disease may also be responsible for recurrent headaches secondary to vascular dilatation.

B. Migraine — The classic pattern is paroxysmal, unilateral headache with preceding visual aura and nausea or vomiting, as well as a family history. In children, however, paroxysmal symptoms overshadowing the headache may be present. Cyclic vomiting, ataxia, hemiparesis, abdomi-

109

nal pain, and diplopia may suggest other disorders. Headache may become a prominent complaint later. A history of motion sickness may be a clue.

C. Hypoxia and Hypercapnia

Vasodilatation is the cause.

D. Anemia

With severe anemia, compensatory increased blood flow may lead to vasodilatation.

E. Aneurysm

One fifth of patients may have a history of recurrent headaches; cranial nerve palsies may be other findings. Coarctation of the aorta and polycystic disease of the kidneys are found in 25% of patients with aneurysms. Unfortunately, the usual presentation is sudden, severe headache, confusion, vomiting, and loss of consciousness associated with massive subarachnoid bleeding.

F. Arterial Inflammation

Systemic lupus erythematosus and subacute bacterial endocarditis are examples. Other systemic clues may be present.

G. Carbon Monoxide Poisoning

Headache and vertigo are early symptoms; with continued exposure, bounding pulse, vomiting, dilated pupils, dusky skin, and convulsions may develop.

H. Hypertension

This is not as common a cause in children as often thought. Headache may be present upon awakening and increases with activity. Renal causes of increased blood pressure are most frequent.

I. Seizures

In convulsive disorders, headache is present most commonly in the postictal state, although occasionally as an aura that may mimic migraine. Vascular dilatation is the probable cause.

J. Cluster Headache

An unusual migraine variant in children. Severe, short-lived, retro- or periorbital pain often associated with signs of sympathetic overactivity on the ipsilateral side of the face.

K. Cerebral Venous Sinus Thrombosis

Initial symptoms may be mild and suggest a functional disorder. Headache, nausea, vomiting, photophobia, blurred vision, diplopia, and lethargy may be present. Birth control pills have been implicated in some cases.

II. Muscular Causes: Tension and Stress

These headaches usually appear in late afternoon; the ache is located posteriorly in and around the neck muscles and is described as "tight." Pain fluctuates with stressful situations but does not interfere with recreation. Muscular causes are common, especially in adolescents.

III. Psychological Causes

A. Depression	Associated symptoms include loss of appetite, sleep disturbances, inability to concentrate, and failure to participate in activities.
B. Conversion	Vivid descriptions of the head pain may be given. There may be other somatic complaints, frequently associated with an indifferent attitude.
C. Mimicry	Headaches may be a common expression of frustration or stress in the family. A parent or other family member may be a role model.

IV. Increased Intracranial Pressure

Headaches are produced by traction on pain-sensitive structures (see Chap. 23, Increased Intracranial Pressure, for additional causes).

A. Brain Tumor	The head pain is generalized but often more severe in the occiput; it is most frequently present early in the morning upon arising but may last all day. Vomiting and increased pain on position change or with coughing may develop later. Papilledema and complaints of diplopia, weakness, and numbness may be other features.
B. Pseudotumor Cerebri	Excessive vitamin A ingestion (as in acne therapy), outdated tetracycline usage, and hypoparathyroidism may be causes.
C. Withdrawal from Steroids	
D. Oral Contraceptives	
E. Hydrocephalus	
F. Electrolyte Disturbances	A wide variety of conditions may lead to inappropriate antidiuretic hormone secretion. Hyponatremia may be associated with nausea, delirium, incoordination, and seizures.

G. Intoxications with Cerebral Edema — Lead poisoning should be considered.

H. Brain Abscess — Symptoms depend on the child's age and on the size and location of the abscess and include headache, fever, lethargy, and seizures, as well as focal neurologic deficits.

I. Intracranial Hemorrhage — The clinical course is usually more acute in epidural hemorrhage, leading to obtundation, than in subdural hemorrhage.

V. Extracranial Disorders

A. Sinusitis — Sinusitis may be infectious or allergic. Rhinorrhea, sinus tenderness, nasal congestion, and fever may be present. Pain is often retroorbital, accentuated on eye movement.

B. Dental Problems — Caries or abscesses may manifest as headache rather than local pain. Malocclusion of teeth or grinding of teeth during sleep (bruxism) may also cause headache.

C. Ocular Disorders — Headache may be an early complaint in glaucoma or uveitis. "Eye strain" is most often a manifestation of stress rather than a primary eye disorder.

D. Aural Disorders — Acute otitis media, serous otitis media, and mastoiditis are more likely to have localized complaints.

VI. Trauma

A. Concussion — Headache may last for days or rarely for years following concussion.

B. Occipital Neuralgia — Pain is usually unilateral and can be induced by palpation over the occiput or second cervical vertebra; it results from root compression due to malformation of the joint space between the first and second cervical vertebrae with intermittent subluxation.

VII. Meningeal Irritation

A. Infection — Meningitis and encephalitis may be associated with headache.

B. Leukemic or Tumor Infiltration

VIII. Miscellaneous Causes

A. Allergy — Allergy may cause the tension–fatigue syndrome with headache. A past history of milk or other allergies suggests this possibility. An elimination diet, especially of milk, chocolate, and eggs, is worthwhile in suspected cases.

B. Environmental Factors — Heat, humidity, noxious fumes, and noise have all been implicated. Tension may be a common factor, because muscle contraction is the pathogenetic mechanism.

C. Hypoglycemia

D. Decreased Intracranial Pressure — Headache may follow lumbar puncture.

E. Hyperventilation — Chest tightness, dizziness, numbness and tingling of arms and legs, and carpopedal spasm may be other findings.

F. Obstructive Sleep Apnea — Children who develop intermittent obstruction of their upper airway during sleep may wake in the morning with a headache, probably the result of chronic hypoxemia. Snoring with obstructive-type breathing patterns may be a clue.

G. Drugs — Amphetamines, for example, may cause headaches as well as irritability, insomnia, and loss of appetite and weight. Nitrates and nitrites produce vasodilatation, which can cause headache.

H. Metabolic Acidosis

I. Basilar Impression — Invagination of margins of the foramen magnum result in posterior displacement of the odontoid and compression of the spinal cord and brain stem. Ataxia, stiff neck, head tilt, nystagmus, and cortical tract signs may occur.

J. Sarcoidosis

SUGGESTED READINGS

Ferry PC: Diagnosis and office management of headaches in children. Clin Pediatr 11:195–200, 1972

Honig PJ, Charney EB: Children with brain tumor headaches. Am J Dis Child 136:121–124, 1982

Ling W, Oftedal G, Weinburg, W: Depressive illness in childhood presenting as severe headache. Am J Dis Child 120:122–124, 1970

Prensky AL: Migraine and migrainous variants in pediatric patients. Pediatr Clin North Am 23:461–471, 1976

21

MACROCEPHALY

Macrocephaly is defined as a head circumference that is greater than two standard deviations above the mean for age, sex, race, and gestation.

In infancy the most common cause of an enlarged head is hydrocephalus produced by various lesions. Chronic subdural hematomas are probably the second most common cause. It is important to remember, however, that the head being measured may be a "chip off the old block." In other words, the child's macrocephaly may reflect a familial trait. Measurements of the head circumference of the parents and other family members are an essential part of evaluation.

Head enlargement in older children may be due to a chronic pseudotumor cerebri; other signs of increased intracranial pressure will predominate, however. In cranial and skeletal dysplasias, other prominent somatic features assist in defining the cause of the macrocephaly and related problems.

Macrocephaly may also be the result of an increase in brain substance rather than of increased intracranial pressure or thickness of the skull. In addition to familial or primary forms of megalencephaly, metabolic disorders, neurocutaneous syndromes, and other disorders must be considered in the differential diagnosis.

I. Disorders Associated with Hydrocephalus

A. Malformations with Obstruction

1. Arnold–Chiari Malformation — This anomaly accounts for 40% of cases of hydrocephalus in infants and children. Obstructive hydrocephalus results from the herniation of the lower brain stem through an enlarged foramen magnum.

2. Aqueductal Stenosis — Stenosis of the cerebral aqueduct is responsible for about 20% of cases of hydrocephalus in children; however, hydrocephalus may develop at any time from birth to adulthood and may be associated with other malformations including spina bifida. In a few cases, sex-linked recessive inheritance has been reported.

3. Dandy–Walker Syndrome — The fourth ventricle becomes greatly dilated and acts as a cyst; onset of symptoms may be delayed until after infancy. Presenting signs

	include a bulging occiput, nystagmus, ataxia, and cranial nerve palsies.
4. Holoprosen-cephaly	Failure of division of the cerebral hemispheres is usually associated with midline facial defects. Hydrocephalus is rare; microcephalus is more common.
B. Aqueductal Gliosis	Obstruction of the aqueduct is a result of an inflammatory response to a perinatal infection or hemorrhage.
1. Congenital Infections	Rubella, cytomegalovirus, toxoplasmosis, and syphilis are the most frequently recognized infections.
2. Perinatal Hemorrhage	Intraventricular hemorrhage, especially in hypoxic premature infants, or vascular malformations or trauma may result in obstruction to cerebrospinal fluid flow.
C. Communicating Hydrocephalus	Normal absorption of the cerebrospinal fluid may be impaired in various disorders. This form accounts for 30% of all childhood hydrocephalus.
1. Intracranial Hemorrhage	
2. Bacterial or Granulomatous Meningitis	
3. Obstruction of Vein or Sinuses	Any number of disorders that result in an increased intracranial venous pressure may cause diminished cerebrospinal fluid absorption.
4. Diffuse Meningeal Malignant Tumors	Rarely, lymphomas or leukemias may produce this problem.
D. Excess Cerebrospinal Fluid Secretion: Choroid Plexus Papilloma	Head enlargement is usually not seen until after infancy, with signs of increased intracranial pressure.
E. Tumors	
1. Neoplasms	Various primary and metastatic tumors may cause increased intracranial pressure and head enlargement. Headache and vomiting are the most constant signs.
2. Arteriovenous Malformations	As the lesions enlarge, obstruction of cerebrospinal fluid flow may occur. Cranial bruits and unexplained congestive heart failure are possible associated findings.

3. Brain Abscess   An abscess generally causes acute symptoms, and its clinical course is rarely prolonged enough to result in head enlargement.

4. Cysts   Porencephalic cysts may enlarge to produce a clinical picture resembling that of hydrocephalus. Since the cysts are usually unilateral, focal neurologic problems are common.

F. Hydranencephaly   The cerebral tissue is minimal and replaced by a sac filled with cerebrospinal fluid. Infants with this disorder appear normal at birth but then have progressive head enlargement. Primitive reflexes persist. Hypertonia, hyperreflexia, and later, decerebration follow.

II. Disorders Associated with Pseudotumor Cerebri

Various disorders may cause increased intracranial pressure without obstruction of cerebrospinal fluid flow. If the disorders are long-standing, some increase in head circumference may be seen. Symptoms of increased intracranial pressure predominate the clinical picture, however.

A. Lead Poisoning

B. Drug Reactions   The most frequently implicated drugs are tetracycline, sulfonamides, penicillin, nalidixic acid, and oral contraceptives.

C. Corticosteroids (Administration or Withdrawal)

D. Cyanotic Congenital Heart Disease

E. Hypoparathyroidism

F. Hypervitaminosis or Hypovitaminosis A

G. Adrenal Insufficiency

H. Galactosemia

III. Intracranial Hemorrhage

A. Subdural Hematoma   Chronic subdural collection of fluid may produce slowly progressive head enlargement, seizures, developmental delay, and sometimes anemia. Subdural effusions may develop following meningitis.

B. Intraventricular or Subarachnoid Hemorrhage	Symptoms are almost invariably acute. Head enlargement may develop in infants following hemorrhage as a result of aqueductal stenosis or diminished CSF absorption.

IV. Skeletal and Cranial Dysplasias

A. Achondroplasia	In short-limbed dwarfism, head enlargement is secondary to increased brain size. Hydrocephalus may be a complication.
B. Osteogenesis Imperfecta	Brittle bones, bowing of the legs, blue sclerae, and wormian bones of the skull are classic features.
C. Rickets	Findings include frontal and parietal bossing, epiphyseal enlargement, bowing of the legs, and swelling of the costochondral junctions.
D. Craniosynostosis	The head may appear enlarged because of a distortion of shape.
E. Cleidocranial Dysostosis	There is congenital absence or hypoplasia of the clavicles. The skull is soft at birth; fontanels are large, and sutures remain open. Short stature is a common finding.
F. Metaphyseal Dysplasia	Progressive enlargement of the skull, hypertelorism, and a broad flat nose are characteristic. Cranial nerve deficits may occur secondary to obliteration of foramina by bony overgrowth.
G. Osteopetrosis	There is early onset of generalized bone sclerosis with thickening of the skull, delayed development, cranial nerve deficits, pancytopenia, and occasionally hydrocephalus.
H. Hyperphosphatasia	Bowed tubular bones, flared ribs, a protruding sternum, and marked dwarfism are characteristic.
I. Conradi Syndrome (Chondrodystrophia Calcificans Congenita)	Scoliosis, cataracts, asymmetrical limb shortening, joint contractures, short stature, and stippled epiphyses on roentgenograms are found.
J. Marshall Syndrome	In this rare disorder, linear growth and skeletal maturation are accelerated; other features are prominent eyes, blue sclerae, and motor and mental delay.
K. Camptomelic Dwarfism	This is a prenatal growth deficiency characterized by markedly bowed legs, a flat facies, macrocephaly, and many other skeletal anomalies.
L. Craniofacial Dysostosis	Premature synostosis of the lambdoid suture and the posterior part of the sagittal suture

results in a prominent forehead and a flat occiput. Short stature, hypoplastic supraorbital ridges, and micrognathia are other features.

M. Robinow Syndrome

This condition has also been called the "fetal face syndrome" because of the disproportionately large cranium. Midface hypoplasia, a short upturned nose, short forearms, and genital hypoplasia are other features.

N. Pycnodysostosis

Findings include short stature, frontal and occipital skull prominence, delayed closure of the anterior fontanel, and wormian bones.

O. Kenny Syndrome

This syndrome is a rare cause of growth retardation with delayed closure of the anterior fontanel, hyperopia, episodic hypocalcemic tetany, internal cortical thickening, and medullary stenosis of tubular bones. Intelligence is normal.

P. Proteus Syndrome

Other features include asymmetric rapid growth, macrodactyly, and an unusual thickening of the skin and subcutaneous tissues.

Q. Osteopathia Striata and Cranial Sclerosis

This is a rare autosomal dominant disorder in which striae replace the normal appearance of trabecular bone.

V. Megalencephaly

A. Primary Megalencephaly

Macrocephaly may be familial without associated anomalies. Measurement of the head circumference of other family members is mandatory.

B. Metabolic Diseases

1. Tay–Sachs Disease

Macrocephaly may be a feature in children surviving beyond about 2 years of age. Hypertonia, hyperreflexia, psychomotor retardation, and blindness, are earlier findings.

2. Metachromatic Leukodystrophy

Several forms occur; age of onset is variable. Progressive neurologic and mental deterioration are present in all.

3. Canavan Disease (Spongy Degeneration of Central Nervous System)

Megalencephaly is striking. Onset is between 3 and 9 months of age with initial hypotonia and progressive dementia followed by spasticity and blindness.

4. Alexander Disease (Infantile Leukodystrophy)	Deterioration begins in the first year of life, with progressive psychomotor retardation, seizures, spasticity, and macrocephaly.
5. Mucopolysaccharidoses	Both Hurler and Hunter syndromes are characterized by progressive mental retardation and coarse features. Macrocephaly is occasionally seen in the Maroteaux–Lamy syndrome, as well as coarse features, stiff joints, and hepatosplenomegaly, but without mental retardation.
6. Generalized Gangliosidosis	Coarse features, joint stiffness, and hypotonia are present in early infancy.
7. Methylmalonic Acidemia	Microcephaly or macrocephaly may be seen in the vitamin B_{12}–responsive form, characterized by difficulty in nursing, vomiting, failure to thrive during the neonatal period, and episodic metabolic acidosis.
8. Maple Syrup Urine Disease	Macrocephaly is an uncommon feature. In the first few weeks of life, the infants have seizures, episodes of opisthotonos, and intermittent hypertonia, followed usually by an early death.

C. Neurocutaneous Syndromes

1. Neurofibromatosis	Multiple café-au-lait spots and, later, neurofibromas in the skin are key features. Cranial enlargement may be due to hydrocephalus or intracranial tumors as well as megalencephaly.
2. Tuberous Sclerosis	Hypopigmented macules and shagreen and ashleaf patches precede the development of adenoma sebaceum.
3. Riley–Smith Syndrome	Cutaneous hemangiomas, macrocephaly, and pseudopapilledema are found in this rare autosomal-dominant disorder.
4. Klippel–Trenaunay–Weber Syndrome	Unilateral hemangiomatoses, varicosities, and bony overgrowth are characteristic.
5. Sturge–Weber Syndrome	Port-wine stain of the face involving the upper eyelid and forehead may be associated with ipsilateral cerebral hemangiomatosis.
6. Cutis Marmorata Telangectatica Congenita	Macrocephaly has been described in CMTC which gives a reticulated vascular appearance to the skin.

7. Macrocephaly, Lipomatosis, and Angiomatosis

8. Disseminated Hemangiomatosis

9. Bannayan Syndrome — Subcutaneous hamartomas, lipomas, and hemangiomas with early linear growth acceleration are part of this autosomal dominant disorder.

10. Basal Cell Nevus Syndrome — Multiple nevi (actually hamartomas) increase with age. Basal cell carcinomas are a major problem. Other features include a square jaw, tiny pits in the skin of the palms and soles, rib and vertebral anomalies as well as multiple jaw cysts.

D. Anemia — Any severe chronic anemia may result in skull enlargement secondary to bone marrow expansion. Beta-thalassemia major is best recognized for this phenomenon.

E. Miscellaneous Syndromes

1. Cerebral Gigantism (Soto Syndrome) — There is excessive somatic growth during the first few years of life. Children are usually large at birth, have acromegalic features including large hands and feet and a large jaw, and are mentally retarded.

2. Beckwith–Wiedemann Syndrome — Characteristic features include macroglossia, an omphalocele or umbilical anomaly, macrosomia, and often severe hypoglycemia in the neonatal period.

3. Histiocystosis X — Children with Hand–Schüller–Christian disease may appear to have macrocephaly.

4. Weaver Syndrome — Only two cases have been reported. Features include macrosomia, camptodactyly, an unusual facies, and accelerated skeletal maturation.

5. Fetal Alcohol Syndrome — Although most affected children have microcephaly, two with enlarged cranial vaults have been described.

VI. Benign Subdural Effusion in Infants

The development of computed tomography has allowed identification of children with rapid head growth who appear to have areas of cortical atrophy resembling subdural effusion. Features include some ventricular enlargement, wide cerebral sulci, large sylvian cisterns, prominent interhemispheric fissures, and decreased density over the cerebral convexities. In some infants, initial developmental delay disappears with time.

SUGGESTED READINGS

Asch AJ, Myers GJ: Benign familial macrocephaly. Pediatrics 57:535–539, 1976

Menkes JH: Textbook of Child Neurology. Philadelphia, Lea & Febiger, 1980

Mori K, Handa H, Itoh M et al: Benign subdural effusion in infants. J Comput Assist Tomography 4:466–471, 1980

National Foundation—March of Dimes: Birth Defects Compendium, 2nd ed. Bergsma D (ed). New York, AR Liss, 1979

Robertson WC Jr, Chun RWM, Orrison WW et al: Benign subdural collections of infancy. J Pediatr 94:382–385, 1979

Smith DW: Recognizable Patterns of Human Malformation, 3rd ed. Philadelphia, WB Saunders, 1982

Stephan MJ, Hall BD, Smith DW et al: Macrocephaly in association with unusual cutaneous angiomatosis. J Pediatr 87:353–359, 1975

22

MICROCEPHALY

There is some disagreement about the clinical definition of microcephaly. The criterion of a head circumference more than 2 standard deviations below the mean for age, sex, and gestational age has been used; measurements 3 or more standard deviations below the mean have also been recommended. Whatever the definition, microcephaly describes a small head, and a small head generally denotes a small brain, since it is brain growth that produces head enlargement. (A notable and perhaps the only exception is microcephaly secondary to craniosynostosis.)

There seems to be a linear relationship between head size and intellectual capacity: The smaller the head, the less likely intelligence will be normal. Some children with microcephaly may be exceptions to this rule, but the association cannot be ignored in the differential diagnosis.

Primary microcephaly is caused by anomalous development of the brain during the first 7 months of gestation. Familial factors, congenital infections, chromosomal abnormalities, syndromes of dysmorphogenesis, anatomic defects of the brain produced by insults to the fetus during early gestation, drugs, and toxins, and metabolic disorders, as well as craniosynostosis, are the most common causes. Secondary microcephaly follows injuries to the growing rather than to the developing brain; these include anoxia, trauma, and hypoglycemia occurring any time in the last 2 months of gestation or during early infancy.

The lists of dysmorphogenetic syndromes and chromosomal abnormalities are exceptionally long; undoubtedly, they are not comprehensive but they are offered as an aid to further evaluation of these disorders, in which distinctions may be subtle. Although the possible causes of microcephaly are many, most are rarely seen in clinical practice. It is important to measure the head size of all family members, and to obtain a careful history of the gestational period, including maternal infections and drug or alcohol ingestion. In the infant who does not have an unusual phenotype or evidence of premature closure of the cranial sutures, serologic tests for congenital infections may be in order.

I. Genetic or Familial Microcephaly

A. Autosomal-Dominant Form	The microcephaly is generally not as severe as in the autosomal-recessive form. Affected children may have receding or small foreheads, upslanted palpebral fissures, and prominent ears.

B. Autosomal-Re- cessive Form	The phenotype is usually striking. Height is less than normal, the forehead inclines acutely, and the chin may be hypoplastic and the nose and ears prominent; the scalp may be furrowed. Spastic diplegia and seizures are frequently found. Severe mental retardation occurs in most cases.

II. Congenital Infections

Intrauterine infections with rubella, cytomegalovirus, toxoplasmosis, herpes simplex, syphilis, and others may result in microcephaly. Many infants may have other signs and symptoms in the newborn period including thrombocytopenia, low-birth weight, hepatospleno-megaly, and jaundice. Some infections, however, are subclinical and manifest as psychomotor retardation, microcephaly, or deafness later.

III. Chromosomal Abnormalities

Many chromosomal abberrations are associated with anomalous brain development. Usually many phenotypic abnormalities are present, some of which are listed with each defect.

A. Down Syn- drome	The most common of the chromosomal defects is associated with a mild microcephaly.
B. Trisomy 18 Syn- drome	Features include hypertonia, failure to thrive, prominent occiput, a short sternum, congenital heart disease, micrognathia, and limited hip abduction.
C. Trisomy 13 Syn- drome	The triad of microphthalmia, cleft lip and palate, and polydactyly suggests this defect. Literally hundreds of other anomalies have also been reported.
D. Cri du Chat Syndrome	A weak, cat-like cry in an infant with micro-cephaly, hypertelorism, growth failure, microphthalmia, and hypotonia suggests this syndrome.
E. 18 p⁻ Syndrome	Low birth weight, webbed neck, lymphedema, shield chest, short stature, hypertelorism, ptosis, epicanthal folds, strabismus, and stubby hands are prominent features.
F. 19 q⁻ Syndrome	Low birth weight, midfacial dysplasia, carp-shaped mouth, atretic ear canals, long finger tips, and hypotonia are characteristic.
G. 11 q Partial Tri- somy	Features include short nose with a long philtrum, growth retardation, micropenis, micrognathia, and congenital heart disease.

H. 4 p⁻ Syndrome	Retardation, hypertelorism, downward-slanted palpebral fissures, cleft palate, beaked nose, and a carp-like mouth are seen.
I. 14 q Distal Partial Trisomy	Normal birth weight, hypertonia or hypotonia, high forehead, epicanthal folds, low-set ears, micrognathia, and camptodactyly are findings.
J. 14 q Proximal Partial Trisomy	Features are low birth weight, seizures, hypertonia, low anterior hairline, hypotelorism or hypertelorism, low-set and malformed ears, and a short neck.
K. 13 q⁻ Syndrome	Broad nasal bridge, low-set abnormal ears, ptosis, and microphthalmia are characteristic.
L. Triploidy	Incidence is rare. Variable features include very low birth weight, coloboma, and cutaneous syndactyly.
M. 21 Monosomy	Low birth weight, prominent nose, wide nasal bridge, large and low-set ears, microcephaly, micrognathia, and hypertonia are the features.
N. 22 Monosomy	Low birth weight, seizures, hypotonia, ptosis, and hypertelorism are found.

IV. Syndromes of Dysmorphogenesis

A. Pierre Robin Anomalad	This triad of cleft palate, micrognathia, and glossoptosis may be seen in other disorders.
B. De Lange Syndrome	Severe mental retardation, a growling-like cry, long philtrum, anteverted nares, hirsutism, and deformities of the extremities are common.
C. Cockayne Syndrome	Infants appear normal for the first year but then become dwarfed. The face appears thin with a prominent nose and deep-set eyes; other features include neurologic deficits, cataracts, and a photosensitive dermatitis.
D. Smith–Lemli–Opitz Syndrome	Infants demonstrate failure to thrive with anteverted nostrils, ptosis, cryptorchidism, and hypospadias.
E. Hallermann–Streiff Syndrome (Oculomandibulofacial Syndrome)	Short stature, microphthalmia, cataracts, micrognathia, sparse hair, and a small, pinched nose are common.
F. Focal Dermal Hypoplasia (Goltz Syndrome)	Hypoplastic areas of skin with protrusions of fat, reddish streaks, papillomas, sparse hair, deformities of fingers, and short stature are characteristic.

G. Seckel Syndrome (Bird-Headed Dwarfism)	Features include marked growth deficiency, prominent nose, low-set malformed ears, and dislocated hips.
H. Laurence–Moon–Biedl Syndrome	Obesity, mental deficiency, polydactyly and syndactyly, hypogonadism, and retinitis pigmentosa are common.
I. Williams Syndrome	Microcephaly is mild, with short stature, prominent lips, a hoarse voice, and, often, cardiac abnormalities.
J. Fanconi Syndrome (Pancytopenia)	Hypoplastic or absent thumb, short stature, hyperpigmentation, and the later development of pancytopenia are characteristic.
K. Meckel–Gruber Syndrome	The key feature is a posterior encephalocele. Polydactyly, microphthalmia, micrognathia, and a short neck are frequently present.
L. Langer–Giedion Syndrome (Trichorhinophalangeal Syndrome)	Mild microcephaly with large protruding ears and a large bulbous nose is characteristic.
M. Bloom Syndrome	Short stature, facial telangiectasia, light photosensitivity, and microcephaly of variable degree are features.
N. De Sanctis–Cacchione Syndrome	Growth deficiency, mental deterioration, sun sensitivity, and hypogonadism are found.
O. Johanson–Blizzard Syndrome	Deafness, retardation with hypoplastic alae nasi, and hypothyroidism are characteristic.
P. Rubinstein–Taybi Syndrome	Features include broad thumbs and toes, often with angulation, retardation, a beaked nose, and downward slant to palpebral fissures.
Q. Prader–Willi Syndrome	Hypotonia, hypogonadism, short stature, obesity, and small hands and feet characterize this syndrome.
R. Coffin–Siris Syndrome	Features include hypotonia, mild microcephaly, sparse scalp hair, and hypoplasia or absence of the fifth finger and toenails.
S. Rhizomelic Chondrodysplasia Punctata	Proximal shortening of extremities with stippled epiphyses on roentgenograms, flat facies, and low nasal bridge are characteristic.
T. Roberts Syndrome	There is severe retardation with significant deformities of the extremities.

U. Cerebrocosto-mandibular Syndrome	Severe micrognathia and rib deformities with pronounced respiratory difficulties are findings.
V. Cerebrooculofacioskeletal Syndrome	Sloping forehead, cataract, microphthalmia, narrow palpebral fissures, large ears, scoliosis, and kyphosis are features of this syndrome.
W. Craniofacial Dysostosis with Diaphyseal Hyperplasia	Findings include premature craniosynostosis, exophthalmos, maxillary hypoplasia, hypertelorism, strabismus, short stature, and short hands.
X. Craniofacial Dyssynostosis	Features are a prominent forehead and a small, flat (or bulging) occiput due to premature closure of the lambdoid and posterior part of the sagittal sutures.
Y. Craniooculodental Syndrome	Affected children have a low hairline, nasal septum deviation, brachydactyly, ptosis, facial asymmetry, and beaked nose.
Z. Dubowitz Syndrome	Low birth weight, sparse hair, high sloping forehead, flat supraorbital ridges, broad nasal bridge, and ptosis are characteristic.
AA. Dyggve–Melchior–Clausen Syndrome	Findings include short-trunk dwarfism, protruding sternum, barrel chest, restricted joint mobility, and flat vertebral bodies.
BB. Ectrodactyly and Ectodermal Dysplasia with Clefting	Absence of fingers or hand clefts, cleft lip or palate, and sparse scalp hair are the findings.
CC. Happy Puppet Syndrome	Affected children have jerking movements and a pleasant laughing demeanor with retardation and seizures.
DD. Leprechaunism (Donohue Syndrome)	Prenatal growth and adipose tissue deficiency are characteristic, as well as thick lips, wide eyes, hirsutism, and genital enlargement.
EE. Megalocornea and Mental Retardation	Short stature, hypotonia, ataxia, seizures, and enlarged corneas are features.
FF. Microphthalmis with Digital Anomalies	One or both eyes are small, the ears are misshapen, and rudimentary sixth digits are present.
GG. Oculodentoosseous Dysplasia	Features include a thin nose with hypoplastic alae nasi, microcornea, syndactyly of fourth and fifth fingers, and enamel hypoplasia.

HH. Opticocochleo-dentate Degeneration — Optic atrophy and deafness occur with spastic quadriplegia.

II. Orocraniodigital Syndrome — Bilateral or unilateral cleft lip, thumb anomalies, and curvature or syndactyly of the toes are characteristic features.

JJ. Osteoporosis and Pseudoglioma — Recurrent fractures from minor injuries and blindness from retinal detachment are problems.

V. Anatomic Defects Secondary to Early Insults to the Developing Brain

A. Schizencephaly (Schizencephalic Porencephaly) — Clefts are placed symmetrically within the cerebral hemispheres; there are profound neurologic and developmental defects, with symmetric spastic and rigid quadriparesis and seizures.

B. Macrogyria — The gyri of brain are too few and are coarse. Neurologic deficits tend to be lateralized.

C. Polymicrogyria — There are small, numerous gyri. The clinical picture is one of retardation, spasticity, or hypotonia with active deep tendon reflexes.

D. Agenesis of Corpus Callosum — Two forms are seen: In one, patients have seizures with mild to moderate mental retardation and impaired vision and motor coordination. In the X-linked form, severe retardation and seizures are found.

E. Lissencephaly (Miller–Dieker Syndrome) — The cortex of the brain is smooth and lacks sulci. Spastic quadriplegia with severe retardation and seizures is present.

VI. Drugs and Toxins

Fetal exposure to drugs or toxins ingested by the mother or to which the mother was exposed may affect brain growth.

A. Fetal Alcohol Syndrome — Growth deficiency, microcephaly, short palpebral fissures, and maxillary hypoplasia are characteristic.

B. Fetal Hydantoin Syndrome — Growth deficiency, large fontanel, hypertelorism, cleft lip and palate, hypoplastic distal phalanges, and coarse hair are among the many features.

C. Fetal Trimethadione Syndrome — Midfacial hypoplasia, short upturned nose, upslant to eyebrows, broad nasal bridge, and cleft lip and palate may be seen.

D. Aminopterin
   Syndrome

Growth deficiency, hypoplasia of facial bones, upswept frontal scalp hair, micrognathia, and short limbs are found.

E. Irradiation

Exposure to ionizing radiation during the first 2 trimesters may cause interference with brain growth.

F. Methadone

VII. Craniosynostosis

Premature closure of sutures usually occurs *in utero*. Only 10% of cases are associated with dysmorphic syndromes. The shape of the skull depends on which sutures are closed.

VIII. Metabolic Disorders

A. Phenylketonuria

Features include mental retardation, seizures, and imperfect hair pigmentation. Vomiting and irritability are frequent in the first few months of life. The skin is rough and dry.

B. Maternal
   Phenylketonuria

Growth retardation, both before and after birth, microcephaly, and severe intellectual delay are common.

C. Citrullinemia

Infants may appear normal for a few months and then have severe vomiting with coma and seizures; a rapidly fatal course is the rule.

D. Maple Syrup
   Urine Disease

Infants usually die in the first few weeks. Opisthotonos, respiratory irregularities, and seizures are common.

E. Hyperglycinemia

Profound retardation and seizures are present from the time of birth.

F. Maternal Diabe-
   tes Mellitus

Infants of diabetic mothers may have microcephaly if the mother's diabetes has been poorly controlled.

G. Glycogen Syn-
   thetase Defi-
   ciency

Hepatomegaly, lethargy, and poor weight gain are the result of a severe neonatal hypoglycemia.

IX. Miscellaneous Disorders

A. Incontinentia
   Pigmenti

This hereditary disorder is seen predominantly in females. Vesiculobullous linear skin lesions are present at birth or appear shortly thereafter, followed by verrucous lesions and then hyperpigmented swirls. Seizures, cataracts, and dental and renal abnormalities may also be found.

B. Riley–Day Syndrome (Familial Dysautonomia)	Recurrent aspiration, absent lacrimation, unexplained fevers, absent deep tendon reflexes, and insensitivity to pain are among the unusual features of this syndrome.
C. Beckwith–Wiedemann Syndrome	Microcephaly is occasionally seen. Postnatal gigantism associated with an omphalocele or umbilical anomaly, macroglossia, and visceromegaly suggests the diagnosis.
D. Myotonic Dystrophy	Microcephaly is sometimes a feature of this disorder of difficulty of muscle relaxation. Infants are usually hypotonic. The facies is immobile.
E. Schwachman Syndrome	Pancreatic insufficiency and leukopenia are prominent features.

X. Secondary Microcephaly

Several insults to the growing brain may occur prior to delivery or in the early neonatal period.

A. Meningitis
B. Birth Trauma
C. Anoxia
D. Severe Dehydration
E. Hypoglycemia
F. Acquired Immune Deficiency Syndrome

SUGGESTED READINGS

Haslam RHA, Smith DW: Autosomal dominant microcephaly. J Pediatr 95:701–705, 1979

Menkes JH: Textbook of Child Neurology, 2nd ed. Philadelphia, Lea & Febiger, 1980

National Foundation—March of Dimes: Birth Defects Compendium, 2nd ed. Bergsma D (ed). New York, AR Liss, 1979

Smith DW: Recognizable Patterns of Human Malformation, 3rd ed. Philadelphia, WB Saunders, 1982

23

INCREASED INTRACRANIAL PRESSURE AND BULGING FONTANEL

Increased intracranial pressure (IIP) may be of sudden onset with characteristic symptoms or may develop gradually and be relatively asymptomatic. The type of symptoms often depends on the age of the child. In the older child who complains of headaches and has papilledema, the diagnosis of IIP is almost assured. In the infant or toddler, who may not be able to express the presence of headache, signs and symptoms including irritability, colic, head-holding, and of course a tense or bulging fontanel suggest IIP. Nausea, vomiting, strabismus, personality changes, head enlargement, and lethargy progressing to coma may be part of the clinical picture, and all are important clues in the differential diagnosis.

In this chapter, IIP and bulging fontanel are considered together, since most of the disorders listed below may produce a bulging or tense fontanel if it is open.

I. Space-Occupying Lesions

A. Brain Tumor	Presenting signs are usually the result of IIP. Headache and vomiting are the most constant signs. Increasing head size occurs in long-standing cases. Convulsions are rarely a part of the picture. Spinal cord tumors and, much less commonly in children, metastatic tumors, (particularly neuroblastoma) may also be causes.
B. Intracranial Hemorrhage	In the neonate, hemorrhage is usually due to birth trauma or anoxia.
1. Intraventricular Hemorrhage	Decreased movement and tone, seizures, and a decreasing hematocrit with a tense fontanel are suggestive signs.
2. Cerebral Bleeding	Diffuse parenchymal bleeding with secondary brain swelling may produce signs similar to those seen with intraventricular hemorrhage.

3. Subarachnoid Hemorrhage	Lacerations of the tentorium or falx in newborns, trauma in children of any age, or a ruptured aneurysm may be the initiating event. Symptoms are generally sudden in onset.
4. Subdural Hemorrhage	Changes in consciousness, vomiting, convulsions, papilledema, and retinal hemorrhages may be found. In young children, child abuse should be considered. If there is no external evidence of trauma, a shaking insult may have produced the bleeding. Children with chronic subdural hematomas may present with slowly progressive head enlargement, seizures, developmental delay, and sometimes anemia.
C. Brain Abscess	Early symptoms are nonspecific. Most children have no fever. This diagnosis must be considered in the child with cyanotic congenital heart disease, or with a primary infection such as mastoiditis, who develops headaches, vomiting, and convulsions, followed by localized neurologic signs.

II. Hydrocephalus

Several disorders may cause ventricular enlargement as a consequence of increased pressure of the cerebrospinal fluid (CSF). Most cases are secondary to obstruction of the normal flow and egress of the CSF. In young infants, in addition to progressive cranial enlargement, other symptoms include irritability, poor feeding, and developmental delay in severe cases. The scalp veins may appear distended, and eventually the disproportion between the size of the face and the head becomes apparent. The fontanel may bulge later. Older children, with closed cranial sutures, demonstrate the usual signs of IIP.

III. Infectious Causes

A. Meningitis	A bulging fontanel in a sick child demands immediate examination of the CSF.
B. Encephalitis	
C. Roseola	Bulging of the fontanel occasionally occurs during this common infection.
D. Shigella	Central nervous system symptoms including convulsions and IIP may precede the development of diarrhea.
E. Guillain–Barré Syndrome	The development of an ascending paralysis or paresis suggests this possibility.
F. Poliomyelitis	

G. Cysticercosis

The larval form of the pork tapeworm may invade the CNS resulting in seizures and signs of increased intracranial pressure.

H. Other Infections

Several infections may cause IIP, the mechanism of which is unclear: otitis media, paranasal sinusitis, ethmoiditis, upper-lobe pneumonia, and pyelonephritis.

IV. Endocrine Causes

A. Hypoparathyroidism

Repetitive convulsions, particularly at the time of fever, may be the presenting sign. Tetany may be the primary sign in older children.

B. Pseudohypoparathyroidism

Affected children have short stature with short hands, especially the fourth and fifth metacarpals, a round face, and sometimes intracranial calcifications seen on roentgenograms.

C. Addison Disease

Hypoadrenocorticism is another rare cause of IIP. Vomiting, muscle weakness, increased skin pigmentation, or patches of vitiligo may be seen.

D. Hypothyroidism

E. Hyperthyroidism

F. Ovarian Dysfunction

The cause of the IIP is unclear; it is most frequently seen in adult women.[1]

V. Cardiovascular Causes

A. Dural Sinus Thrombosis

Ear, pharyngeal, or sinus infections or in some cases trauma or tumor invasion may cause the thrombosis.

B. Hypertensive Encephalopathy

C. Congestive Heart Failure

The cause is probably increased venous pressure.

D. Obstructed Vena Cava

Obstruction is by an intrathoracic mass. Blockage of venous return produces increased venous pressure.

VI. Hematologic Disturbances

A. Polycythemia

Polycythemia may result in cerebral infarction and swelling or dural sinus thrombosis.

B. Anemia

Severe iron-deficiency anemia has been described as a cause.

C. Leukemia

Central nervous system involvement may produce pressure symptoms.

VII. Metabolic Causes
A. Uremia

B. Galactosemia

C. Hypophospha-
tasia

In severe cases, the fontanel may be large and tense and the skull soft. Anorexia, vomiting, and irritability are other prominent symptoms. Serum alkaline phosphatase levels are low.

D. Osteopetrosis

As a cause of IIP, osteopetrosis is rare. The bones become sclerotic and thickened. Head enlargement, hepatosplenomegaly, pancytopenia, and multiple cranial nerve palsies are highly suggestive findings.

E. Maple Syrup Urine Disease

F. Electrolyte Dis-
turbances

Water intoxication secondary to inappropriate antidiuretic hormone secretion may result from a number of disorders.

VIII. Drugs and Toxins
A. Tetracycline

Infants on tetracycline therapy may develop IIP by an unknown mechanism after only a few doses. This phenomenon occasionally occurs in adolescents being treated for acne with this drug.

B. Nalidixic Acid

C. Hypervitamin-
osis A

High doses of vitamin A may cause an IIP picture. The vitamin may have been taken for the treatment of acne, ichthyosis, or other skin disorders. The ingestion of polar bear liver, which has a high vitamin A content, is a favorite "roundmanship" cause.

D. Lead Encepha-
lopathy

The prodrome of lead poisoning may have been overlooked. This possibility should always be considered in the child with pica who has central nervous system signs and symptoms.

E. Steroid With-
drawal

F. Steroid Therapy

G. Oral Contracep-
tives

H. Aluminum Tox-
icity

Infants receiving aluminum containing phosphate binders may develop an osteodystrophy with delayed closure of the fontanel, poor muscle tone, and a ricket-like picture.

IX. Miscellaneous Causes

A.	Craniostenosis	Coronal synostosis, as seen in Crouzon syndrome, may produce signs of IIP and a bulging fontanel.
B.	Status Epilepticus	Cerebral edema results in IIP.
C.	Reye Syndrome	
D.	Chronic Pulmonary Disease	Chronic hypoxia is felt to be the pathogenetic mechanism.
E.	Obesity	Obesity may be a cause of IIP in adolescents and adults, but the pathogenesis is unclear.
F.	Hypovitaminosis A	
G.	Vitamin B$_2$ (Riboflavin) Deficiency	
H.	Rapid Brain Growth Following Starvation	This finding has been reported after nutritional improvement in cystic fibrosis.
I.	Food or Drug Allergies	
J.	Congenital Subgaleal Cyst over the Anterior Fontanel	
K.	Lupus Erythematosus	

REFERENCE

1. Hagberg B, Sillanpää M: Benign intracranial hypertension. Acta Paediatr Scand 59:328–339, 1970

SUGGESTED READINGS

Bell WE, McCormick WF: Increased Intracranial Pressure in Children. Philadelphia, WB Saunders, 1972

Griffith JL, Brasfield JC: Increased intracranial pressure. Pediatr Rev 2:269–276, 1981

Smith DW: Introduction to Clinical Pediatrics, 2nd ed. Philadelphia, WB Saunders, 1977

24

ENLARGED ANTERIOR FONTANEL

An enlarged anterior fontanel may indicate increased intracranial pressure or any of several disorders affecting calcification and development of the calvarium.

The first step in the evaluation of an apparently enlarged anterior fontanel is measurement for comparison with the range of normal size consistent with age. Popich and Smith[1] have developed a graph for normal size of the anterior fontanel based on their study of normal newborn infants. The fontanel size was calculated as length plus width divided by 2. In these infants, anterior fontanel size ranged from 0.6 cm to 3.6 cm, with a mean of 2.1 cm. These measurements are recommended as limits of normal size in newborns, with 0.6 cm defined as 2 standard deviations below and 3.6 cm as 2 standard deviations above the mean.

In this chapter disorders that may be associated with an enlarged anterior fontanel are listed. Short descriptors of many of these disorders are included to aid in the differential diagnosis.

I. Increased Intracranial Pressure

Any disorder resulting in increased intracranial pressure may produce an abnormally large anterior fontanel (see Chap. 23, Increased Intracranial Pressure and Bulging Fontanel).

II. Skeletal Disorders

A. Achondroplasia — Short stature, short limbs, and a large head with a prominent forehead and depressed nasal bridge are characteristic features.

B. Osteogenesis Imperfecta — Affected children usually are short in stature and have a history of multiple bone fractures. The sclerae are bluish. In infants, there is a soft feel to the skull caused by wormian bones, as well as a large fontanel.

C. Vitamin D-Deficiency Rickets — In addition to the large fontanel there may be frontal and parietal bossing. Other findings include bowed legs, enlarged epiphyses, prominent costochondral junctions, and scoliosis.

D. Cleidocranial Dysostosis — This disorder, with autosomal-dominant inheritance, features partial to complete aplasia of the clavicles, brachycephaly with frontal bossing, wormian bones, late dentition, and irregular finger length.

E. Apert Syndrome (Acrocephalo-syndactyly) — Inheritance is also autosomal dominant; craniosynostosis with a short anteroposterior diameter, a high forehead and flat occiput, flat facies with hypertelorism, and syndactyly of fingers and toes are findings.

F. Hypophosphatasia — This rare disorder, characterized by hypoplastic fragile bones, bowed lower extremities, short ribs with a rachitic rosary, and defective dentition, is inherited as an autosomal-recessive trait.

G. Pyknodysostosis — Features include short stature, osteosclerosis with a tendency to fracture, frontal and occipital prominence, a persistent anterior fontanel with delayed suture closure, wormian bones, and irregular teeth.

H. Kenny Syndrome — The main findings are short stature, myopia, and a late closure of the fontanel.

III. Chromosomal Abnormalities
   A. Down Syndrome
   B. Trisomy 13 Syndrome
   C. Trisomy 18 Syndrome

IV. Endocrine Disorders
   A. Athyrotic Hypothyroidism — In addition to a large fontanel other findings include an immature facies, macroglossia, umbilical hernia, dry skin, neonatal jaundice, and constipation. These features may not be prominent in the neonate.

V. Congenital Infections
   A. Rubella — The classic major abnormalities, in various combinations, are deafness, microcephaly, congenital heart disease, psychomotor retardation, and cataracts.

   B. Syphilis

VI. Drugs and Toxins

A. Fetal Hydantoin Syndrome

Infants born to mothers who are taking this anticonvulsant may manifest several dysmorphogenic abnormalities including failure to thrive, cleft lip or palate, hypoplastic nails, hypertelorism, broad nasal bridge, and mental deficiency.

B. Aminopterin-Induced Malformation

Exposure to this folic acid antagonist *in utero* results in severe hypoplasia of facial and skull bones, micrognathia, and clubfoot.

VII. Dysmorphogenetic Syndromes

A. Russell–Silver Syndrome

Prenatal onset of growth deficiency with short stature, small triangular facies, short incurved fifth fingers, and occasionally limb asymmetry are characteristic features.

B. Rubinstein–Taybi Syndrome

A large anterior fontanel is occasionally seen in this syndrome in which the main features are short stature, broad thumbs and great toes, antimongoloid slant to the palpebral fissures, and cryptorchidism

C. Hallermann–Streiff Syndrome (Oculomandibulofacial Syndrome)

Small stature, brachycephaly with frontal and parietal bossing, micrognathia, cataracts, a small thin nose, and hypoplastic teeth are found.

D. Zellweger (Cerebrohepatorenal) Syndrome

There is marked hypotonia from birth, as well as a high forehead, flat occiput, redundant skin of the neck, hepatomegaly, and an early death.

E. Robinow Syndrome (Fetal Face Syndrome)

Mild-to-moderate short stature, macrocephaly, frontal bossing, hypertelorism, small upturned nose, long philtrum, short forearms, and hypoplastic genitals are findings in this disorder inherited as an autosomal-dominant trait.

F. Cutis Laxa

Inheritance is autosomal recessive; in affected children, loose skin creates a "bloodhound" appearance. Short stature and laxity of joints are other features.

G. Progeria

In this rare but striking syndrome, early onset of premature aging is seen, with alopecia, loss of subcutaneous fat, and short stature.

H. VATER Association

This group of anomalies may occur in various combinations: vertebral defects, ventricular septal defect, anal atresia, tracheoesophageal fistula, and radial dysplasia.

I. Opitz–Frias Syndrome

Swallowing problems with recurrent aspiration, stridor, a weak hoarse cry, hypertelorism, and hypospadias are characteristic findings.

J. Beckwith–Wiedemann Syndrome

VIII. Miscellaneous Causes

A. Malnutrition

B. Hydranen-cephaly

The head is enlarged at birth with a large fontanel. The skull vault is thin, and primitive reflexes are preserved. Transillumination verifies the diagnostic suspicion.

C. Intrauterine Growth Retardation

Term newborns, who are small for gestational age, may have large anterior fontanels, particularly if their epiphyseal ossification is delayed.[2]

D. Mucopolysac-charidoses

A large fontanel is most likely to be found in Hurler syndrome (type I mucopolysaccharidosis).

E. Hyperpipecolic Acidemia

Additional features include developmental delay, hypotonia, and retinopathy with visual impairment.

REFERENCES

1. Popich GA, Smith DW: Fontanels: Range of normal size. J Pediatr 80:749–752, 1972
2. Philip AGS: Fontanel size and epiphyseal ossification in neonates with intrauterine growth retardation. J Pediatr 84:204–207, 1974

25

DELAYED CLOSURE OF ANTERIOR FONTANEL

In Chapter 24, disorders associated with a large fontanel were presented. In many of these disorders, delayed closure of the anterior fontanel is subsequently seen. Descriptions of conditions associated with a large fontanel as well as delayed closure are not repeated here.

The anterior fontanel generally closes by 12 to 18 months of age; however, normal closure time may range from 4 to 26 months. Most conditions associated with delayed closure have dysmorphic features that should facilitate their recognition.

I. Increased Intracranial Pressure

In addition to causing an enlarged anterior fontanel, increased intracranial pressure from a wide variety of causes may result in delayed closure of the fontanels.

II. Skeletal Disorders

A. Achondroplasia

B. Osteogenesis Imperfecta

C. Vitamin D–Deficiency Rickets

D. Cleidocranial Dysostosis

E. Apert Syndrome (Acrocephalosyndactyly)

F. Hypophosphatasia

G. Pyknodysostosis

H. Kenny Syndrome

I. Pseudodeficiency Rickets (Vitamin D-Resistant Rickets)   Bony changes similar to those in rickets are found but are unresponsive to treatment with vitamin D. Additional findings are hypotonia, growth deficiency, susceptibility to fractures, and hypocalcemia.

  J. Stanesco Dysos-   In this unusual form of dwarfism, features
     tosis   include a thin skull, shallow orbits, and a
                         small mandible.

III. Chromosomal Abnormalities
  A. Down Syndrome
  B. Trisomy 13 Syn-
     drome
  C. Trisomy 18 Syn-
     drome

IV. Endocrine Disorders
  A. Athyrotic Hypo-
     thyroidism

V. Drugs and Toxins
  A. Fetal Hydantoin
     Syndrome
  B. Aminopterin-
     Induced Malfor-
     mation
  C. Aluminum Toxic-   Infants receiving aluminum-containing phos-
     ity   phate binders may develop an osteodystrophy
                       with a bulging fontanel, poor muscle tone,
                       and a ricket-like picture.

VI. Dysmorphogenetic Syndromes
  A. Russell–Silver
     Syndrome
  B. Rubinstein–   Occasional late closure may be seen.
     Taybi Syndrome
  C. Hallermann–
     Streiff Syndrome
     (Oculomandib-
     ulofacial Syn-
     drome)
  D. Zellweger Syn-
     drome (Cerebro-
     hepatorenal Syn-
     drome)
  E. Robinow (Fetal
     Face) Syndrome
  F. Cutis Laxa   Occasional late closure may be seen.
  G. Progeria

H. VATER Associa-
tion
Occasional late closure may be seen.

I. Aase Syndrome
Triphalangeal thumbs, congenital anemia, narrow shoulders, and mild growth deficiency are features.

J. Melnick–Nee-
dles Syndrome
Infants fail to gain well; physical findings include exophthalmos, full cheeks, micrognathia, marked malocclusion, and large ears.

K. Conradi–Hüner-
mann Syndrome
Occasional late closure may be seen. Features include mild-to-moderate growth deficiency, asymmetrical limb shortening, downslanting palpebral fissures, and frequently scoliosis.

L. Otopalatodigital
Syndrome
Late closure of the anterior fontanel is occasionally seen. Prominent findings are frontal prominence, hypertelorism, small nose and mouth, broad distal digits, conduction deafness, and mild mental retardation.

M. Saethre–Chotzen
Syndrome

VII. Miscellaneous Causes

A. Primary Megal-
encephaly
Macrocephaly may be familial without associated anomalies. Measurement of the head circumference of other family members is mandatory. The macrocephaly may be related to idiopathic hydrocephalus.

B. Malnutrition
C. Congenital Syph-
ilis

SUGGESTED READING

Smith DW: Recognizable Patterns of Human Malformation, 3rd ed. Philadelphia, WB Saunders, 1982

26

EARLY CLOSURE
OF ANTERIOR
FONTANEL

The conditions associated with delayed closure of the anterior fontanel are considerably more numerous than those associated with early closure. What constitutes early closure? The definition is not clear, but if the anterior fontanel is no longer palpable at 4 to 5 months of age, further investigation is in order. In some children, roentgenographic examination discloses that the fontanel is still open despite clinical evidence to the contrary. If the fontanel is truly closed, the following conditions should be considered in the differential diagnosis.

I. Normal Variation
Although the mean age of closure of the anterior fontanel is about 18 months, closure as early as 4 to 5 months of age may still be a normal variation. Subsequent head growth must be closely monitored.

II. Microcephaly
Abnormal brain development may be accompanied by microcephaly and early fontanel closure. Causes of failure of development include prenatal and postnatal insults.

III. Craniosynostosis
A. Idiopathic Causes

B. Hyperthyroidism — Premature closure has been reported in idiopathic hyperthyroidism as well as with the administration of excessive amounts of thyroid hormone in replacement therapy.

C. Hypophosphatasia — In this rare inherited disorder, skeletal changes are similar to those in rickets. Hypercalcemia is frequently found, the serum alkaline phosphatase is low, and excessive amounts of phosphoethanolamine are excreted in the urine. The fontanel closure may be early or late.

D. Rickets — Craniosynostosis may occur in as many as one third of cases of rickets.

E. Hyperparathyroidism — Two cases of premature fontanel closure have been described in this disorder. Hypercalcemia, generalized bone rarefraction, and failure to thrive suggest hyperparathyroidism in infancy.

27

PAROTID GLAND SWELLING

The normal parotid gland is not palpable. Enlargement of this salivary gland is most commonly due to infection by mumps virus, whose symptoms usually are well recognized, even by most laymen.

In this chapter, other causes of parotid swelling are enumerated. In some cases, swelling is recurrent, and careful evaluation of the amount and nature of the glandular secretions is required. Secondary or recurrent infections often develop in glands with deficient saliva production. "Wind parotitis," swelling of the gland as a result of air forced into Stensen's duct, may be mistaken for recurrent infections.

I. Infection
A. Viral Infections
1. Mumps — Mumps is the most common and easily recognized cause of parotid gland swelling. The gland is usually tender to touch, but the overlying skin is not erythematous. There is some debate about whether mumps parotitis can be recurrent.
2. Parainfluenza Types 1 and 3 — Parainfluenza types 1 and 3 are probably the second most common causes of acute parotitis.
3. Other — Less common viruses implicated include Coxsackie A, echovirus, varicella, cytomegalovirus, and lymphocytic choriomeningitis.

B. Bacterial Infections
1. Acute Suppurative Infections — These infections are most frequently seen in neonates or infants under 1 year of age and in those with debilitating diseases. *Staphylococcus aureus* is the most common pathogen while *H. influenzae* is an occasional cause. The gland is tender and red, and there may be significant systemic symptoms. In some cases pus can be expressed from Stensen's duct.

144

2. Abscess of
   Parotid
   Gland
C. Other Infections
   1. Tuberculosis   As a cause of swelling, tuberculosis is rare at present. Infection is not as acute as with viral and bacterial causes.
   2. Actinomy-
      cosis   Swelling is usually the result of direct extension from infection elsewhere.
   3. Sarcoidosis   Swelling of the parotid gland occurs in less than 10% of the cases of sarcoidosis. The swelling is firm, painless, and often nodular. Heerfordt syndrome is an unusual form characterized by febrile uveitis and parotitis, preauricular swelling, and occasional paralysis of the facial nerve.
   4. Cat-Scratch
      Disease   Granulomas may develop in the parotid gland following scratches about the face. Recurrent facial swelling due to preauricular lymphadenitis may simulate parotid gland disease.
   5. Tularemia   Swelling is part of the uveoparotid syndrome.
   6. Histoplas-
      mosis   Consider this possibility particularly if hilar adenopathy is present.

II. Chronic or Recurrent Sialadenitis

A. Nonobstructive,
   Intermittent
   Sialadenitis
   1. Benign Lym-
      phoepithelial
      Lesion   Decreased salivary flow and stasis due to changes in the salivary ducts predispose the gland to recurrent inflammation. The lesion generally occurs in children over 5 years of age. The swelling is recurrent, may be slightly tender, and is nonerythematous. The diagnosis is confirmed by sialography, which shows punctate sialectasia. This lesion has been thought to represent a localized form of Sjögren syndrome.
   2. Idiopathic
      Causes   Enlargement is usually unilateral. It is associated with mild pain and lasts 1 to 2 weeks. The recurrences resolve at puberty.
   3. Functional
      Hypersecre-
      tion   This is a rare cause of enlargement.

B. Allergic Reactions

The presence of eosinophilic plugs in the parotid duct with swelling has been documented in allergic reactions. In a significant number of patients, there are other allergic symptoms. The onset of the swelling is sudden and it lasts hours to several days.

C. Drug Sensitivities

Iodides in drugs or food are the best-known cause of parotid swelling from drugs. Other medications that may cause swelling are rarely used in children. Phenothiazines in large doses may cause xerostomia (dry mouth) and repeated infections, resulting in swelling.

III. "Wind Parotitis"

Air may be forced into the parotid duct and cause glandular swelling, especially in children learning to play wind instruments or blowing up balloons. More rarely, the child may learn how to force air into Stensen's duct as an attention-getting device.

IV. Tumors

A. Hemangioma

The swelling is soft and nontender. There may be a bluish hue to the overlying skin. When the infant cries, the swelling may become more tense.

B. Lymphangioma

The swelling tends to be more diffuse than with hemangiomas and not confined to a specific salivary gland.

C. Mixed Tumor

This form is the most common of the benign tumors and is first seen as a firm, painless mass.

D. Mucoepidermoid Tumor

This is the most common of the malignant tumors. The usual presenting feature is a firm, mobile mass in the parotid fascia. A sudden growth of a mass or facial nerve palsy raises the suspicion of malignancy.

V. Metabolic and Endocrine Disorders

A. Endocrine Disturbances

The parotid enlargement seen with endocrine disturbances is benign, slowly progressive, painless, and lacking inflammation.

1. Hypothyroidism

2. Cushing Syndrome

Enlargement is due to fatty infiltration.

B. Metabolic Disorders
   1. Diabetes Mellitus — Salivary gland swelling as a result of diabetes is unusual in childhood.
   2. Starvation — Parotid hypertrophy is the cause and it may be secondary to hypoproteinemia.
   3. Anorexia Nervosa — If starvation is severe enough, salivary gland hypertrophy may occur.
   4. Postnecrotic Cirrhosis

VI. Obstructive Enlargement

A. Strictures — Strictures may be congenital or secondary to poor oral hygiene, dental or external trauma, recurrent infection, or calculi. The swelling usually occurs suddenly with eating and is painful. Secondary infection is common. Sialography is diagnostic.

B. Calculi — Calculi rarely occur in the parotid gland. Symptoms are the same as in strictures. Calculi occur more commonly in teenagers than in younger children and may follow recurrent infection.

VII. Miscellaneous Causes

A. Cystic Fibrosis — Parotid enlargement rarely occurs, but the submaxillary gland is enlarged in 90% of affected children.

B. Autoimmune Disorders
   1. Sjögren Syndrome — Dry mouth and eyes are characteristic. The swelling may be related to intermittent blockage of the parotid duct by mucus plugs or to repeated infection.
   2. Mixed Connective Tissue Disease — Children with this disorder have various symptoms of various connective tissue disorders.
   3. Systemic Lupus Erythematosus — Recurrent swelling may occasionally be the initial clue.

C. Impaction of Stensen's Duct with a Food Particle

D. Acquired Immune Deficiency Syndrome   Chronic parotid swelling may be part of the picture usually characterized by recurrent infection and poor growth.

VIII. Disorders That Mimic Parotid Swelling

A. Lymphadenopathy

B. Masseter Muscle Hypertrophy   Hypertrophy may occur as a result of teeth grinding, while awake or sleep. In some cultures, such as that of the Alaskan Eskimo, hypertrophy is normal and is associated with a diet of foods requiring prolonged chewing.

SUGGESTED READINGS

Banks P: Nonneoplastic parotid swellings: A review. Oral Surg 25:732–745, 1968

Strome M: Differential Diagnosis in Pediatric Otolaryngology. Boston, Little, Brown & Co, 1975

28
FACIAL PARALYSIS

Facial paralysis is a relatively uncommon disorder in general pediatric practice. Otolaryngologists, naturally, have written most about this problem, and they suggest that any child with facial palsy be examined thoroughly by someone specifically trained to evaluate facial nerve function, to uncover potentially remediable causes. Nevertheless, a brief review of possible causes is included for perusal. Some causes will be obvious to the "unspecialized" eye.

Although the list of causes is long, only a few disorders account for most cases. Idiopathic facial paralysis (Bell palsy) has been reported to cause anywhere from one third to two thirds of the cases seen in children. Traumatic causes make up 8% to 25%; otitis media, about 10%; and congenital causes, 5% to 20%.

The following classification has been modified from Swaiman and Wright.[1]

I. Congenital Causes

A. Congenital Facial Paralysis (Möbius Syndrome)	Absence of seventh nerve nuclei, usually evident at birth, is bilateral and associated with bilateral involvement of the sixth nerve. The face is expressionless, the eyes do not close completely, and the infant drools constantly. Mental retardation is frequent.
B. Temporal Bone Malformation	A unilateral paralysis may result.
C. Supranuclear Facial Nerve Lesion	This lesion is associated with anoxia before or during birth. The lower half to two thirds of the face is affected on the side opposite the lesion.
D. Hypoplasia of the Depressor Anguli Oris Muscle	Asymmetric movements of the face, noted especially on crying, may suggest facial nerve paralysis, but in fact there is a congenital absence or hypoplasia of this muscle. The forehead wrinkles, the eyes close, and nasolabial folds appear equal. Although Cayler described an association with only cardiac anomalies,

renal and musculoskeletal abnormalities also occur.[2]

II. Trauma

A. Birth Trauma Facial paralysis not uncommonly results from pressure on the peripheral portion of the nerve during forceps application, by the maternal sacral promontory, or occasionally by bone fragments in skull fractures.

B. Facial Trauma Injuries to the facial nerve may occur from accidents or missiles.

C. Skull Fracture Temporal bone fracture may result in a delayed paralysis. Cochlear function is lost in a large percentage of cases.

III. Idiopathic Causes

A. Bell Palsy The exact pathogenetic mechanism is unclear, but the paralysis is thought to follow vasospasm of the blood vessels supplying the facial nerve, leading to edema and resultant loss of function. Onset is usually sudden and often around the time of an upper respiratory infection. Paralysis is usually unilateral and may be complete or partial. Ear pain may be an early symptom. Vertigo, loss of taste, and hyperacusis may also occur.

B. Melkersson Syndrome This hereditary syndrome is characterized by recurrent facial paralysis that is often bilateral, relapsing, and familial, angioneurotic edema, especially of the lips, and in some cases a furrowing of the tongue.

IV. Infectious Disorders

A. Otitis Media Acute otitis media may produce a transient palsy, treated best with antibiotics and a myringotomy. Chronic otitis media may result in suppuration of the apex of the petrous portion of the temporal bone, resulting in sixth and seventh nerve paralysis. Fever, ear pain, and chronic otorrhea may be present. Gradenigo syndrome is the name given to the petrositis with cranial nerve involvement.

B. Guillain–Barré Syndrome Up to one third of patients with this ascending peripheral neuropathy have a facial paralysis.

C. Mastoiditis	Incidence is much less today than in the pre-antibiotic era. The auricle may be pushed forward, and the mastoid area is swollen and tender.
D. Herpes Zoster Oticus (Ramsay Hunt Syndrome)	This disorder is much more common in adults. Severe, deep-seated ear pain followed by the appearance of vesicles on the tympanic membrane, in the external auditory canal, or on the auricle is characteristic.
E. Meningitis	
F. Encephalitis	Various encephaliditides may result in facial palsy, including varicella, mumps, rubella, poliomyelitis, and other enteroviral infections.
G. Osteomyelitis of Temporal Bone	
H. Mumps Parotitis	
I. Brain Abscess	Central paralysis may occur, but this sign is overshadowed by central nervous system signs and symptoms.
J. Miscellaneous Infections	Infectious mononucleosis, influenza, tuberculosis, tetanus, trichinosis, and syphilis are examples.
K. Lyme Arthritis	Total paralysis of the facial nerve has been described in some patients with this unusual form of arthritis.

V. Metabolic Disorders

A. Hypothyroidism	
B. Osteopetrosis	Overgrowth of bone may compress cranial nerves. Bones are brittle; the head is square; and anemia, blindness, and deafness develop.
C. Diabetes	Diabetes is a rare cause in children.
D. Uremia	

VI. Tumors and Neoplasia

A. Acoustic Neuroma	A neuroma rarely produces paralysis and is rare in children. Suggestive symptoms include unilateral progressive hearing loss, unilateral tinnitus, and intermittent vertigo or unsteadiness.
B. Gliomas of Brain Stem	Facial paralysis may be a presenting complaint. Sixth nerve palsy, with or without headache and ataxia, is common.
C. Leukemia	

D. Metastatic Tumors   Neuroblastoma may be a cause in children.

E. Eosinophilic Granuloma, Teratoma, Hemangioma, Rhabdomyosarcoma   Paralysis may result when the middle ear is involved.

F. Neurofibromatosis

G. Parotid Gland Tumors

H. Facial Nerve Tumors   A slowly progressive paralysis results.

VII. Miscellaneous Causes

A. Vascular Lesions   Thrombosis of the carotid artery or of the middle cerebral or pontine branches of the basilar artery may produce paralysis. Aneurysms may also be responsible, but in both lesions, central nervous system signs are evident.

B. Hypertension   Facial paralysis is an uncommon finding in severe hypertension.

C. Polyarteritis Nodosa

D. Postictal Paralysis   Paralysis is brief if it occurs.

E. Myotonic Dystrophy   Ptosis, immobile facies with eventual facial muscle atrophy, and muscle weakness with myotonia are found.

F. DPT Immunization Reaction

G. Hydrocephalus

H. Drug Reactions   Vincristine is best known.

I. Freeman–Sheldon Syndrome (Craniocarpotarsal Dystrophy)   Mask-like facies with a small mouth gives a "whistling face" impression; the chin is dimpled and the tongue is small.

J. Schwartz Syndrome   Myotonia with a mask-like face, joint motion limitation, and short stature are findings.

K. Goldenhar Syndrome (Oculo-auriculovertebral Dysplasia)   Multiple facial anomalies, with hemifacial microsomia, small or atretic ears, and epibulbar dermoids, are characteristic.

L. Kawasaki Disease (Mucocutaneous Lymph Node Syndrome)	
M. Henoch–Schönlein Purpura	Compression of the seventh nerve from edema has been reported.
N. Sarcoidosis	Facial paralysis is the most common neurologic complication of sarcoidosis. It is generally associated with parotid swelling and, less commonly, with uveitis.

REFERENCES

1. Swaiman KF, Wright FS: Pediatric Neuromuscular Diseases. St. Louis, CV Mosby, 1979
2. Caylor GE: Cardiofacial Syndrome. Arch Dis Childh 44:69–75, 1969

SUGGESTED READINGS

Manning JJ, Adour KK: Facial paralysis in children. Pediatrics 49:102–109, 1972
Maran AGD, Stell PM: Clinical Otolaryngology. Oxford, Blackwell Scientific Publications, 1979
Pape KE, Pickering D: Asymmetric crying facies: An index of other congenital anomalies. J Pediatr 81:21–30, 1972

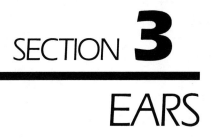

SECTION **3**

EARS

29

EARACHE

Earache, or otalgia, is a common symptom in the pediatric age group. Earache in most cases is the result of acute middle ear infections or chronic accumulations of fluid in the middle ear. Otitis externa is more common in the summer months. Self-induced trauma to the ear canal or tympanic membrane occurs more frequently than generally thought; children (and adults) stick all sorts of matter into their ear canals.

In this chapter causes of otalgia are divided into two groups: disorders involving the ear primarily, and those in which ear pain is referred from disease in another region.

I. Primary Otalgia
  A. External Ear

1. Otitis Externa	The pain associated with infection of the ear canal is intensified by pulling on the auricle. *Pseudomonas aeruginosa* is the most common pathogen.
2. Foreign Body	Irritation and pain may result from the presence of foreign material in the canal.
3. Ear Trauma	The ear canal or auricle may be injured by self-induced trauma with sticks, paper clips, and similar objects used to scratch the ear or remove cerumen, or by falls, blows, and other forms of trauma.
4. Impacted Cerumen	Occlusion of the ear canal by cerumen may cause loss of hearing and, occasionally, ear pain.
5. Cellulitis	The auricle may become acutely red, tender, and swollen owing to a bacterial infection. Frequently an external otitis has preceded the cellulitis.
6. Furuncle or Abscess	Furuncles or abscesses of the external canal are exquisitely painful.
7. Chronic Eczema	Pruritus of the auricular skin induces chronic rubbing with resulting irritation. Fissuring of the auricle and canal may occur, and secondary infections are common.

8. Herpes Simplex	The finding of grouped vesicles suggests this infection.
9. Herpes Zoster	In mild cases the inner ear may not be involved. Painful vesicles may be present on the auricle and in the external canal.
10. Relapsing Polychondritis	Recurrent attacks of inflammation of the auricular cartilage is characteristic of this condition, which is rare in children. It is usually bilateral, and the auricle becomes swollen, red, and quite tender.

B. Middle and Inner Ear

1. Acute Otitis Media	This is by far the most common cause of ear pain. The tympanic membrane is dull, often bulging, and sometimes erythematous.
2. Serous Otitis Media	Fluid in the middle ear may cause intermittent acute sharp or dull aching pain. Hearing is often diminished. Ear "popping" or cracking sensations may be reported.
3. Barotrauma	Sudden changes in air pressure cause acute ear pain.
4. Bullous Myringitis	Vesicles, often hemorrhagic, may be noted on the tympanic membrane.
5. Eustachian Tube Obstruction	Swelling of the lining tissues of the eustachian tube by infection or allergies may prevent equalization of air pressure between the middle ear and the environment. Serous otitis media may follow long-standing obstruction.
6. Mastoiditis	Untreated middle ear infection may extend to the mastoid air cells. The mastoid area becomes swollen, erythematous, and tender to touch. The auricle may be pushed out and forward away from the head.
7. Bell Palsy	A deep earache may accompany acute peripheral facial nerve paralysis.
8. Temporal Bone Neoplasms	Tumors are a rare cause of ear pain. Embryonal rhabdomyosarcoma may be associated with excruciating ear pain with hearing loss and tinnitus.
9. Petrositis	Infection of the petrous ridge, secondary to otitis media, may cause a sixth nerve palsy by entrapment of the nerve. Facial nerve paralysis is less frequent.

II. Secondary Otalgia

A. Pharyngeal Lesions

1. Acute Pharyngitis

2. Tonsillitis — Peritonsillar abscess may cause ear pain.

3. Retropharyngeal Abscess

4. Following Tonsillectomy or Adenoidectomy

5. Nasopharyngeal Fibroma — This lesion occurs most commonly in adolescent boys. The presenting symptoms are usually recurrent nose bleeds and unilateral or bilateral nasal obstruction.

B. Oral Cavity Lesions

1. Acute Stomatitis or Glossitis

2. Dental Problems — Dental abscesses and impacted molars may produce referred ear pain.

C. Laryngeal and Esophageal Causes

1. Laryngeal Ulceration

2. Cricoarytenoid Arthritis — Rarely, a child with juvenile rheumatoid arthritis may develop hoarseness, stridor, a feeling of fullness in the throat, and referred ear pain.

3. Esophageal Foreign Body — Difficulty in swallowing and throat pain are much more common symptoms than ear pain.

4. Esophageal Reflux — Rarely, reflux may be so forceful that esophagitis and pain referral to the ear occur.

D. Miscellaneous Causes

1. Mumps — Ear pain may precede or accompany overt parotid gland swelling.

2. Postauricular Lymphadenopathy — Pain is localized to the area of the adenopathy.

3. Sinusitis

4. Acute Thyroiditis — The thyroid is usually enlarged and tender to palpation.

5. Temporoman-   Pain associated with arthritis of this joint
   dibular Arthritis   rarely is referred to the ear.
6. Temporoman-   Suspect in children who have recurrent facial
   dibular Joint   or ear pain for which no etiology can be deter-
   Dysfunction   mined. It is strikingly associated with depres-
      sion.

SUGGESTED READINGS

Belfer ML, Kaban LB: Temporomandibular joint dysfunction with facial pain in children. Pediatrics 69:564–567, 1982

Cody DTR, Kern EB, Pearson BW: Diseases of the Ears, Nose and Throat. Chicago, Year Book Medical Publishers, 1981

Paparella MM, Shumrick DA: Otolaryngology, Vol 2. Philadelphia, WB Saunders, 1973

30

DEAFNESS AND HEARING LOSS

It has been estimated that 2000 to 4000 profoundly deaf infants are born in the United States each year. If acquired causes of hearing loss are added to this number, it becomes readily apparent that deafness is a major problem for various health, educational, and social reasons.

The list of possible causes in this chapter is long in order to illustrate the many types of disorders that should be considered in the differential diagnosis of deafness in children. Too often during evaluation little attempt is made to uncover the precise cause of a hearing disability; or, when children have other abnormalities, testing for hearing loss may be delayed or not done at all. The monograph *Genetic and Metabolic Deafness* by Konigsmark and Gorlin[1] is a literal treasure of such disorders. The hereditary causes are too numerous to include in this chapter. Careful physical examination of the deaf child may reveal characteristics suggestive of one of these hereditary conditions. Some of the major abnormalities of hereditary nature associated with deafness are listed in this chapter as headings, for example, deafness with anomalies of the external ear; deafness associated with eye disorders; and so forth.

Various studies have estimated that the genetic causes account for 30% to 50% of cases of deafness in children. Approximately one third of these are associated with other abnormalities, but two thirds are not. A careful family history is important to disclose hereditary causes. Some of the more common genetic causes of deafness associated with other abnormalities include the syndromes of Pendred, Usher, Jervell and Lange–Nielsen, Waardenburg, and Alport.

Acquired causes of deafness account for approximately half of all cases. Excluded from this group are the most common causes of acquired deafness, serous otitis media and purulent otitis media. These disorders usually result in a transient conductive hearing loss, but chronic infections may lead to permanent damage. Fraser,[2] in a review of thousands of cases of deafness in children, estimated that deafness in close to 10% is perinatally acquired (associated with prematurity, cerebral palsy, and hyperbilirubinemia) and that in another 25%, deafness is postnatally acquired (following meningitis, viral infections, and head trauma).

A few rare causes of congenital deafness associated with prominent phenotypic abnormalities are also listed here.

I. Acquired Causes of Hearing Loss

A. Prenatally Acquired Deafness

  1. Infections

    a. Rubella   Epidemic rubella is a leading cause of deafness.

    b. Cytomegalovirus Infection   Infections may be asymptomatic or symptomatic.

    c. Toxoplasmosis   Deafness is rare, but retinal changes are common.

    d. Herpes Simplex

    e. Varicella

    f. Syphilis   Formerly, prenatal infection was an important cause of deafness.

  2. Exposure to Drugs Taken by Mother

    a. Streptomycin

    b. Quinine

    c. Chloroquine

    d. Trimethadione

    e. Thalidomide

B. Perinatally Acquired Deafness   Usually the deafness is not an isolated finding. Associated abnormalities include cerebral palsy, epilepsy, blindness, and mental retardation.

  1. Prematurity   Perhaps as many as 2% of premature infants suffer some hearing loss. Several factors may be involved, including hereditary predisposition, anoxia during birth, trauma, drugs, and possibly incubator noise.

  2. Kernicterus   The classic signs of kernicterus—shrill cry, opisthotonos, and spasticity followed by hypotonia, may not have been obvious in the neonatal period. Deafness is usually detected much later. Hyperbilirubinemia has been implicated in some cases, but there may have been many factors involved.

  3. Hypoglycemia

  4. Anoxia and Hypoxia

5. Trauma	Deafness may be a result of hemorrhage or skull fractures, especially of the temporal bone.
6. Meningitis and Encephalitis	
C. Deafness Acquired in Infancy or Childhood	
1. Otitis Media	Serous fluid collections in the middle ear are the most common cause of transient hearing loss in children. Chronic infections may cause permanent damage to the inner ear, with perforations and cholesteatoma formation. Mastoid infection resulting in hearing loss is less commonly seen today.
2. Other Infections	
a. Mumps	Mumps most commonly causes unilateral hearing loss.
b. Measles	
c. Rubella	
d. Poliomyelitis	
e. Scarlet Fever	
f. Infectious Mononucleosis	
g. Varicella	
h. Herpes Zoster	
i. Adenovirus	
j. Diphtheria	
k. Influenza	
3. Meningitis	Acute bacterial or tuberculous meningitis is an important cause of deafness. All children should have hearing evaluations following these infections.
4. Trauma	Deafness may follow head trauma, as in destruction of the middle ear by hemorrhage or severance of the acoustic nerve by fractures. Noise injury from prolonged or sudden loud noise may also result in deafness.
5. Drugs	Various drugs have been implicated as causes of hearing loss.

a. Strepto-
   mycin
b. Kanamycin
c. Gentamicin
d. Neomycin
e. Furosemide
f. Quinine
g. Nortryp-
   tyline Hy-
   drochlo-
   ride
h. Acetylsali-   The ingestion of excessive amounts of aspirin
   cylic Acid   is an important cause of transient deafness.

6. Tumors
   a. Acoustic   These tumors generally occur in young adult-
      Neuromas   hood but may occur in childhood. Some may
                      be familial and associated with neurofibroma-
                      tosis. A central form of neurofibromatosis
                      characterized by deafness and one or more
                      café-au-lait spots has been described.

   b. Cholestea-
      tomas
   c. Meningi-
      omas
7. Obstruction of   Cerumen, foreign bodies, and polyps may
   the Auditory   cause obstruction with hearing loss.
   Canal
8. Cogan Syn-   The diagnostic triad is interstitial keratitis,
   drome   bilateral sensorineural hearing deficit, and
                     nonreactive serologic tests for syphilis. Other
                     systemic symptoms include headaches, ar-
                     thralgias, myalgias, fever, abdominal pain,
                     and aortic insufficiency.

9. Psychogenic
   Deafness

II. Congenital Causes of Deafness
Occurrence is sporadic.
Turner Syndrome
Noonan Syndrome   The phenotype resembles that of Turner syn-
                     drome, but the defect is nonchromosomal.

Trisomy 13 Syndrome
Goldenhar Syndrome   Microtia, hemifacial microsomia, and hemiver-
   (Oculoauriculover- tebrae are present.
   tebral Dysplasia)

Frontonasal Dysplasia	Features include median cleft face, hypertelorism, and cleft palate.
Langer–Giedion Syndrome (Trichorhinophalangeal Syndrome)	Affected infants have mild postnatal growth deficiency, large protruding ears, and a bulbous nose.
De Lange Syndrome	
Frontometaphyseal Dysplasia	Features include a pronounced supraorbital ridge, pointed chin, and wasting of muscles of the arms and legs with contraction of fingers, as well as conductive hearing loss.

III. Hereditary Deafness

A. Deafness Without Associated Abnormalities — In the following descriptions, the inheritance pattern is indicated in brackets as appropriate: AD = autosomal dominant; AR = autosomal recessive; X = sex-linked; XR = sex-linked recessive.

1. Congenital Severe Deafness — [AD]

2. Progressive Deafness — [AD] Onset of mild high-tone hearing loss is in childhood, progressing slowly to moderate to severe deafness.

3. Unilateral Deafness — [AD] Deafness is usually severe and may be bilateral.

4. Low-Frequency Hearing Loss — [AD] Early onset of hearing loss in low frequencies is followed by high-tone loss in later life.

5. Mid-Frequency Hearing Loss — [AD] Progressive mid-frequency loss begins in childhood.

6. Otosclerosis — [AD] Otosclerosis is one of the most common causes of hearing loss in the elderly. There is variable penetration of the trait. Onset is in the second or third decade.

7. Congenital Severe Deafness — [AR] In one series, 26% of cases of profound childhood deafness was the result of recessive inheritance.

8. Early-Onset Sensorineural Deafness — [AR] Hearing loss becomes severe by 6 years of age.

9. Congenital Moderate Hearing Loss — [AR] This form is noted usually when the child first starts school.

10. Congenital
Sensorineural
Deafness

[X] Severe deafness is the rule.

11. Early-Onset
Sensorineural
Deafness

[X] Deafness is severe.

12. Moderate
Hearing Loss

[X] Hearing loss is slowly progressive and
moderately severe.

13. Hereditary
Meniere's
Disease

[AD and AR] Vertiginous attacks are a common finding.

14. Atresia of
External Au-
ditory Canal
and Conduc-
tive Deficits

[AD]

B. Deafness Associ-
ated with External
Ear Malforma-
tions
    1. Preauricular
       Pits
    2. Lop Ears
    3. Microtia
    4. Cup-Shaped
       Ears
C. Deafness Associ-
ated with Eye
Disorders
    1. Cataracts

Examples are Cockayne and Marshall syndromes and Norrie disease.

    2. Retinitis
       Pigmentosa

Usher, Refsum, Laurence–Moon–Biedl syndromes, plus others with neurologic defects.

    3. Myopia

Myopia occurs particularly with skeletal deformities or hypertelorism.

    4. Optic Atrophy

Optic atrophy occurs with juvenile diabetes
mellitus and polyneuropathy.

    5. Iris Dysplasia
    6. Corneal De-
       generation
D. Deafness Associ-
ated with Skeletal
Disorders
    1. Cranial Synos-
       tosis

Crouzon; Apert

2. Facial Bone Hypoplasia — Treacher–Collins

3. Poly- or Syndactyly — Orofaciodigital; ectrodactyly.

4. Bony Overgrowth — Osteopetrosis; Craniodiaphyseal dysplasia; van Buchem sclerosteosis; Stickler syndrome; craniometaphyseal dysplasia; Camurati–Engelmann disease.

5. Joint Fusion — Proximal symphalangism; with mitral stenosis.

6. Dwarfism — Weill–Marchesani; Kniest; metaphyseal dysostosis; spondyloepiphyseal dysplasia, diastrophic dwarfism; Fanconi syndrome.

E. Deafness Associated with Disorders of the Integument

1. Waardenburg Syndrome — This autosomal dominant condition may account for 2% of cases of congenital deafness. Prominent findings include heterochromia (25%), white forelock (20%), lateral displacement of the medial canthi and lacrimal puncta, broad nasal root (75%), and congenital unilateral or bilateral hearing loss, mild to severe (50%).

2. Leopard Syndrome — This is also an AD inherited disorder. Freckle-like skin lesions are the classic finding; hearing loss occurs in 50% of the cases. Cardiac abnormalities (pulmonary stenosis or subaortic stenosis), electrocardiographic abnormalities (including conduction defects), growth retardation, and, occasionally, hypogonadism, delayed puberty, and cryptorchidism are other findings.

3. Neurofibromatosis — Hearing loss owing to acoustic neuromas develops in the second or third decade. A central type has been described with occasional café-au-lait spots.

4. Albinism

5. Piebaldism

6. Vitiligo

7. Anhidrosis

8. Knuckle Pads

9. Nail Dystrophies

10. Alopecia

11. Twisted hair (Pili Torti)
12. Ichthyosis
F. Deafness Associated with Renal Disease
   1. Alport Syndrome

   This is an autosomal-dominant disorder in which progressive nephritis (hematuria and proteinuria) begins in the first or second decade. Deafness begins by about 10 years of age. Changes in the ocular lenses have been described. This syndrome may account for up to 1% of cases of congenital deafness.

   2. Other Nephritides
   3. Renal Tubular Acidosis
   4. Renal Hypoplasia
G. Deafness Associated with Central Nervous System Disease
   1. Acoustic Neuroma
   2. Sensory Neuropathy
   3. Ataxia
   4. Bulbar Palsy
   5. Myoclonic Epilepsy
H. Deafness Associated with Metabolic and Endocrine Disorders
   1. Thyroid
      a. Pendred Syndrome
      b. Johanson–Blizzard Syndrome
      c. With Goiters

2. Mucopolysac-   Most children with Hurler syndrome (type I),
   charidoses   and some with other forms of this disorder,
                        have deafness.
3. Mannosidosis
4. Progressive
   Lipodystrophy
5. Wilson disease
I. Miscellaneous
   Causes
   1. Cardioauditory   This autosomal recessive disorder is character-
      Syndrome of   ized by deaf mutism, a prolonged Q-T interval
      Jervell and   with Stokes–Adams syncope, and sudden
      Lange–Nielson   death. Attacks of unconsciousness begin at
                       about 3 to 5 years of age.
   2. Sickle Cell
      Anemia
   3. Otodental Dys-
      plasia

REFERENCES

1. Konigsmark BW, Gorlin RJ: Genetic and Metabolic Diagnosis. Philadelphia, WB Saunders, 1976
2. Fraser GR: The Causes of Profound Deafness in Childhood. Baltimore, Johns Hopkins University Press, 1976

SUGGESTED READINGS

Coplan J: Deafness: Ever heard of it? Delayed recognition of permanent hearing loss. Pediatrics 79:206–213, 1987
Kanter WR, Eldridge R, Fabricant R et al: Central neurofibromatosis with bilateral acoustic neuroma: Genetic, clinical, and biochemical distinctions from peripheral neurofibromatosis. Neurology 30:851–859, 1980
Konigsmark BW: Hereditary childhood hearing loss and integumentary system disease. J Pediatr 80:909–919, 1972

31

TINNITUS

Tinnitus is the sensation of a noise or ringing in the ear. It is a relatively uncommon symptom in the pediatric age group and is almost never a verbalized complaint in young children.

In this section the causes of tinnitus have been divided into nonpulsatile and pulsatile types: Nonpulsatile tinnitus is a steady, uninterrupted noise, whereas pulsatile tinnitus usually has a rhythmic quality, often coinciding with the heart beat. The most common cause of tinnitus is hearing loss.

I. Nonpulsatile Tinnitus

A. Hearing Loss — Tinnitus may be the first symptom of hearing loss, especially of sensorineural causes. The hearing loss generally begins in the high tones and may be detectable only by an audiometric examination.

B. Perforation of Tympanic Membrane

C. Physiologic Tinnitus — In extremely quiet rooms some people may note the presence of a noise in their ears.

D. Drug-Induced Tinnitus — Various drugs with ototoxic properties may produce tinnitus; the most frequently recognized are kanamycin, gentamicin, streptomycin, neomycin, and quinine. Tinnitus is a sign of salicylate toxicity and is sometimes used in determining the salicylate dosage in therapy for chronic diseases such as arthritis. Arsenic poisoning may also cause tinnitus secondary to cochlear damage.

E. Noise Injury — A sudden loud blast or exposure to loud background noise over a period of years may produce tinnitus. The tinnitus is a warning of impending hearing loss.

F. Convulsive Disorders — Tinnitus may be an aura, preceding the onset of the seizure.

G. Migraine — In rare cases tinnitus may precede the headache phase of attacks of migraine.

H. Acoustic Neuroma	Tinnitus may precede or accompany the hearing loss associated with this and other lesions of the cerebellopontine angle. The tinnitus and hearing loss are unilateral.
I. Menière Disease	Attacks of labyrinthitis of sudden onset are characterized by vertigo, a distorted hearing loss, and often a roaring tinnitus. Nausea is constant, and vomiting is common.
J. Functional Tinnitus	Tinnitus may be a subjective complaint. If the noise description is bizarre, a psychiatric problem should be considered.
K. Hypoxia and Ischemia	Episodes of decreased blood and oxygen supply to the cells in the organ of Corti may result in tinnitus.
L. Labyrinthine Concussion	Tinnitus may follow a head injury.
M. Temporomandibular Joint Dysfunction	Tinnitus may accompany temporomandibular joint disorders.
N. Brain Stem Tumors	

II. Pulsatile Tinnitus

A. Serous Otitis Media	Conductive hearing loss secondary to fluid or acute or chronic infections of the middle ear is the most common cause of pulsatile tinnitus.
B. Cerumen	Occlusion of the external ear canal by cerumen or a foreign body may result in tinnitus.
C. Foreign Bodies	Hair, grains of sand or stone, and other foreign bodies may scratch the tympanic membrane, causing tinnitus.
D. Physiologic Causes	Compression of the ear on a pillow may occlude the external canal and produce a pulsatile tinnitus.
E. Patent Eustachian Tube	This is an uncommon cause in children. The eustachian tube may remain open, particularly while the person is upright, resulting in rushes of air into the middle ear during respiration. The breath sounds may be heard with a stethoscope placed in the external auditory canal. Causes include sudden weight loss, adhesions around the nasopharyngeal opening secondary to adenoidectomy, and paralysis of the fifth nerve.

F. Glomus Jugulare Tumor	This benign but locally invasive tumor arises from tissue in the middle ear histologically similar to that of carotid and aortic bodies. The earliest symptom is a pulsatile tinnitus.
G. Intracranial Arteriovenous Fistula	The bruit may also be heard by the examiner's stethoscope.
H. Hypertension	Pulsatile tinnitus may fluctuate with the blood pressure elevation.
I. Aberrant Internal Carotid Artery	In this rare congenital abnormality, the artery lies on the medial wall of the middle ear and may be seen as a bluish mass behind the tympanic membrane.
J. Carotid Artery Lesions	Turbulence in the carotid artery produced by internal lesions or severe stenotic lesions may result in a pulsatile tinnitus.
K. Palatal Myoclonus	The muscles of the palate may undergo rhythmic contractions, producing a clicking sound in the ear. The clicking may be heard by placing a stethoscope over the auditory canal.
L. Functional Tinnitus	

SUGGESTED READING

Cody DTR, Kern EB, Pearson BW: Diseases of the Ears, Nose and Throat. Chicago, Year Book Medical Publishers, 1981

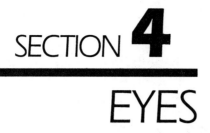

SECTION 4

EYES

32

PERIORBITAL EDEMA

Periorbital edema may be a reflection of local or systemic disorders. Often the cause of the swelling is obvious, either from accompanying local findings or from systemic signs and symptoms. Many disorders that cause edema in other parts of the body (see Chap. 11) may also cause swelling of the tissues around the eye, especially because these tissues are so loose.

I. Inflammatory Causes

A. Dacryocystitis	The swelling and tenderness are greatest below the lid margin at the side of the nose.
B. Chalazion or Stye	The swelling is at the lid margin in the meibomian gland.
C. Erysipelas	This is a rapidly expanding cellulitis secondary to group A streptococcal infection. Children usually have fever and other signs of toxicity.
D. Orbital and Periorbital Cellulitis	Signs of infection are present: fever, erythema, and pain. Both types require parenteral antibiotic therapy. Orbital cellulitis is associated with proptosis and decreased extraocular muscle movement. The ethmoid sinus may be the initial site of infection.
E. Herpes Zoster	Vesicles develop in a dermatome distribution and do not cross the midline. When the cornea is involved, serious damage to the eye often results.
F. Vaccinia	The edema is secondary to a local lesion caused by autoinnoculation.
G. Anthrax	The swelling is painless. An ulcer with a central eschar develops. Patients usually have a history of contact with animal hides.
H. Syphilis	
I. Conjunctivitis	Various types—bacterial, viral, chlamydial, and chemical—may be responsible.
J. Tularemia	The swelling is nearly always unilateral. Small yellowish white areas of necrosis occur in the

upper conjunctival folds. The preauricular glands are swollen. A history of contact with rabbits is common.

K. Cat-Scratch Fever   Preauricular adenopathy is associated with the swelling. A history of contact with cats—usually kittens—should be sought.

L. Iridocyclitis   Periorbital swelling is associated with the acute form; eye pain, photophobia, and flushing of ciliary vessels are present. The pupil is small.

M. Contact Dermatitis   Erythema of the skin, usually with pruritus and some scaling, may be present. Other areas of dermatitis are often present.

N. Sinusitis   There may be tenderness over the sinuses, but the infection may be "silent."

O. Cavernous Sinus Thrombosis   Affected children are acutely ill; proptosis develops. The disorder may follow a facial infection.

P. Myiasis   The swelling increases as the fly larva develops.

Q. Dental Abscess   Toothache may not be present, but there may be pain when the affected tooth is tapped. Dental radiographs will support this diagnosis. The swelling may wax and wane.

R. Chronic Epstein–Barr Virus Infection   Affected individuals may have recurrent episodes of pharyngitis, fever, cervical lymphadenopathy, and malaise, often with periorbital and finger edema.

II. Noninflammatory Causes

A. Angioneurotic Edema

1. Hereditary Form   The swelling is often precipitated by trauma. A family or personal history of recurrent extremity swelling, abdominal pain, or (most serious) laryngeal edema should be sought.

2. Drug-Induced Swelling   Swelling may follow the administration of antibiotics, aspirin, barbiturates, or other drugs.

3. Allergic Reaction to Foods

4. Other Allergens   Inhalants and contactants are examples.

B. Serum Sickness   Symptoms include urticaria, arthritis or arthralgia, and fever.

C. Foreign Proteins from Parasites	The intestinal infestation may be occult. Stool examination for ova and parasites is required in suspected cases.
D. Acute Glaucoma	Features include pain, photophobia, lacrimation, and a steamy large cornea.

III. Systemic Disorders (see also Chap. 11, Edema)

A. Renal Diseases	Causes include acute glomerulonephritis and nephrosis.
B. Thyroid Disorders	Puffiness of eyelids, often subtle, is a common feature of acquired hypothyroidism. Hyperthyroidism may be associated with a prominence of the eyes simulating edema.
C. Cardiac Disease	Swelling of soft tissues occurs early in congestive heart failure.
D. Collagen–Vascular Diseases	Swelling may be seen especially with dermatomyositis, lupus erythematosus, and scleroderma.
E. Localized Scleroderma	Periorbital edema has been described as the presenting finding in a case with coup-de-sabre linear scleroderma of the scalp.
F. Infectious Diseases	
1. Infectious Mononucleosis	
2. Roseola	
3. Diphtheria	
4. Scarlet Fever	
5. Trichinosis	Periorbital swelling may be an early manifestation; muscle pain and eosinophilia may be marked.
6. Rocky Mountain Spotted Fever	
7. Malaria	
8. Trypanosomiasis	
9. Onchocerciasis (Filariasis)	

IV. Traumatic Causes

A. Injuries	A history and signs of trauma are diagnostic.
B. Insect Sting	A papule is present at the site of the bite.
C. Foreign Bodies	Corneal pain and lacrimation are usually present.

V. **Tumors and Malignancies**

A. Neuroblastoma — Metastatic neuroblastoma has a propensity for the orbit. Ecchymoses and proptosis are usually present.

B. Leukemia — Pallor, lymphadenopathy, and splenomegaly are clues.

C. Neurofibromas — Café-au-lait macules and the family history suggest this possibility.

D. Hemangiomas

E. Lymphangiomas

VI. **Miscellaneous Causes**

A. Melkersson–Rosenthal Syndrome — This condition is characterized by recurrent facial and lid edema, furrowed tongue, and facial nerve paresis.

B. Vasociliary Syndrome (Charun Syndrome) — Unilateral lid edema, conjunctivitis, rhinorrhea, and in some cases, keratitis are primary features. Pain is a prominent symptom.

C. Dermatochalasis (Cutis Laxa) — Lax skin of the upper eyelids may hang over the lid margins simulating swelling.

D. Subcutaneous Emphysema — This disorder may follow fractures of the sinuses. Palpation of the swelling elicits a crackling sensation.

E. Superior Vena Cava Syndrome — Periorbital puffiness, especially in the morning, is often the first sign.

F. S–C Disease — An orbital infarction crisis is characterized by the rapid onset of exophthalmos, marked edema of the eyelids, and a severe, localized headache.

G. Rifampin Toxicity — A striking red discoloration of the skin occurs in addition to facial and periorbital edema.

33

PTOSIS

Ptosis, or drooping of one or both eyelids, is not a common pediatric complaint or finding. Nevertheless, this sign cannot be ignored, for it may be a subtle presentation of a number of disorders. A careful examination of the child may disclose other diagnostic clues. The age at onset of the condition is particularly important, because several conditions associated with ptosis are congenital; photographs of the child as an infant may be very helpful. A family history of ptosis is also important to uncover genetic causes.

I. Congenital Ptosis

A. Genetic Trait — Most often bilateral; inherited as an autosomal dominant. Some weakness of the superior rectus muscle may be present.

B. Traumatic Origin — If unilateral, the ptosis may be secondary to birth trauma or an intracranial third cranial nerve lesion.

C. Marcus–Gunn Phenomenon — In this condition, also called the jaw-winking syndrome, opening of the mouth or movement of the jaw laterally causes elevation of the ptotic eyelid. A misdirected cross-innervation between the oculomotor and pterygoid nerves is thought to be the cause. The disorder may be inherited as an autosomal-dominant trait.

D. Hereditary External Ophthalmoplegia — In this rare disorder, there is total paralysis of extraocular eye movements; other findings include bilateral ptosis, convulsions, ataxia, mental impairment, and retinitis pigmentosa.

E. Möbius Syndrome — Affected children usually have bilateral facial paralysis and sixth cranial nerve palsy. The face is expressionless; ptosis is not always present.

F. Syndromes and Chromosomal Abnormalities — Congenital ptosis is part of a host of other findings in these disorders. For further definition, David Smith's classic text,[1] from which the following list was modified, is recommended.

1. Chromosomal Disorders	Turner syndrome, Trisomy 18 syndrome, and deletions of short arm 4 or 18 and of long arm 13 may be associated with ptosis.
2. Fetal Drug Exposure	Alcohol, hydantoin, and trimethadione have been implicated.
3. Inherited Syndromes	Aarskog syndrome, familial blepharophimosis, Dubowitz syndrome, Freeman–Sheldon syndrome, Schwartz syndrome, pachydermoperiostosis, Saethre–Chotzen syndrome; Crouzon syndrome; Apert syndrome, Smith–Lemli–Opitz syndrome, Fanconi pancytopenia, Noonan syndrome, and the craniooculodental syndrome.
4. Syndromes of Unidentified Etiology	The Coffin–Siris and Rubinstein–Taybi syndromes are examples.

II. Neuromuscular Disorders

A. Migraine	Unilateral ptosis or a complete third nerve palsy may be seen in ophthalmoplegic migraine. Paralysis usually lasts only a few hours, but with repeated attacks it may persist for weeks or months or even become permanent.
B. Myasthenia Gravis	Ptosis is the most common presenting sign. Other findings include diplopia, facial weakness, dysphonia, weakness of arms or legs, external ophthalmoplegia, and respiratory difficulties. Increased weakness generally develops during the day.
C. Myotonic Dystrophy	Congenital ptosis may precede involvement of other muscle groups or generalized myotonia (failure of relaxation of voluntary muscles). The distinctive "hatchet face" (sharp facial features) is eventually produced by facial muscular atrophy. In infants, hypotonia, weak sucking reflex, elevated diaphragm, and arthrogryposis may be present as well as facial weakness.
D. Hydrocephalus	Ptosis may be present. Other findings include a large forehead and head circumference and a tense fontanel (if open); there may be a unilateral or bilateral sixth nerve palsy.
E. Oculomotor Nerve Involvement	Trauma, intracranial aneurysms, diabetes mellitus, and other disorders may affect the third nerve. Ocular muscle palsy as well as ptosis is

present. The eye is displaced outward and downward with impaired adduction and elevation.

F. Dermatomyositis
In addition to skin changes and muscle weakness, there may be extraocular muscle myositis with ptosis.

G. Ocular Muscular Dystrophy
Onset of symptoms of this autosomal-dominant condition is generally delayed until adulthood. Findings include diplopia, ptosis, and strabismus, as well as weakness of facial muscles, particularly of the upper face.

H. Myotubular (Centronuclear) Myopathy
Ptosis and weakness of the extraocular muscles are characteristic. Progressive weakness of limb girdle and neck muscles is most prominent during acute respiratory illnesses but may have been present from birth.

I. Horner Syndrome
Ptosis is mild; there may be unilateral miosis, enophthalmos, and absence of facial sweating due to involvement of cervical sympathetic ganglion.

III. Poisoning

A. Botulism
Ptosis may be an early sign. Progressive neurologic symptoms include blurring of vision, impaired pupillary reaction to light, diplopia, difficulty in swallowing, respiratory difficulties, and paralysis.

B. Lead, Arsenicals, Carbon Monoxide, and Dichlorodiethylsulfide
Ptosis may be part of the clinical picture.

IV. Lesions of the Eyelid

Ptosis may be the result of local inflammation, edema, styes, tumors, conjunctival scarring, deposition of amyloid, or trauma.

V. Tumors

A. Orbital Tumors
Orbital tumors, primary or metastatic, may be associated with ptosis. Neurofibromatosis, hemangiomas, neuroblastoma, and rhabdomyosarcoma should be considered in the differential diagnosis.

B. Pinealoma
Paralysis of upward gaze is the classic localizing sign. Bilateral ptosis may be the presenting symptom. Signs of increased intracranial pressure eventually follow.

VI. Inborn Errors of Metabolism

A. Carnitine Defi-
ciency

Myopathic facies with ptosis may be present, but extraocular muscle movement is normal. Other findings are progressive muscular weakness, greater in the proximal muscles, and impaired liver function.

B. Abetalipoprotein-
emia

Abdominal distension and steatorrhea begin after 1 to 2 months of age. By 7 or 8 years of age, ataxia, muscle weakness, and awkward gait have developed. Affected children eventually lose visual acuity, deep tendon reflexes, and vibratory and position sense, and develop nystagmus.

C. Tangier Disease

Ptosis may be present in this disorder characterized by hepatosplenomegaly and marked orangish yellow tonsillar enlargement with a variable peripheral neuropathy.

VII. Miscellaneous Causes

A. Cutis Laxa   Excessive skin folds may stimulate ptosis.
B. Addison Disease
C. Cushing Syn-
drome

D. Thiamine Defi-
ciency

Onset in infancy is characterized by anorexia, vomiting, lethargy, pallor, ptosis, edema of the extremities, and cardiac failure.

E. Vitamin E Defi-
ciency

Hyporeflexia is the initial sign. Ptosis and mild ataxia occur later.

F. Familial Posterior
Lumbosacral
Fusion

REFERENCE

1. Smith DW: Recognizable Patterns of Human Malformation, 3rd ed. Philadelphia, WB Saunders, 1982

34

STRABISMUS

The term *strabismus* comes from the Greek word meaning "a squinting." It refers to an imbalance of movements of the eyes causing a lack of parallel movements.

Strabismus has been estimated to occur in about 3% of children. There are various types of strabismus, named according to the direction of the abnormal eye movement, including esotropia (turning in), exotropia (turning out), and hypertropia and hypotropia (upward and downward, respectively). Some classifications divide strabismus into concomitant types or nonparalytic causes, which are most common in children, and nonconcomitant types of paretic causes, which comprise most of the cases with onset in adulthood.

Probably 50% of cases of strabismus in children are hereditary. The exact anatomic cause is unknown. In this chapter the causes of strabismus have been divided into three main groups: congenital, acquired, and those associated with syndromes. If the cause of strabismus in a child of any age is not apparent, an ophthalmologist should be consulted for further evaluation.

I. Congenital Strabismus

A. Pseudostrabismus	In young infants and children, a broad, flat nasal bridge and epicanthal folds may create a false impression of strabismus. The reflection of light on the corneas from a source held $2\frac{1}{2}$ to 3 feet in front of the child is symmetrically placed, however.
B. True Congenital Strabismus	Nonparalytic esotropia or exotropia may be noted before 6 months of age. Esotropia is much more common than exotropia; both are frequently genetically determined. The cause of this problem, which accounts for a large percentage of cases of childhood strabismus, is unclear.
C. Duane Syndrome	This hereditary disorder features decreased abduction of one or both eyes. The palpebral fissure widens on attempted abduction and narrows on adduction.
D. Möbius Syndrome	In this unusual disorder, there is hypoplasia or agenesis of several cranial nerve nuclei. The face is mask-like because of facial paralysis;

sixth nerve palsies are also present. Several other deformities may also be found.

E. Strabismus Fixus
This is a rare disorder involving both medial rectus muscles, which are taut. The eyes cannot be abducted past the midline.

F. Double Elevation Palsy
This is a congenital weakness of both the superior rectus and inferior oblique muscles. The eye cannot be rotated upward.

G. Congenital Familial External Ophthalmoplegia
In this autosomal-dominant disorder, bilateral ptosis with partial to complete paralysis of the external ocular muscles causes affected children to walk with the chin held up.

H. Congenital Third Nerve Paralysis
Paralysis is usually unilateral. Ptosis, hypotropia, and exotropia are found. The palsy has been observed to occur in families.

I. Central Nervous System Insults
Various insults to the developing central nervous system, whether hypoxic, vascular, or infectious, may result in strabismus, as well as other signs such as microcephaly and cerebral palsy.

II. Acquired Strabismus

A. Accommodative Strabismus
Strabismus occurs during visual accommodation and may be due to hyperopia or high accommodation : convergence ratios or both. Refractive errors are common. This form usually develops between $1\frac{1}{2}$ to 4 years of age and may be hereditary; it accounts for about one third of all esotropias. Amblyopia commonly occurs.

1. Orbital Injury
Fracture of orbital bones may cause entrapment of eye muscles, so that full range of movement is impossible. The eye often appears sunken, and the palpebral fissure is narrowed.

2. Head Trauma

B. Interference with Foveal Vision
Eye disorders such as cataracts may prevent fusion of sight on the fovea, resulting in strabismus.

C. Tumors
Tumors involving the orbit, either primary or metastatic, as well as primary eye tumors, such as retinoblastoma, may cause strabismus. Exophthalmos and hemorrhages of retina, conjunctivae, and lids may suggest orbital tumors. A white pupillary reflex is the most

common sign of a retinoblastoma. Intracranial tumors may cause increased intracranial pressure or entrap the ocular nerve, with resulting strabismus.

D. Increased Intracranial Pressure

Any cause of increased intracranial pressure may affect cranial nerves, especially the sixth, resulting in strabismus. Many children with hydrocephalus have sixth nerve palsies.

E. Neuromuscular Disorders

1. Myasthenia Gravis

Ocular complaints and signs are often early findings. Ptosis, ophthalmoplegias, and facial weakness, especially if intermittent, suggest this disorder.

2. Ocular Myopathy

Progressive, symmetrical external opththalmoplegia with ptosis, occasionally involving the facial muscles, appears in infancy to late adulthood. A family history is positive in most cases.

3. Multiple Sclerosis

Childhood onset is unusual. Neurologic signs and symptoms are often rapid in onset but initially may regress quickly.

4. Guillain–Barré Syndrome

5. Botulism

Ptosis, diplopia, and difficulty in swallowing usually precede other signs of progressive weakness.

6. Fisher Syndrome

This rare disorder is characterized by the acute onset of ophthalmoplegia, ataxia, and hyporeflexia, and often follows an upper respiratory infection.

7. Acquired Postganglionic Cholinergic Dysautonomia

This rare disorder of unknown cause is characterized by bilateral internal ophthalmoplegia, lack of tears, saliva and sweat, atony of the bowel and bladder, and normal adrenergic function. It may appear at any age.

F. Vascular Disorders

1. Cerebral Hemorrhage

2. Ophthalmoplegic Migraine

Strabismus is an unusual occurrence in migraine. Third nerve palsy most frequently occurs 6 to 24 hours after the onset of the migraine attack.

G. Infections

Strabismus may occur in a variety of infections

including encephalitis, meningitis (both bacterial and tuberculous), measles, diphtheria, poliomyelitis, and other enteroviruses. Orbital cellulitis usually results in loss of full ocular mobility, whereas periorbital cellulitis does not. Gradenigo syndrome is a sixth nerve palsy resulting from entrapment of this nerve as it crosses the petrous ridge in children with chronic otitis media.

H. Drugs and Toxins — Strabismus has been described in lead and other heavy metal poisonings and also with the use of tricyclic antidepressants.

I. Miscellaneous Causes

1. Endocrine Disorders — An ocular myopathy may occur with thyrotoxicosis and diabetes mellitus, but these are both rare in children.

2. Metabolic Disorders — Transient strabismus may occur during episodes of hypoglycemia.

3. Cyclic Esotropia — Esotropia is cyclic, coming and going in 48 hour cycles. Seizures, personality changes, excessive sleepiness, and increased urination have been reported in some patients.

4. Inborn Errors of Metabolism — Strabismus commonly occurs in Hurler syndrome and in Niemann–Pick and Gaucher diseases.

III. Dysmorphogenetic Syndromes with Strabismus

Strabismus is a feature in a rather large number of syndromes. In some, anatomic abnormalities of the orbits are the cause, but in most cases the exact cause is unknown. (For more detailed information, the book by David Smith listed in Suggested Readings is recommended.)

Albright Hereditary Osteodystrophy
Apert Syndrome
Cri du Chat Syndrome
Down Syndrome
Fanconi Syndrome
Fetal Alcohol Syndrome
Fetal Hydantoin Syndrome
Goltz Syndrome (Focal Dermal Hypoplasia)
Hemifacial Microsomia

Incontinentia Pigmenti
Laurence–Moon–Biedl Syndrome
Marfan Syndrome
Noonan Syndrome
Onychodystrophy and Deafness
Osteopetrosis
Pierre Robin Syndrome
Prader–Willi Syndrome
Pseudohypoparathyroidism

Rubinstein–Taybi Syndrome
Smith–Lemli–Opitz Syndrome
Williams Syndrome
Trisomy 18 Syndrome
Turner Syndrome
18 p$^-$ Syndrome
18 q$^-$ Syndrome
5 p$^-$ Syndrome

SUGGESTED READINGS

Harley RD: Pediatric Ophthalmology, Philadelphia, WB Saunders, 1975

Smith DW: Recognizable Patterns of Human Malformation, 3rd ed. Philadelphia, WB Saunders, 1982

35

NYSTAGMUS

Nystagmus is defined as rhythmic oscillations of the eyes occurring involuntarily. Neurologic and ophthalmologic texts describe various types of nystagmus, such as pendular, jerky, vertical, and downbeat; these designations may offer some help in localization of the causative lesion. Harley's textbook, listed at the end of this chapter, is suggested for further reading.

This chapter presents an overview of causes of nystagmus, rather than a comprehensive listing. The most common causes include disorders affecting central vision, drugs, hereditary conditions, and disorders affecting the vestibular apparatus of the ear. Neoplasms, particularly those involving the brain stem, must always be included in the differential diagnosis.

I. Ocular Causes

Nystagmus is secondary to poor central vision. If a child is born blind or becomes blind before the age of 2 to 3 years, nystagmus usually follows. Some children may develop nystagmus after visual loss up to age 6. Defective vision acquired later in childhood or in adult life is not associated with nystagmus unless macular vision is affected. For a more complete listing, see Chapter 39, Loss of Vision and Blindness.

A. Congenital Optic Atrophy

B. Optic Atrophy of Early Onset

C. Septo-optic Dysplasia — This is a congenital optic nerve hypoplasia with hypopituitarism. Hypoglycemia may be a clue in the neonatal period. Growth retardation, recurrent hypoglycemia, seizures, and diabetes insipidus may appear.

D. Chorioretinitis

E. Aniridia

F. Coloboma

G. Macular Abnormalities

H. Cortical Blindness

I. Albinism
    1. Generalized Albinism — Inheritance pattern is autosomal recessive.
    2. Ocular Albinism — This disorder is inherited as a sex-linked recessive trait. Affected boys may have light skin and hair, decreased visual acuity, photophobia, and nystagmus.

J. Congenital Cataracts

K. Total Color Blindness — Findings in this autosomal-recessive condition include poor vision, prominent photophobia, nystagmus, and normal or near-normal fundi.

II. Drugs and Toxins
    A. Anticonvulsants — Barbiturate and hydantoin intoxication are well-known causes of nystagmus.

    B. Antihistamines

    C. Alcohol

    D. Lead Poisoning

    E. Codeine

    F. Salicylates

    G. Bromides

    H. Nicotine

    I. Quinine

III. Congenital Nystagmus
    1. Hereditary Nystagmus — A family history is often present; inheritance may be autosomal dominant or sex-linked recessive. Nystagmus either is present at birth or appears shortly thereafter. The nystagmus is horizontal, not vertical, and may be associated with bobbing of the head, and it tends to lessen with age.

    2. Latent Nystagmus — This form is often associated with strabismus but is not apparent on examination unless vision in one eye is occluded. It must be considered when a child's binocular vision is much better than monocular vision.

    3. Congenital Jerking Nystagmus — This horizontal nystagmus is more pronounced in one direction of gaze than in the other. The nystagmus may interfere with vision so that the child will turn the head to achieve the position with least nystagmus.

IV. Spasmus Nutans

This poorly understood disorder, with an onset at between 4 and 18 months of age, is characterized by the triad of nystagmus, head nodding, and torticollis. These signs may not all be present at the same time; they disappear usually within months and invariably by 2 years of age. It is important to look for other neurologic signs suggestive of an intracranial neoplasm.

V. Disorders Affecting the Vestibular System

A. Trauma	The most common cause is head trauma, especially with fracture of the petrous portion of the temporal bone. Vertigo is a common accompanying symptom.
B. Labyrinthitis	Labyrinthitis is an uncommon cause of nystagmus in children but may follow middle ear infections. Vertigo usually accompanies the nystagmus.
C. Benign Paroxysmal Vertigo	Attacks of vertigo are brief but recurrent, with an onset before 5 years of age. After the attack the child appears normal. Nystagmus may be present during the episodes.
D. Tumor	Neoplasms and other tumors of the brain stem or upper spinal cord may involve the vestibular nuclei and associated tracts, causing nystagmus.
E. Arnold–Chiari Malformation	With a type I defect, the onset of symptoms may be delayed until late childhood or adolescence. Symptoms may include headache, neck pain, and ataxia.
F. Basilar Impression	In this skeletal malformation inherited as an autosomal-dominant trait, pressure on the medulla and upper cervical spinal cord produces neck stiffness, progressive leg weakness, head tilt, and a short neck; occasionally, nystagmus may be seen.

VI. Other Neurologic Disorders

A. Encephalitis	
B. Tuberculous Meningitis	
C. Acute Cerebellar Ataxia	There is an acute onset of truncal ataxia followed by extremity involvement. The cause is unclear, but there appears to be an association with viral illnesses.

D. Brain Tumors — Tumors in various locations may produce nystagmus. Signs of increased intracranial pressure, headache, vomiting, diplopia, strabismus, and papilledema are often present.

E. Demyelinating and Degenerative Disorders — A wide variety of disorders may have nystagmus as an associated feature. Friedreich ataxia, Pelizaeus–Merzbacher disease, ataxia–telangiectasia, metachromatic leukodystrophy, and multiple sclerosis are but a few.

F. Ataxic Cerebral Palsy — Hypotonia, nystagmus, dysmetria, and a wide-base gait are characteristic.

G. Ocular Muscle Paresis — Nystagmus may occur in the affected eye when the direction of gaze requires action by the paretic muscle.

H. Cerebellar Abscess — Coordination disturbances, ataxia, and dysmetria, with signs of increased intracranial pressure, are common.

I. Extradural Hematoma — This injury most commonly follows a severe blow to the occiput. There are persistent diminished consciousness, headache, vomiting, stiff neck, and in some cases, nystagmus, ataxia, and cranial nerve palsies.

VII. Miscellaneous Disorders

A. Hyperpipecolatemia — In the few cases described, hepatomegaly and hypotonia were present. A horizontal nystagmus is usually apparent by 1 year of age.

B. Hypervalinemia — Mental and physical retardation, recurrent vomiting, and nystagmus are prominent symptoms.

C. Trembling Chin Syndrome — This inherited disorder is characterized by episodes of chin trembling that may be associated with nystagmus.

D. Scorpion Bite

VIII. Physiologic Types of Nystagmus

A. Optokinetic Nystagmus — This type may be induced when a series of objects is followed across the field of vision.

B. Evoked Vestibular Nystagmus — Rotation of the body or irrigation of the ear with cold or warm water can induce this type.

C. End-Position Nystagmus — This type occurs in normal children on extreme lateral gaze.

IX. Opsoclonus

Opsoclonus is a condition characterized by nonrhythmic, chaotic, rapid eye movements that often occur in bursts. This special type of movement has received most notoriety for its association with occult neuroblastoma in young children. In adults and older children it may be seen as a consequence of postinfectious encephalopathy.

SUGGESTED READING

Harley RD: Pediatric Ophthalmology, 2nd ed. Philadelphia, WB Saunders, 1983

36

CATARACTS

Cataracts, or opacities of the lens, are not a common pediatric problem; nevertheless, they occur frequently enough that a differential diagnosis is warranted. A large number of syndromes may have cataracts as a feature. The pediatrician should work in concert with the ophthalmologist, particularly in attempting to uncover any recognizable etiologic pattern.

In most cases, cataracts are hereditary or sporadic, not associated with other underlying problems. In this chapter, disorders in which cataracts may develop are grouped according to the age at which the cataracts are most likely to appear; however, there is often some overlap among age groups. In some disorders, the cataracts may be present at birth, or they may not appear until much later, whereas in others, cataracts may not appear until late childhood or adolescence.

I. Hereditary Conditions
From 10% to 25% of congenital cataracts have been reported to be hereditary. Autosomal-dominant inheritance is most common. These cataracts occur as an isolated finding, unlike those associated with syndromes listed below.

II. Sporadic Occurrence
Another one third of all congenital cataracts are sporadic in occurrence and are not associated with other systemic abnormalities.

III. Congenital Infections
The cataracts may be present at birth or appear later in the first year of life.

A. Rubella	Maternal rubella infection was the first (reported in 1941) and is the most widely recognized cause of congenital cataracts in this group. The most common associated defects are growth retardation, microcephaly, deafness, and congenital heart lesions.
B. Varicella	Maternal varicella in the first trimester of pregnancy may result in low birth weight, cortical atrophy with seizures, cicatricial skin lesions, and atrophic limbs in the affected infant.

C. Herpes Simplex, Toxoplasmosis, Cytomegalovirus Infection
: Variable sequelae of these infections include growth retardation, mental retardation, hydrocephalus, microcephaly, cerebral calcifications, chorioretinitis, jaundice, hepatosplenomegaly, and petechiae.

D. Other Infections
: Cataracts have been reported following rubeola, poliomyelitis, influenza, hepatitis, infectious mononucleosis, syphilis, and smallpox.

IV. Cataracts Associated with Prematurity

Transient cataracts may be noted in low-birth-weight infants. Generally they appear during the second week of life and disappear over a 4-month period.

V. Cataracts Present at Birth

A. Primary Persistent Hyperplastic Vitreous
: White pupillary reflex is present; the defect is usually unilateral.

B. Hallermann–Streiff Syndrome (Oculomandibulofacial Syndrome)
: Cataracts are a primary feature of this disorder characterized by short stature, a small thin nose, micrognathia, and sparse hair.

C. Norrie Syndrome
: In this X-linked recessive disorder, congenital microphthalmia, retinal dysplasia, and cataract are often associated with mental retardation and sometimes deafness.

D. Smith–Lemli–Opitz Syndrome
: Cataracts are occasionally present. Key features include microcephaly, anteverted nose, ptosis of eyelids, micrognathia, and, in males, cryptorchidism and hypospadias.

E. Cerebrooculofacioskeletal Syndrome
: Affected children have microcephaly, sloping forehead, cataracts, microphthalmia, large ears, scoliosis, hip dislocation, and flexion contractures.

F. Trisomy 13 Syndrome
: Cataracts have rarely been described in this chromosomal disorder associated with myriad other abnormalities. Microcephaly, cleft lip or palate, scalp defects, apneic episodes, and cardiac abnormalities are important features.

G. Trisomy 18 Syndrome
: Cataracts are unusual in this trisomy also. Infants are generally of low birth weight and have low-set ears, micrognathia, a short sternum, and cardiac defects.

H. Treacher Collins Syndrome — Antimongoloid slant of eyes, malar hypoplasia, malformed ears, and deafness are prominent findings. Cataracts are uncommon.

I. Pierre Robin Syndrome — Micrognathia, cleft soft palate, and glossoptosis create neonatal feeding and breathing difficulties. Cataracts are uncommon.

J. Rubinstein–Taybi Syndrome — Broad thumbs and great toes with downward slanting palpebral fissures and a beaked nose are common features. Cataracts are rare.

K. Goldenhar Syndrome (Oculoauriculovertebral Dysplasia) — Auricular deformities, malar hypoplasia, macrostomia, and, occasionally, epibulbar dermoids are present. Cataracts are uncommon.

L. Craniosynostosis — Cataracts have been rarely reported in Apert syndrome and Crouzon syndrome.

M. Osteogenesis Imperfecta — Cataracts are rarely seen in this syndrome characterized by brittle bones, blue sclerae, and wormian bones of the skull.

VI. Cataracts Present at Birth or of Later Onset

A. Down Syndrome — Cataracts are a relatively common finding. On slit-lamp examination, most children with Down syndrome are found to have cataracts.

B. Turner Syndrome — Approximately one third of patients may develop cataracts at some time. Key features include short stature, webbed neck, cardiac anomalies, and lymphedema of the hands and feet in the neonatal period.

C. Noonan Syndrome — The phenotype is similar to that in Turner syndrome but without an abnormal karyotype. The heart defect is right-sided, pulmonic stenosis, rather than left-sided as in Turner syndrome.

D. Galactosemia — Vomiting, diarrhea, jaundice, hepatosplenomegaly, and failure to thrive are important features. Cataracts tend to develop early.

E. Galactokinase Deficiency — Cataracts are the only known manifestation. They may rarely be present at birth but generally appear in the first decade.

F. Lowe Syndrome (Oculocerebrorenal Syndrome) — Hypotonia, hyporeflexia, short stature, mental retardation, and cataracts are the characteristic findings. Renal tubular acidosis, proteinuria, and aminoaciduria are common.

G. Conradi Syndrome (Chondrodystrophica Calcificans Congenita) — Associated features include asymmetrical shortening of long bones, a flat nasal bridge, and the diagnostic feature of stippled epiphyses on roentgenographic examination.

H. Incontinentia Pigmenti — This condition, primarily seen in girls, is characterized by linear vesiculobullous lesions at birth that become verrucous, then flatten out, and are later replaced by hyperpigmentation. Seizures and dental anomalies are also common.

I. Cerebrohepatorenal Syndrome — Affected infants have severe neonatal hypotonia with a narrow facies, hepatomegaly, and cardiac anomalies, and usually die in the first year.

J. Marinesco–Sjögren Syndrome — Mental retardation, ataxia, and cataracts are primary features.

K. Anhidrotic Ectodermal Dysplasia — Lack of sweating with sparse hair, missing teeth and thick lips create a striking appearance.

L. Shafer Syndrome — Disseminated cutaneous follicular hyperkeratosis, retardation, short stature, microcephaly, cicatricial alopecia and thick nails accompany the congenital cataracts.

M. Clouston Syndrome — This syndrome is characterized by thick dyskeratotic palms and soles; areas of hyperpigmentation over the knuckles, elbows, and axillae; sparse hair; absent or dysplastic nails; retardation; and short stature.

N. Warburg Syndrome — This is an autosomal recessive disorder with many ocular anomalies including megalocornea, coloboma, microopthalmos, as well as central nervous system defects: agyria, cerebellar dysplasia, encephalocele, and hydrocephalus.

VII. Cataracts with Onset in Early Infancy

A. Retrolental Fibroplasia

B. Neonatal Hypocalcemia

C. Niemann–Pick Disease — Symptoms begin in the first year of life and include persistent early jaundice, enlarging abdomen, and psychomotor retardation. Seizures, hypotonia, a cherry red retinal spot, and hepatosplenomegaly may be found. Cataracts are common.

D. Mannosidosis — This defect is characterized by macroglossia, hepatosplenomegaly, hypotonia at birth, repeated infections, and lens opacities.

E. Otooculomusculoskeletal Syndrome — Some cases in children with early deafness, cataracts, muscular atrophy, and growth retardation have been described.

VIII. Cataracts with Onset in Late Infancy or Early Childhood

A. Retinoblastoma — Cataract is secondary to tumor involvement.

B. Aniridia — All or part of the iris is absent at birth. Cataracts occur in two thirds of cases. Sporadic cases have been associated with Wilms tumor, hemiatrophy, and genitourinary tract anomalies. A chromosome 11 p 13 deletion with a 50% incidence of Wilms tumor has been described.

C. Hurler Syndrome — Gradual development of coarse features, with stiff joints, visceromegaly, retardation, and corneal clouding is seen.

D. Cockayne Syndrome — Onset of symptoms is delayed until after the first year of life. Short stature, neurologic defects, a photosensitive dermatitis, deafness, and cataracts are found.

E. Rothmund–Thomson Syndrome — The clinical picture includes an unusual cutaneous atrophy, telangiectasia, alopecia, and nail and dental defects.

F. Refsum Disease — A peripheral neuropathy with motor weakness, cerebellar ataxia, and retinitis pigmentosa is usually found. Some affected children develop an ichthyotic skin disorder, and almost half have cataracts. The cerebrospinal fluid protein is increased.

G. Osteopetrosis — Thick, dense bone results in obliteration of cranial nerve foramina, pancytopenia, and usually, early death.

H. Maroteaux–Lamy Syndrome — Growth deficiency becomes apparent by 3 years of age. Coarse facies, mild joint stiffness, macrocephaly, and macroglossia are present, but affected children are not retarded.

I. Stickler Syndrome — Features include a flat facies, midfacial hypoplasia, myopia, a marfanoid habitus, promi-

	nence of large joints, and in rare cases, cataracts.
J. Congenital Retinal Degeneration (Leber Disease)	Signs of poor vision are noted shortly after birth. Pupillary reflexes are minimal or absent. Nystagmus, cataracts, strabismus, pigmentary stippling of the fundus, and optic atrophy may occur.
K. Alstrom Syndrome	Only 3 cases have been reported. Obesity develops in infancy along with nystagmus, photophobia, progressive visual impairment, and cataracts.
L. Deafness, Myopia, Cataract, and Saddle Nose	This is another rarely described combination of defects.

IX. Cataracts with Onset in Late Childhood or Adolescence

A. Diabetes Mellitus	
B. Hypoparathyroidism	Muscle aches, tetany, dry skin, patchy alopecia, and occasionally increased intracranial pressure may be signs.
C. Pseudohypoparathyroidism and Pseudopseudohypoparathyroidism	Affected children have a short, stocky build with a round facies, short hands, bowing of legs, and the characteristic shortened fourth and fifth metacarpals.
D. Myotonic Dystrophy	In this disorder inherited as an autosomal-dominant trait, myotonia, muscle wasting, and immobile myopathic facies are features; cataracts are found on slit-lamp examination.
E. Sex-Linked Ichthyosis	
F. Alport Syndrome	Familial nephritis and nerve deafness are findings; cataracts may develop later.
G. Prader–Willi Syndrome	Features include hypotonia, short stature, mental retardation, small hands and feet, and later obesity. Cataracts are rare.
H. Marshall Syndrome	This is a variant of anhidrotic ectodermal dysplasia with features of saddle nose, myopia, and the late appearance of cataracts.
I. Cerebrotendinous Xanthomatosis	Slowly progressive cerebellar ataxia with myoclonus or spasticity, xanthomas of tendons, and bilateral cataracts are features.

J. Basal Cell Nevus Syndrome	Multiple basal cell carcinomas develop later in adolescence; jaw cysts, vertebral defects, and occasionally cataracts may be found.
K. Weill–Marchesani Syndrome	Short stature, myopia, ectopic lens, spherophakia, and brachydactyly are findings.
L. Nail–Patella Syndrome (Arthro-onycho-dysplasia)	The patellae are absent or hypoplastic; renal abnormalities develop later.
M. Fabry Disease (Angiokeratoma Corporis Diffusum)	Attacks of burning pain of the hands and feet begin in childhood. Angiectases are noted on the skin at about 10 years of age, and corneal opacities may develop.
N. Wilson Disease (Hepatolenticular Degeneration)	Cataracts rarely develop. The initial clinical picture may suggest a hepatitis, a hemolytic anemia, portal hypertension, or dystonia.
O. Marfan Syndrome	Cataracts may develop secondary to dislocated lenses.
P. Homocystinuria	The clinical picture in this aminoaciduria may resemble that of Marfan syndrome. Cataracts may occur secondary to a dislocated lens.
Q. Werner Syndrome	Onset is usually in early adulthood with signs of premature aging. Cataracts develop later.
R. Head Banging	A bizarre association of cataracts in children who are habitual head bangers has been reported.
S. Retinitis Pigmentosa	This disorder may be seen in several other syndromes or may occur without other systemic features. A progressive loss of night vision and constricted visual fields are the first symptoms. Cataracts may develop.

X. Cataracts with Variable Onset (at Any Age)

A. Atopic Dermatitis	Anterior subcapsular cataracts are common in children with eczema but are rarely significant.
B. Trauma	
C. Glaucoma	Cataracts may develop in the presence of increased intraorbital pressure.
D. Retinal Detachment	
E. Ionizing Radiation	

F. Endophthalmitis	Inflammation of various layers of the eye may cause cataract formation.
G. Hemolytic Anemias	Cataracts are rare but have been reported to occur in hereditary spherocytosis and glucose-6-phosphate dehydrogenase deficiency.
H. Scleroderma	
I. Laurence–Moon–Biedl Syndrome	Cataracts are rare. Features include mental retardation, obesity, hypogenitalism, polydactyly, and retinitis pigmentosa.
J. Cataracts Secondary to Intraocular Inflammatory Disease	Cataracts may develop during the course of intraocular inflammation. Juvenile rheumatoid arthritis, tuberculosis, sarcoidosis, syphilis, Behçet syndrome, and the Vogt–Koyanagi syndrome are included in this group of disorders.
K. Varicella	Cataracts may develop rapidly when they follow acquired infection.

XI. Drug-Induced Cataract

A. Corticosteroids	Prolonged treatment with systemic steroids almost invariably results in the formation of posterior subcapsular cataracts.
B. Chlorpromazine	The condition is reversible on withdrawal of the drug.
C. Ergot	
D. Vitamin D in Excessive Doses	
E. Other Drugs	Cataracts have been reported to occur with these drugs or chemicals: triparanol, dinitrophenol, and naphthalene.

SUGGESTED READINGS

Goldberg MF: Genetic and Metabolic Eye Disease. Boston, Little, Brown & Co, 1974

Kohn BA: The differential diagnosis of cataracts in infancy and childhood. Am J Dis Child 130:184–192, 1976

National Foundation—March of Dimes: Birth Defects Compendium, 2nd ed. Bergsma D (ed). New York, AR Liss, 1979

37

UNEQUAL PUPILS

Anisocoria, or unequal pupils, may be physiologic or indicative of underlying disease of the eye or central nervous system. It may be difficult at times to decide which eye is the one with the abnormal response—the larger or the smaller. Associated signs and symptoms are important, and usually the expertise of an ophthalmologist is required for the complete evaluation. The inequality may be familial.

I. Physiologic Causes

A. Familial Trait — One form of anisocoria is inherited as an autosomal dominant trait. Other members of the family should be examined.

B. Sporadic Occurrence — Mild degrees of anisocoria are common and of no pathologic significance.

C. Anisometropia — When the visual acuity of the eyes is different, the more myopic eye may have a larger pupil.

II. Primary Eye Disorders

A. Amblyopia — Failure of binocular fusion results eventually in suppression of the visual image from one eye. The pupils may appear unequal.

B. Iritis — Inflammation of the iris, ciliary body, or uveal tract causes reduction in reactive capacity of the iris and inequality of pupils.

C. Ocular Trauma — The pupil may be mydriatic following trauma.

D. Corneal Abrasion

E. Keratitis — Inflammation of the cornea, from various causes, produces dilation of limbic vessels and a flush around the cornea. Herpes simplex virus is a common pathogen.

F. Cataract — Any opacity of the cornea, lens, or vitreous may result in pupil inequality.

G. Glaucoma — Pupillary size may vary as a result of increased intraocular pressure. The cornea is enlarged and sometimes "steamy," and the eye is photophobic with increased lacrimation.

H. Blindness — Disorders causing blindness may result in unequal pupillary size.

III. Central Nervous System Disorders

A. Horner Syndrome

This syndrome is characterized by miosis, ptosis, and decreased facial sweating on the affected side. The affected pupil constricts on exposure to light but fails to dilate fully in darker conditions. In children, the most common cause is a birth injury affecting the brachial plexus; in these cases the affected iris may be hypopigmented. Several other lesions may cause Horner syndrome including lesions with systemic effects, such as tumors, hemorrhage, and syringobulbia; neck lesions such as from trauma, cervical ribs, and enlarged cervical nodes; and mediastinal lesions, including tumors, aortic aneurysms, and thyroid adenomas.

B. Hutchinson Pupil

The dilated pupil results from third nerve compression, usually caused by an expanding supratentorial lesion such as tumor or hematoma. Decreasing levels of consciousness are usually found as intracranial pressure increases.

C. Adie Pupil (Tonic Pupil)

The pupil reacts slowly or not at all to light, and in a delayed manner to accommodation of near gaze, and it redilates slowly. A distinctive feature of this condition is constriction following administration of methacholine chloride (Mecholyl). Adie's pupil may occur in women up to 30 years of age for unknown reasons, sometimes with depressed knee- and ankle-stretch reflexes; with lesions of the ciliary ganglion, often attributed to viral infections such as varicella or herpes zoster, and with familial dysautonomia (Riley–Day syndrome).

D. Encephalitis and Meningitis

Unequal pupils may occur during central nervous system infections. The pupils are usually miotic.

E. Epilepsy

Rarely, unilateral mydriasis may be found following seizures.

F. Multiple Sclerosis

Unequal pupil size may occur as one of the signs of this disorder, which is rare in children.

IV. Drugs
Miotic or mydriatic and cycloplegic drugs may cause anisocoria.

SUGGESTED READING

Harley RD: Pediatric Ophthalmology, 2nd ed. Philadelphia, WB Saunders, 1983

38

PROPTOSIS AND EXOPHTHALMOS

The forward protrusion of an eye or eyes is a relatively uncommon finding in the pediatric age group. Orbital cellulitis is the most common cause of proptosis of acute onset, usually secondary to an ethmoid sinusitis. In cases with gradually increasing degrees of exophthalmos, orbital masses—particularly neoplasms—must be considered. The advent of computed tomography has greatly assisted in the evaluation of the proptotic eye, but the history and physical examination remain the most important elements in the successful delineation of the problem.

I. Infection

A. Orbital Cellulitis — This infection is most commonly the result of acute ethmoiditis; however, it may follow trauma or the spread of local infection. Periorbital cellulitis, which is far more common but does not cause true proptosis, must be ruled out. Extraocular movements are lost in orbital cellulitis but not in periorbital cellulitis.

B. Osteomyelitis of Orbit

C. Orbital Tuberculosis — Periostitis may produce proptosis. Ocular tuberculosis is more common and may be associated with ocular protrusion.

II. Endocrine

A. Hyperthyroidism — Hyperthyroidism is a relatively common cause of proptosis. Affected women outnumber men with this disorder, which may be present at any age, including at birth. Tachycardia, irritability, nervousness, and tremors are common.

III. Neoplasia

A. Primary Orbital Tumors

1. Dermoid Tumor — This is the most common benign orbital tumor; it is congenital but presenting signs may

	appear at any age. An external component may be visible.
2. Rhabdomyo-sarcoma	Rhabdomyosarcoma is the most common malignant orbital tumor and must be considered in any eye rapidly becoming proptotic.
3. Optic Nerve Glioma	This tumor may be associated with proptosis and unilateral visual loss.
4. Teratoma	The tumor is obvious at birth.
5. Retinoblastoma	Proptosis is rare; a white pupillary reflex and strabismus are much more common signs.
6. Lacrimal Gland Tumors	These tumors are a rare cause of proptosis.
7. Juvenile Xanthogranuloma	Surprisingly, the yellowish skin nodules that are a characteristic finding with this tumor are rarely associated with those affecting the orbit.

B. Metastatic and Secondary Tumors

1. Neuroblastoma	Metastatic neuroblastoma must be considered in any young child who presents with the spontaneous development of purpura of the eyelids with or without proptosis.
2. Neurofibromatosis	The skin should be examined carefully for café-au-lait spots. The eye may be pulsating. Optic gliomas are also more common in this disorder.
3. Hodgkin Disease	
4. Lymphoma	
5. Metastatic Sarcomas	
6. Juvenile Angiofibroma of the Nasopharynx	This locally invasive tumor usually produces epistaxis or symptoms of nasal obstruction.
7. Intracranial Tumors Involving the Orbit	

IV. Vascular Disturbances

A. Hemangiomas	Cavernous hemangiomas may involve the orbit and create a proptotic eye as they enlarge during infancy and early childhood.

B. Lymphangioma	The associated masses are usually noncompressible.
C. Cavernous Sinus Thrombosis	Signs and symptoms usually develop rapidly. The lids are edematous; there is paresis of extraocular movement; and the eye is injected.
D. Sturge–Weber Syndrome	The ipsilateral facial hemangiomatosis may involve orbital structures, creating glaucoma or a proptotic eye.
E. Carotid–Cavernous Sinus Fistula	A progressive exophthalmos, ophthalmoplegia, secondary glaucoma, retinal edema, and unilateral headaches are associated findings.
F. S–C Disease	Rapid onset of exophthalmos may be seen in an orbital infarction crisis. A severe, localized headache and marked edema of the eyelids are also found.

V. Bony Disturbances

A. Craniostenosis	Early closure of sutures may cause shallow orbits and prominent eyes. Apert and Crouzon syndromes are typical examples.
B. Metaphyseal Dysostosis	Bony overgrowth of the orbits may cause proptosis and optic atrophy as the optic foramina close.
C. Infantile Cortical Hyperostosis (Caffey Disease)	Onset is invariably before 6 months of age. Soft-tissue edema is prominent over the involved bones.
D. Osteopetrosis	In this lethal disorder, the bones become dense, and obliteration of the marrow leads to pancytopenia.
E. McCune–Albright Syndrome	Key features are fibrous dysplasia of bone, pigmented skin patches, and precocious puberty. Unilateral proptosis rarely occurs.
F. Rickets	
G. Hypertelorism	In severe hypertelorism the eyes may appear proptotic.
H. Encephalocele	Protrusion of brain tissue through a defect in the orbital vault may occur.
I. Progressive Diaphyseal Dysplasia (Engelmann Disease)	Leg pain and muscle weakness are the most prominent presenting features of this autosomal dominant disorder.

VI. Hemorrhage

The following conditions may cause proptosis as a result of orbital hemorrhage.

A. Scurvy
B. Leukemia   Cellular infiltration may also cause proptosis.
C. Hemophilia
D. Trauma   Fracture of the orbital floor may result in ex-
                           ophthalmos, diplopia, and superior maxillary
                           pain.

VII. Syndromes with Proptosis or Prominent Eyes

A. Incontinentia   An orbital mass may occur as one of the many
   Pigmenti   systemic effects of this disorder, in which skin
                          lesions are prominent during infancy.
B. Möbius Syn-   Facial diplegia is the most prominent finding.
   drome
C. Progeria
D. Turner Syn-
   drome
E. Seckel Syn-
   drome (Bird-
   headed Dwarf-
   ism)
F. Leprechaunism
G. Leopard Syn-
   drome
H. Pyknodysostosis

VIII. Miscellaneous Causes

A. Congenital Hy-
   drocephalus
B. Histiocytosis X   Proptosis may be a sole finding without clini-
                          cally apparent diabetes insipidus or punched-
                          out bony lesions on roentgenograms.
C. Foreign Body in
   Orbit
D. Collagen–Vas-   Proptosis may occur as part of the vasculitis in
   cular Diseases   periarteritis nodosa and systemic lupus erythe-
                          matosus.
E. Sarcoidosis   Orbital granulomas may cause proptosis.
F. Cystic Fibrosis   Unilateral proptosis has been reported as an
                          early sign of cystic fibrosis.
G. Myasthenia
   Gravis
H. Acrodynia   In mercury poisoning, symptoms of hypoto-
                          nia, irritability, photophobia, recurrent ery-

thematous rashes, and profuse sweating overshadow proptosis if it occurs.

I. Crohn Disease   An orbital pseudotumor has been described in
                        inflammatory bowel disease.

SUGGESTED READINGS

Harley RD: Pediatric Ophthalmology, 2nd ed. Philadelphia, WB Saunders, 1983
Ophthalmic Staff of the Hospital For Sick Children, Toronto: The Eye in Childhood.
  Chicago, Year Book Medical Publishers, 1967
Roy FH: Ocular Differential Diagnosis. Philadelphia, Lea & Febiger, 1975

39

LOSS OF VISION AND BLINDNESS

Although the evaluation of subnormal vision in children requires the aid of an ophthalmologist, the physician who cares for children should have a good general knowledge of causes of loss of vision and blindness in order to approach the problem systematically. The referring physician can supply valuable information disclosed by the history and physical examination that may provide important diagnostic clues.

No attempt has been made in this chapter to enumerate all of the possible causes of subnormal vision. Ophthalmologic textbooks are better suited for that purpose. The aim of the following classification is to present general categories of visual loss that serve as a guide in evaluation.

I. Sudden Loss of Vision

A. Trauma	Loss of vision is most apt to occur after trauma to the occiput. The visual loss is sudden and complete, but vision usually returns in a matter of hours.
B. Migraine	Vision may become blurred or distorted or may be characterized by the appearance of flashing lights; the loss may occasionally be complete. The visual loss may last minutes or hours. Headache, nausea, and vomiting are common but not always present. Ophthalmoplegias occur in some cases. The attacks tend to be repetitive.
C. Arterial Hypotension	Episodes may be accompanied by a temporary loss of vision that may or may not be followed by a loss of consciousness. Lightheadedness and a feeling of weakness occur in most cases.
D. Increased Intracranial Pressure	Transient visual loss or blurring of vision usually lasts less than 30 seconds. The loss may be precipitated by sudden changes in posture or by excitement. Flashes of light are occasionally associated with the visual loss.
E. Hysterical Blindness	Most commonly the visual loss is characterized by tunnel vision, in which the visual field

loss has distinct sharp margins that do not vary over distances. Complete blindness is less common but is characterized by sudden onset with normal pupillary responses and a normal funduscopic examination.

F. Arteriovenous Malformations

The visual loss is unilateral and short-lasting.

G. Cerebral Embolization

Air may be introduced into the vascular system during cardiac or thoracic surgery or into the dural sinus during neurosurgical procedures. Coma, convulsions, and hemiplegia may occur as well as the visual loss. Fat emboli may enter the pulmonary circulation and reach the brain. Dyspnea, tachypnea, and cerebral signs are present.

H. Optic Neuritis

Unilateral or bilateral optic or retrobulbar neuritis are relatively common causes of sudden loss of vision. The optic disc is usually swollen, and retinal vessels are engorged. Although the condition is usually painless, there may be localized pain above the eye. Systemic signs of other disease are more likely to be found in children than in adults.

1. Acute Meningitis
2. Encephalitis
3. Exogenous Drugs or Toxins
   a. Lead Poisoning
   b. Chloramphenicol Toxicity
4. Multiple Sclerosis

Occurrence is rare in childhood. The onset is usually fairly sudden, often with gait disturbances, paresthesias, and dysesthesias. The course is characterized by remissions and exacerbations.

5. Neuromyelitis Optica (Devic Disease)

Visual changes or symptoms of transverse myelitis may occur, as well as various exanthems.

I. Metabolic Disorders

Sudden cortical blindness has been reported to occur during hypoglycemia.

J. Systemic Lupus Erythematosus

K. Cerebral Venous Sinus Thrombosis — Headache, diplopia, nausea, vomiting, blurred vision, and photophobia may be symptoms. Birth control pills may be implicated.

II. Congenital Blindness

A. Congenital Malformations

1. Retinal Aplasia — Pupillary responses are absent.

2. Congenital Optic Atrophy — Signs of this disorder, inherited as an autosomal recessive trait, are evident at birth or shortly thereafter. Nystagmus is generally present.

3. Septo-optic Dysplasia — A congenital optic nerve hypoplasia with hypopituitarism. Hypoglycemia may be a clue in the neonatal period.

4. Congenital Hydrocephalus

5. Hydranencephaly — Failure of development and blindness become evident over the first few months of life. Transillumination of the skull is striking.

6. Porencephalic Cysts — Cysts may involve the visual cortex.

7. Occipital Encephalocele

B. Perinatal Anoxia or Hypoxia

C. Congenital Infections — The TORCH complex of infections may produce blindness present at birth or evidence of visual loss later in life.

III. Congenital Cataracts

Cataracts may be extensive enough to interfere with vision (see Chap. 36, Cataracts).

IV. Optic Atrophy

Optic atrophy may be the result of various disorders, both congenital and acquired.

A. Traumatic Causes:

Chronic Subdural Hematoma — In addition to effects on vision, focal or generalized seizures, an enlarged abnormally shaped head, vomiting, developmental delay, and other signs are common.

B. Degenerative Disorders

A wide variety of neurodegenerative disorders may be associated with optic atrophy, retinitis pigmentosa, and other ophthalmologic signs. A few are listed here (see Harley's text listed at the end of this chapter for a more complete classification).

1. Tay–Sachs Disease

Symptoms begin in the first few months of life with hyperacusis and irritability. Delayed motor development and decreased visual acuity become apparent by 6 months of age.

2. Krabbe Disease

The course is similar to that in Tay–Sachs disease, with onset at 4 to 6 months of age, with irritability, failure of motor development, and progressive deterioration. Blindness is usually complete by 1 year of age.

3. Canavan Disease (Spongy Degeneration of Central Nervous System)

Degeneration of the white matter produces signs and symptoms in the first year of life. Hypotonia, seizures, marked psychomotor retardation, enlarging head size, and decreased visual acuity are prominent features.

4. Metachromatic Leukodystrophy

Deterioration of psychomotor development follows an initially normal period of development. Optic atrophy occurs late in the course of the disease.

5. Menkes Kinky Hair Syndrome

This condition is characterized by the early onset of seizures, episodes of hypothermia, marked psychomotor retardation, and striking sparse, short, depigmented hair.

6. Behr Syndrome

Boys between 3 and 11 years of age are those usually affected; increased extremity tone, hyperreflexia, mild ataxia, and bladder disturbances are found.

7. GM_2 Gangliosidosis

Psychomotor retardation, seizures, and hepatosplenomegaly occur early.

8. Leber Hereditary Optic Atrophy

This condition may develop at any age but is characterized by progressively increasing central blindness. Early in the course, the eye grounds are normal, but optic atrophy and retinal pigmentary changes develop later.

9. Neuronal Ceroid-Lipofuscinosis

The abrupt onset of seizures resistant to therapy, progressive retardation, and regression to a vegetative state are characteristic features. Optic atrophy occurs later in the course.

10. Infantile Neuroaxonal Dystrophy	Onset of symptoms in this autosomal-recessive condition is in late infancy, with loss of ability to walk and failure of speech development, and either hypertonia or hypotonia. Late in the course nystagmus and loss of vision occur.
11. Infantile Optic Atrophy	In this disorder inherited as an autosomal-dominant trait, progressive visual loss occurs during the school-age years. Central scotomata are most common.

C. Neoplastic Lesions

1. Optic Gliomas	Pressure by the tumor on the optic nerve may result in optic atrophy. Visual field cuts and unilateral visual loss are most frequent.
2. Craniopharyngioma	Visual loss is usually due to compression of the optic chiasm. Visual field defects are the earliest findings.
3. Other Brain Tumors	Visual defects may occur with other central nervous system tumors depending on their location.

D. Vascular Lesions	Unilateral blindness may result from compression of the optic nerve by an intracranial aneurysm.

E. Bony Overgrowth

1. Osteopetrosis	In this inherited disorder, generalized sclerosis of bone causes decreased size of the cranial nerve foramina, with resulting nerve compression; facial palsy, strabismus, blindness, and deafness may ensue. Hepatosplenomegaly and severe anemia are the result of marrow replacement by bone.
2. Craniodiaphyseal Dysplasia	Thickening of the cranial bones creates increasing facial distortion. Cranial nerve palsies result from compression by the bony overgrowth.

V. Retrolental Fibroplasia

Varying degrees of retinal scarring and visual loss may be found. Infants at risk should be observed carefully for early signs.

VI. Congenital Nystagmus

Visual acuity may be impaired because of nystagmus (see Chap. 35, Nystagmus).

VII. Chorioretinitis

A. TORCH Complex — Any of the congenital infections may produce chorioretinitis and resultant impaired vision, although toxoplasmosis has been implicated as the most common cause of this lesion.

VIII. Macular Degeneration

A. Amaurotic Familial Idiocy — In the late infantile form (Bielschowsky–Jansky disease) and the juvenile form (Batten–Mayou disease), macular degeneration and loss of vision may occur prior to neurodegeneration with dementia, paralysis, and death.

B. Familial Degeneration of the Maculae — In this disorder inherited as an autosomal recessive trait, loss of central vision begins during the second decade. Peripheral vision is maintained for years before total blindness occurs.

IX. Glaucoma

A loss of visual acuity may be the result of glaucoma, which may be unilateral or bilateral. (An extensive list of causes may be found in Harley's text, listed at the end of this chapter.) Clinical signs of glaucoma include photophobia, increased tearing, corneal enlargement, and later, clouding of the cornea.

X. Retinitis Pigmentosa

This condition is characterized by progressive disorganization of the pigment of the retina, usually accompanied by a decrease in the number of retinal vessels and some degree of optic atrophy. Night blindness is often the fist symptom of visual loss. A progressive loss of vision may occur over decades. Many heredofamilial disorders feature retinitis pigmentosa, only a few of which are listed here.

A. Abetalipoproteinemia (Bassen–Kornzweig Syndrome) — Steatorrhea appears early with acanthocytosis of red blood cells. Ataxia and retinitis occur later.

B. Laurence–Moon–Biedl Syndrome — Prominent features include short stature, obesity, mental retardation, hypogonadism, and polydactyly.

C. Refsum Disease — Main symptoms include ichthyosis, an unsteady gait, polyneuritis, and deafness.

D. Usher Syndrome — Retinitis pigmentosa and deafness are the two major signs.

XI. Other Neurodegenerative Diseases

A. Schilder Disease	Progressive loss of vision is associated with spastic hemiparesis, seizures, and intellectual deterioration.
B. Leigh Subacute Necrotizing Encephalomyelopathy	Onset is usually in infancy; the course is rather rapid and includes deterioration of psychomotor development with feeding difficulties, vomiting, seizures, and ataxia.
C. Progressive Multifocal Leukoencephalopathy	Generalized cerebral and motor function deterioration is associated with major motor seizures. Affected children usually die within 3 to 12 months of onset. A relationship to Papovavirus infection has been suggested.
D. Progressive Infantile Cerebral Cortical Atrophy	Onset is during the first 6 years of life, with deceleration of development, seizures, spasticity, and cerebral blindness.

XII. Uveitis

Inflammation of the uveal tract (iris, ciliary body, and choroid) may be acute or chronic. In chronic uveitis the symptoms may be subtle and late—predominantly loss of vision—whereas in acute uveitis, pain, photophobia, and increased tearing may be prominent. Some of the important causes are listed below.

A. Toxoplasmosis	
B. Juvenile Rheumatoid Arthritis	Chronic iridocyclitis is most common in young girls with pauciarticular disease who have positive antinuclear antibody titers.
C. Sarcoidosis	
D. Ankylosing Spondylitis	Acute inflammation is most common.
E. Peripheral Uveitis	The pathogenetic mechanism is unknown, but the peripheral form is a common cause of uveitis in children. Onset is usually between 6 and 10 years of age.

XIII. Miscellaneous Causes

A. Retinoblastoma	Although it may be inherited as an autosomal-dominant trait, this condition in most cases appears to be a spontaneous mutation. The tumor may be unilateral or bilateral. The most common presenting signs are a white pupillary reflex and strabismus.
B. Retinal Detachment	Trauma is the most common cause in children.

C. Drugs and Tox-
   ins

Effects of various drugs and toxins may impair vision. Potential toxins include methanol, steptomycins, quinine, isoniazid, thallium, arsenic, and penicillamine.

SUGGESTED READINGS

Duffner PK, Cohen ME: Sudden bilateral blindness in children. Clin Pediatr 17:705–712, 1978

Harley RD: Pediatric Ophthalmology, 2nd ed. Philadelphia, WB Saunders, 1983

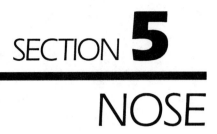

SECTION **5**

NOSE

40

EPISTAXIS

Epistaxis, or nose bleed, is a common occurrence in children. In most cases, the episode is brief in duration and related to minor trauma so that medical attention is not sought. Children who have epistaxis that is difficult to control or recurrent nose bleeds constitute the bulk of cases brought for evaluation. Even among these groups, trauma is still the most common cause; the injury to the nose may be subtle, such as wiping, picking, or excessive blowing. The tendency to bleed is enhanced by low environmental humidity, allergic rhinitis, or venous congestion. Ineffective means are frequently used in an attempt to control epistaxis, such as ice packs placed on the nape of the neck or bridge of the nose. Surprisingly few parents realize that "clothes-pin" constriction of the anterior nares by thumb and finger is effective in most cases. Failure to apply pressure may create a false impression of excessive bleeding.

Trauma and irritation account for most cases of epistaxis. Infections that may cause nose bleeds are usually obvious from systemic symptoms. Bleeding disorders generally have other manifestations of hemostatic problems in addition to the epistaxis.

I. Trauma and Irritation

A. Injury	The most common cause of epistaxis is trauma to the nose, in the form of a direct blow, rubbing, or digital manipulation.
B. Low Environmental Humidity	This condition is likely to occur during the winter. Chronic dryness may lead to crust formation in the nares. Rubbing or blowing may result in tears of underlying superficial blood vessels.
C. Allergic Rhinitis	Chronic rhinorrhea associated with allergies may cause irritation of superficial blood vessels and result in bleeding.
D. Foreign Body	A unilateral nasal discharge, especially if bloody, should always suggest this possibility.
E. Deviated Nasal Septum	A change in normal air flow may produce local irritation to mucous membranes.

II. Infection

Rhinorrhea associated with localized or systemic infections may result in epistaxis. In addition, coughing or sneezing may also traumatize congested vessels leading to bleeding. The infections listed below are known to be associated with epistaxis more often than others.

A. Streptococcosis	Chronic infection of the nasopharynx with β-hemolytic streptococci may produce excoriated nares, generalized lymphadenopathy, and low-grade fever.
B. Scarlet Fever	
C. Rheumatic Fever	Epistaxis is obviously not a reliable sign.
D. Infectious Mono-nucleosis	
E. Pertussis	Epistaxis is most likely to occur during paroxysms of coughing.
F. Measles	
G. Varicella	
H. Diphtheria	A serosanguinous discharge is an early manifestation.
I. Other Infections	Epistaxis may be a sign in malaria, typhoid fever, psittacosis, and syphilis.

III. Bleeding Disorders

A. Thrombocytopenia	Epistaxis may be a finding in any of a variety of disorders associated with a decrease in the number of platelets (see Chap. III, Purpura [Petechiae and Ecchymoses]). Leukemia is often a prime concern of parents.
B. Coagulation Disturbances	Clotting disorders are less likely to be associated with epistaxis than is thrombocytopenia. There may be evidence of bleeding at other sites.
1. Drugs	Aspirin may predispose to an increased likelihood of bleeding.
2. Von Willebrand Disease	Recurrent episodes of epistaxis, especially after ingestion of aspirin, may be a presenting sign.
3. Hepatic Disease	Depletion of clotting factors is responsible.
C. Uremia	Children with renal failure have a propensity toward easy bruising and bleeding.

IV. Tumors

A. Chronic Adenoidal Enlargement	Obstruction of the posterior nasal pharynx may result in chronic rhinorrhea and irritation of the nasal passages. The associated bleeding is usually minimal.

B. Polyps	Irritation of nasal polyps may lead to bleeding. Allergies and cystic fibrosis are among causes to consider.
C. Angiofibroma	This nasopharyngeal tumor occurs most commonly in adolescent boys who present with severe and recurrent nosebleeds and progressive unilateral or bilateral nasal obstruction.
D. Lymphoepithelioma	This uncommon nasopharyngeal tumor produces unilateral, tender cervical lymphadenopathy, epistaxis, and torticollis.

V. Vascular Abnormalities

A. Increased Venous Pressure

1. Exertion	Intense muscular activity with straining may produce vascular congestion, increased pressure, and spontaneous epistaxis.
2. Superior Vena Cava Syndrome	Obstruction of blood flow from the superior vena cava may greatly increase nasal venous pressure.
3. Mitral Stenosis	Severe stenosis may produce increased pressure.
4. Pulmonary Arteriovenous Fistula	Symptoms depend on the size of the arteriovenous shunt. Dyspnea, cyanosis, hemoptysis, epistaxis, and exercise intolerance are common. There may be generalized telangiectasia of the skin and mucous membranes.
B. Hypertension	Systemic arterial hypertension is an uncommon cause of epistaxis although often considered in the differential diagnosis.
C. Rendu–Osler–Weber Syndrome (Hereditary Hemorrhagic Telangiectasia)	Epistaxis is the most common presenting sign. The number of cutaneous and mucous membrane telangiectasia increases with age.
D. Hemangioma	Nasal hemangiomas are uncommon.

VI. Miscellaneous Causes

A. Barometric Changes	Epistaxis may occur especially at high altitudes.
B. β-Thalassemia	Epistaxis is common in Cooley anemia.
C. Associated with Menstruation	Adolescent girls occasionally have epistaxis associated with their menstrual periods, but the mechanism is unknown.

41

CHRONIC RHINITIS/ NASAL OBSTRUCTION

Stuffy or runny noses are common in children and adults. Chronic rhinitis, defined as inflammation of the nasal mucosa that results in discharge, congestion, and sneezing that occurs for some portion of the day for 2 months or longer, is a less frequent problem. Difficulties resulting from nasal obstruction are more profound in infants who are obligatory nose breathers; however, older children may have significant symptoms as well. Chronic mouth breathers may have complaints of recurrent pharyngitis or snoring. Appetite and exercise tolerance may be affected. Chronic cough is not uncommon.

I. Inflammatory Nasal Obstruction

A. Allergic Rhinitis — The rhinorrhea is usually watery and profuse. It is associated with sneezing; an allergic salute (itchy nose); watery and itchy eyes; and cough during sleep or on arising in the morning due to postnasal drip.

B. Infectious Rhinitis — A viral upper-respiratory infection may be complicated by bacterial overgrowth. The discharge is mucopurulent. Streptococcosis, a chronic rhinitis secondary to group A β-hemolytic streptococci, is seen primarily in young children. It is associated with a prolonged low-grade fever, generalized lymphadenopathy, and weight loss. Congenital syphilis is a much less common cause of chronic rhinorrhea today.

C. Sinusitis — A chronic mucopurulent nasal discharge should always suggest sinusitis. Headaches and fever may not be present. A persistent "cold" may reflect involvement of the sinuses.

D. Nonallergic Rhinitis — Profuse watery or mucoid nasal discharge, with marked congestion, paroxysmal sneezing and itching may occur from cigarette smoke, pungent odors, or other irritants.

E. Vasomotor Rhinitis	This appears to be a hyperactive cholinergic response. Alternating nasal congestion and, occasionally, watery rhinorrhea may be present. A postnasal drip is a frequent complaint. Triggers include recumbency and temperature and humidity changes.
F. Atrophic Rhinitis	Atrophic rhinitis is a rare form in childhood with symptoms of severe nasal obstruction with physiologically widely patent nasal passages. A foul odor may be present. The causes include infection, trauma, nasal surgery, and Wegener granulomatosis. There is also an autosomal dominantly inherited form with onset around puberty.
G. Retropharyngeal Abscess	This abscess more commonly presents with pharyngitis, dysphagia, meningismus, and stridor.

II. Acquired or Iatrogenic Obstruction

A. Adenoidal Hypertrophy	This is a common cause of nasal obstruction. Mouth breathing, noisy respirations when awake, and loud snoring during sleep are prominent features. Severe cases may result in obstructive sleep apnea. Rarely, congestive heart failure secondary to pulmonary hypertension from chronic hypoxia may be the presentation. Enuresis has also been described in severely affected children.
B. Foreign Body	A unilateral nasal discharge should always suggest this possibility. Bilateral obstructions are not uncommon. A generalized body odor (bromhidrosis) may be present.
C. Nasal Polyps	A history of progressive nasal obstruction in children with allergic rhinitis, asthma, or chronic purulent nasal discharge may suggest the presence of polyps. Ten percent of children with cystic fibrosis develop polyps. Other causes include Kartagener syndrome (immotile cilia), recurrent sinusitis, and aspirin intolerance. Woake syndrome is a hereditary disorder with severe recurrent nasal polyposis during childhood with broadening of the base of the nose, tenacious secretions, frontal sinus aplasia, and bronchiectasis.

D. Rhinitis Medica-
mentosa

Prolonged use of topical nasal decongestants may cause a rebound phenomenon. Cocaine abuse is a possibility in adolescents. Systemic medications that may cause nasal stuffiness include antihypertensives (*e.g.*, reserpine, hydralazine, guanethidine, and methyldopa), beta blockers (*e.g.*, propranolol, nadolol), and antidepressants (*e.g.*, thioridazine, chlordiazepoxide, amitriptyline, and perphenazine). Oral contraceptives have also been incriminated.

E. Trauma

Dislocation of nasal bones and septum may cause an anatomical obstruction. An untreated septal hematoma may result in dissolution of the nasal septal cartilage in as little as 48 hours.

F. Nasopharyngeal
Stenosis

Fusion of the tonsillar pillars and soft palate to the posterior pharyngeal wall by scar tissue may follow tonsilloadenoidectomy.

G. Hormonal
Rhinitis

Pregnancy and hypothyroidism are rare causes.

III. Congenital Obstruction

A. Choanal Atresia

Bilateral atresia presents at birth with strenuous but unsuccessful attempts at breathing. Unilateral obstruction presents later with rhinorrhea. Bony obstruction accounts for 90% of the cases. Associated anomalies occur in 50%.

B. Posterior Choanal
Stenosis

If posterior choanal stenosis is severe it may mimic true atresia. Less severe cases present with increased symptoms during feeding. An excessive mucoid discharge may be the only symptom.

C. Tornwaldt Cyst

A pharyngeal bursa-diverticulum-like structure is found in 3% of the population. It is a potential space lying in the midline of the posterior wall of the nasopharynx just superior to the adenoidal pad. Symptoms occur when it becomes infected and include a persistent occipital headache accompanied by an annoying postnasal discharge. A lateral soft tissue radiograph may demonstrate this structure.

D. Dermoid

A dermoid is a progressively enlarging mass in the midline of the nose. Suspect this possibility whenever a discrete swelling of the nose

	of a newborn or infant is found. A sinus tract may be present that can extend intracranially.
E. Encephalocele	An encephalocele is an extrusion of meningeal-lined brain tissue. Sixty percent are seen externally over the bridge of the nose and another 30% occur intranasally.
F. Glioma	The presentation of a glioma is similar to that of an encephalocele or dermoid. Most occur intranasally and they are often misdiagnosed as polyps.
G. Teratoma	A teratoma is a tumor containing derivatives of all three germ cell layers which grows rapidly in early infancy.

IV. Neoplasms

A. Hemangiomas	The tumor tends to grow rapidly during the first 6 months of life. Other cutaneous lesions may or may not be present.
B. Juvenile Nasopharyngeal Angiofibroma	This is generally seen in adolescent males. Presenting symptoms include recurrent epistaxis, rhinorrhea, and nasal obstruction.
C. Lymphoma	Hodgkins and nonHodgkins lymphomas are the most common nasopharyngeal malignancies in childhood.
D. Rhabdomyosarcoma	Seventy percent occur in children under 12 years of age. The progression is usually silent until eustachian tube obstruction and nasality to the voice occur.
E. Nasopharyngeal Carcinoma	Nasopharyngeal carcinoma is rare in childhood.
F. Other Neoplasms	Craniopharyngioma, chordoma, lipoma, and chondroma may occur in this area.

V. Miscellaneous Causes

A. Fibrous Dysplasia of Facial Bones	This is a slowly progressive obstruction caused by bony overgrowth. Distortion of the facies and cranial nerve involvement, especially vision, are common.

SUGGESTED READINGS

Myer CM III, Cotton RT: Nasal obstruction in the pediatric patient. Pediatrics 72:766–777, 1983

Simons FER: Chronic rhinitis. Pediatr Clin N Am 31:801–819, 1984

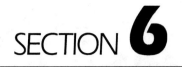

SECTION **6**

MOUTH AND THROAT

42

MACROGLOSSIA

Macroglossia, or enlargement of the tongue, may be caused by tumors, infiltrates, storage products, muscular hypertrophy, or edema, or the tongue may simply appear enlarged because the mouth is too small to accommodate it. In this chapter, disorders associated with macroglossia are grouped according to age and mode of onset.

I. Macroglossia Present at Birth

A. Trisomy 21 Syndrome (Down Syndrome)
The tongue actually may not be enlarged, but the oral cavity is so small that it protrudes.

B. Hypothyroidism
Athyrotic cretinism is usually associated with an enlarged tongue. Affected infants are lethargic and feed poorly. They may have facial edema; run low temperatures; and tend to have prolonged jaundice. Coarse features become more apparent with age.

C. Beckwith–Wiedemann Syndrome
Clinical presentations are variable but macroglossia and omphalocele or umbilical hernia with neonatal hypoglycemia are key features. Postnatal rapid growth, visceromegaly, and ear-lobe grooves are found.

D. Hemihypertrophy
Congenital hemihypertrophy may include enlargement of half of the tongue.

E. Idiopathic Muscular Macroglossia
The tongue may be enlarged without evidence of associated problems or abnormalities.

F. Robinow Syndrome (Fetal Face Syndrome)
Prominent features include macrocephaly, a large anterior fontanel, frontal bossing, hypertelorism, a small upturned nose, short forearms, and a small penis. The small mouth may create an impression of macroglossia.

G. Generalized Gangliosidosis
The main characteristics are coarse features, prenatal onset of growth deficiency, hypotonia, low nasal bridge, alveolar ridge hypertrophy, and joint contractures.

II. Macroglossia Appearing after the Neonatal Period

A. Hemangio-lymphangioma	The tongue becomes progressively enlarged and protuberant, usually with an irregular or papillary surface. Enlargement may be present at birth.
B. Hemangioma	Enlargement may become noticeable during the first few months of life as the vascular tumor grows.
C. Rhabdomyoma	Proliferation of muscle tissue results in enlargement of the tongue. Usually the margins of the tumor are palpable.
D. Neurofibromatosis	Café-au-lait spots usually increase in number with age along with cutaneous tumors. Tongue enlargement may be seen in occasional cases.
E. Mucopoly-saccharidoses	In type I (Hurler Syndrome), striking features are progressive facial coarseness, deceleration of growth, broad claw hands, hepatosplenomegaly, hernias, kyphosis, alveolar ridge hypertrophy, and macroglossia. In type V (Scheie Syndrome), there is a more gradual development of coarse features with a broad mouth, full lips, prognathism, hirsutism, clouding of the corneas, joint limitation, and occasionally, macroglossia. Intelligence is normal. In type VI (Maroteaux–Lamy syndrome), onset is in the first few years of life, with growth deficiency, coarse facies, large nose, thick lips, prominent sternum, umbilical hernia, cloudy corneas, hepatosplenomegaly, and occasionally, macroglossia.
F. Pompe Disease (Glycogen Storage Disease, Type II)	The main features are marked hypotonia, cardiomegaly with early heart failure, and swallowing and respiratory difficulties. Death usually occurs in the first year of life.
G. Multiple Mucosal Neuroma Syndrome	Gradual coarsening of the facies occurs with age, along with prominent lips, thickened anteverted eyelids, and a nodular tongue. Medullary thyroid carcinoma is common.
H. Mucolipidosis II	Alveolar ridge hypertrophy gives the impression of macroglossia. Growth deficiency, developmental retardation, and other features similar to those of Hurler syndrome are apparent.

I. Mannosidosis	In this storage disorder, features include progressively coarsening features, hypotonia, cloudy lenses, and retardation.
J. Aspartyl-glucos-aminuria	Affected infants appear well at birth but develop diarrhea and recurrent respiratory infections after 4 months of age. Mental retardation is apparent by 1 year of age. Protuberant abdomen and coarse features develop later.
K. Primary Amyloidosis	Macroglossia develops in about one third of the cases but is usually not apparent until adulthood.
L. Pachyonychia Congenita	Keratoses of the palms and soles with thickened finger and toenails are striking features. The tongue appears enlarged secondary to a thick white coating.
M. Sandhoff Disease	This inborn error of metabolism has a clinical presentation mimicking that of Tay-Sachs disease. Macroglossia has been described but is not a prominent feature.

III. Macroglossia of Sudden Onset
    A. Angioneurotic
       Edema
    B. Infection

43

SORE THROAT

The symptom of sore throat usually means the presence of an infection, either bacterial or, more commonly, viral. Various other factors may produce irritation and soreness of the throat, including postnasal drip associated with allergies, low environmental humidity, smoke, and foreign bodies.

I. Infection

A. Tonsillopharyn-gitis

1. Bacterial Infection

Primary bacterial tonsillitis is caused by three organisms: group A β-hemolytic streptococci, *Corynebacterium diphtheriae,* and *Neisseria gonorrhoeae.* Gonococcal pharyngitis must be considered in adolescents and young adults with oral or oropharyngeal ulcerations with ragged borders. Diphtheritic pharyngitis may be associated with a grayish membrane, regional adenopathy, and mild fever, but most often its onset is insidious.

2. Viral Infection

Most sore throats are caused by acute viral infection, most commonly adenovirus infections, herpes simplex, influenza, coxsackievirus infections, and infectious mononucleosis. In herpangina, caused by a coxsackie virus, there are tiny vesicles on the anterior tonsillar pillars, whereas in hand-foot-and-mouth disease, shallow ulcers are present in the mouth, and vesicles are found on the hands and feet.

3. Mycoplasma Infection

Mycoplasma infection as a cause of sore throat may be more common that previously recognized.

B. Peritonsillar Abscess or Cellulitis

These conditions are usually a result of extension of a tonsillar infection by group A streptococci. The pharyngeal pain is severe, swallowing is difficult, and the uvula is shifted away from the abscess.

C. Retropharyngeal Abscess	Intense pharyngeal pain and difficulty in swallowing with drooling and hyperextension of the neck are common.
D. Epiglottitis	Acute epiglottitis is usually caused by *Hemophilus influenzae*. The onset and progression of symptoms is rapid.
E. Supraglottitis	Inflammation of the aryepiglottic folds rather than the epiglottis may give the same symptoms as epiglottitis. Group A β-hemolytic streptococci have been implicated.
F. Laryngotracheo-bronchitis	Croup is viral in origin, and a sore throat may precede the barking cough and stridor.
G. Laryngitis	Laryngitis is also viral in etiology. Hoarseness is a prominent symptom.
H. Trench Mouth (Necrotizing Ulcerative Gingivitis	The tonsils may be involved by this infection, which causes ulcerations, friable and bleeding gums, and the formation of a yellow gray pseudomembrane over the involved tissues.
I. Oral Moniliasis	Candidal infections, even if extensive, rarely cause pain.

II. Chronic Pharyngitis

The sore throat is usually milder than in those associated with the infections described above. There may be a feeling of scratchiness with frequent clearing of the throat. The posterior pharyngeal wall is injected and often has a cobblestone appearance because of lymphoid hypertrophy.

A. Repeated Attacks of Acute Pharyngitis	
B. Irritation	Irritation may be caused by dust, smoke, or excessive dryness of the air.
C. Allergy	A chronic postnasal drip may cause pharyngeal irritation.

III. Trauma

A. Vocal Abuse	Excessive shouting, singing, or other forms of vocal abuse may result in throat pain as well as hoarseness.
B. Foreign Body	Sudden onset of throat pain may be caused by the presence of a foreign body. Drooling and difficulty in swallowing are common findings.
C. Burns	The pharynx may be injured by hot food or drink, or by acids and alkalis.

D. Smoke   Children may develop pharyngeal irritation
                            from heavy cigarette smoke in the household.
                            Pharyngitis may follow smoke inhalation asso-
                            ciated with fires.

IV. Pharyngeal Drying

The mouth and pharynx may become dry and sore from mouth
breathing associated with nasal congestion during upper respiratory
infections, allergies, or adenoidal hypertrophy. The problem is more
common in winter months when the environmental humidity is low.

V. Other Causes

A. Neutropenia   In cyclic neutropenia or during episodes of
                            neutropenia associated with drug therapy or
                            leukemia, pharyngeal pain may occur with
                            oral ulcerations or membrane formation.
B. Thyroiditis   A sense of fullness in the throat or true pain
                            may be found in thyroid inflammation. The
                            thyroid gland is enlarged and tender to palpa-
                            tion.
C. Herpes Zoster   Oropharyngeal lesions may occur, but vesicles
                            are usually present on the face.
D. Lethal Midline   Rare in childhood, this unusual disorder is
   Granuloma   marked by ulceration of the palate, base of the
                            tongue, or oropharynx with progressive de-
                            struction. The lungs and kidneys may also be
                            affected by the vasculitis.
E. Pharyngeal Car-   This is mainly a disease of middle or old age
   cinoma   but has been described in adolescents. The
                            classic triad is pain on swallowing, referred
                            ear pain, and hoarseness.

SUGGESTED READING

Cody DTR, Kern EB, Pearson BW: Diseases of the Ears, Nose and Throat. Chicago,
   Year Book Medical Publishers, 1981

44

DYSPHAGIA

The seemingly simple act of swallowing involves a rather complex array of neuromuscular activities that include sucking or taking food into the mouth and propelling it into the stomach, along with mechanisms that prevent food or liquid from entering the trachea. The process of deglutition may be impaired by various disorders.

In this chapter, disorders that may produce dysphagia are divided into two main categories: disorders of the mouth and pharynx and disorders affecting the esophagus.

I. Disorders of Mouth and Pharynx

A. Mechanical Problems
   1. Cleft Palate
   2. Choanal Atresia
   3. Macroglossia   Macroglossia may be caused by cysts, hemangiomas, or lymphangiomas or may be associated with true muscular enlargement (see Chap. 42, Macroglossia).
   4. Temporomandibular Ankylosis   Lack of movement of the joint may be congenital or associated with inflammatory processes.
   5. Micrognathia   Severe receding chin may interfere with feeding.
   6. Pharyngeal Diverticuli
      a. Congenital Diverticulum   The posterior hypopharynx is the usual site of the diverticulum.
      b. Lateral Pharyngeal Diverticulum
      c. Pulsion Diverticulum
      d. Traumatic Pseudodiverticulum of Pharynx
   7. Foreign Bodies

8. Tumors of
   Tongue or
   Pharynx
9. Cysts of Larynx
   or Epiglottis
B. Infections
   1. Oral Infection   Infections of the gums, tongue, tonsils, and
                            buccal mucosa may interfere with swallowing.
   2. Epiglottitis   In this life-threatening infection, there are
                            drooling, fever, and a preference to sit up-
                            right. An acute onset is typical.
   3. Retropharyn-   Children with these abscesses prefer to keep
      geal Abscess   their heads hyperextended.
   4. Peritonsillar   The uvula is usually shifted to one side.
      Abscess
   5. Cervical Ade-
      nitis
   6. Guillain–Barré   Ascending paralysis associated with this post-
      Syndrome   infectious syndrome may involve muscles
                            used in swallowing.
   7. Diphtheria   The pseudomembrane or toxin released from
                            nasopharyngeal infection may cause swallow-
                            ing difficulties.
   8. Tetanus   Muscular spasms may prevent swallowing.
   9. Botulism   The toxin produces paralysis of muscles in-
                            volved in swallowing.
  10. Poliomyelitis   Bulbar paralysis has become uncommon since
                            vaccine development.
C. Neuromuscular
   Disorders
   1. Delayed Matu-   An effective sucking and swallowing coordina-
      ration   tion may be delayed in premature infants and
                            in those with severe mental retardation; occa-
                            sionally, this may be a normal variation.
   2. Cerebral Palsy   Insults to the central nervous system may
                            produce neuromuscular lesions in many areas,
                            including those necessary for coordination of
                            swallowing.
   3. Cranial Nerve   Disorders affecting the fifth, seventh, and
      Palsies   ninth through twelfth cranial nerves—either
                            the nucleus or along the course—may inter-
                            fere with swallowing.
      a. Palatal Paral-   Paralysis involving the tenth cranial nerve is
         ysis   associated with nasal regurgitation as the in-
                            fant attempts to feed.

b. Möbius Syndrome	Facial diplegia occurs along with bulbar palsy. Infants with this uncommon disorder have a striking immobility of the face.
4. Arnold–Chiari Malformation	Displacement of the brain stem and cerebellum through the foramen magnum usually results in hydrocephalus. Stridor and swallowing difficulties may develop.
5. Syringomyelia	Depending on the area of the spinal cord or brain stem involved, bulbar symptoms may be present. Loss of pain and of temperature sensation of the extremities or face is often present early.
6. Cricopharyngeal Incoordination	The disorder is usually present at birth. Muscular spasm prevents effective swallowing. Vomiting, aspiration, and nasal regurgitation are present.
D. Muscular Problems	
1. Werdnig–Hoffman Disease	Severe muscle weakness may interfere with effective swallowing.
2. Myasthenia Gravis	Difficulty in swallowing may be an early sign along with ptosis and strabismus.
3. Myotonic Dystrophy	In the neonatal period sucking difficulties may be prominent along with respiratory distress. Muscle weakness occurs later.
4. Dermatomyositis	
5. Dystonia Musculorum Deformans	Involuntary bizarre posturing may be mistaken for a psychiatric problem.
E. Miscellaneous Disorders	
1. Angioneurotic Edema	Swelling of soft tissues may interfere with swallowing as well as breathing.
2. Familial Dysautonomia	Feeding difficulties occur early. Choking and aspiration episodes are common; delayed development, hypotonia, relative pain insensitivity, decreased tearing, absence of fungiform tongue papillae, thermal instability, and emotional lability are other features.
3. Prader–Willi Syndrome	Feeding difficulties occur early. Hypotonia, growth retardation, cryptorchidism, and later, obesity are characteristic features.
4. Cerebrohepatorenal Syndrome	Affected infants are also hypotonic and have a characteristic facies with a high forehead.

5. Sydenham Chorea	There may be feeding difficulties as well as the choreiform movements.

6. Vitamin Deficiencies
  a. Pellagra
  b. Scurvy	

7. Stevens–Johnson Syndrome	Involvement of the esopharyngeal mucosa and oropharynx with erosive lesions creates swallowing difficulties.
8. Acrodynia	Mercury poisoning produces a diffuse pink rash, hypotonia, painful extremities, and photophobia and may create feeding difficulties.
9. Cricopharyngeal Spasm	Trauma to the posterior pharyngeal wall may produce spasm of this muscle group.
10. Juvenile Rheumatoid Arthritis	Involvement of the cricoarytenoid joint usually manifests as stridor, hoarseness, and dyspnea, but swallowing difficulty may ensue.
11. Infantile Gaucher Disease	Opisthotonus, bulbar paralysis, stridor, strabismus, and spastic paralysis are prominent features.

II. Esophageal Causes
A. Obstruction

1. Tracheoesophageal Fistula	Swallowing is normal, but aspiration, choking, and difficulty in handling secretions are noted at birth.
2. Esophageal Stricture	Stricture may be due to corrosives, reflux esophagitis, or irritation from foreign bodies.
3. Foreign Body	This possibility must always be considered in dysphagia of recent onset.
4. External Compression	
a. Vascular Anomalies	Tracheal compression is usually more severe than esophageal compression. Anomalies include anomalous right subclavian artery, double aortic arch, and right aortic arch.
b. Esophageal Duplication	
c. Mediastinal Tumors	
d. Diaphragmatic Hernia	
e. Atopic Thyroid	
f. Thyroiditis	

g. Congenital
Esophageal
Diverticulum

5. Esophageal
Tumors

Various esophageal tumors have been described including hamartomas, leiomyomas,
neuromas, papillomas, and lipomas.

6. Leukemic Infil-
trates

Chest pain and dysphagia are usually present.

B. Psychological
Causes: Globus
Hystericus

The complaint is usually a lump in the throat
with an inability to swallow. Drooling does
not occur.

C. Inflammation

1. Candidiasis

Oral candidal infection is usually present. The
immunocompromised host is at risk, as well
as patients with hypoparathyroidism and hypoadrenocorticism.

2. Mediastinitis

3. Perforation of
Esophagus

4. Herpes Esopha-
gitis

Some immunocompetent patients have been
described with this infection without obvious
oral involvement.

D. Altered Motility

1. Achalasia

The esophagus is dilated, and the gastroesophageal junction is narrowed. Difficulty in
swallowing and regurgitation after meals are
the main complaints.

2. Gastroesopha-
geal Reflux

Episodes of vomiting, recurrent aspiration,
coughing, wheezing, and failure to thrive may
be symptoms. Esophagitis may cause dysphagia.

3. Esophageal
Spasm

Spasm is usually related to stress, eating rapidly, or reflux. There is generally severe substernal pain with intermittent dysphagia and a
history of regurgitation.

4. Chagas Disease

In the chronic phase of trypanosomiasis, heart
block and esophageal dilatation may take
place.

E. Miscellaneous
Causes

1. Collagen–
Vascular Dis-
eases

a. Scleroderma

Altered esophageal motility is a relatively common systemic complication.

b. Dermato-myositis	
c. Sjögren Syndrome	
d. Behçet Disease	
2. Hyperkalemia	With muscle paralysis, dysphagia may occur but is short-lived.
3. Muscular Hypertrophy of the Esophagus	This is a rare disorder of unknown cause, in which the hypertrophy may be localized or diffuse.
4. Brain Tumors	There may be involvement of cortical motor areas or motor nuclei of the medulla that control sucking and swallowing reflexes.
5. Demyelinating Diseases	
6. Epidermolysis Bullosa Congenita	Esophageal or oral lesions may interfere with swallowing.
7. Lesch–Nyhan Syndrome	Along with choreoathetoid movements and impressive self-mutilation, swallowing difficulties may be present.
8. Wilson Disease (Hepatolenticular Degeneration)	Coordination of swallowing may be affected. Drooling is a late finding.
9. Opitz–Frias Syndrome	Difficulty in swallowing with recurrent aspiration may be fatal in infancy. Hypertelorism and hypospadias along with persistent stridor and hoarseness suggest this diagnosis.
10. Dyskeratosis Congenita	Skin and nail findings are most prominent in this hereditary disorder, but leukoplakia of the mucous membranes including the esophagus leads to dysphagia.

SUGGESTED READINGS

Gryboski J: Gastrointestinal Problems in the Infant. Philadelphia, WB Saunders, 1975
Illingworth RS: Sucking and swallowing difficulties in infancy: Diagnostic problem of dysphagia. Arch Dis Childh 44:655–664, 1969

45

INCREASED SALIVATION

Ptyalism, or increased salivation, is a common physiologic sign of teething and is also commonly present in oropharyngeal infections and irritations. The acute onset of excessive salivation with respiratory, gastrointestinal, and central nervous system symptoms suggests the possibility of a poisoning, particularly with organophosphate pesticides.

The sialorrhea or drooling that occurs in many central nervous system or muscular disorders should not be confused with increased salivation.

I. Physiologic Factors

A. Teething — Irritation of the gums associated with eruption of teeth causes increased salivation.

B. Reaction to Foods — Ingestion or smell of certain foods, particularly spicy or heavily seasoned ones, may increase salivary flow.

C. Nausea — Any condition causing the sensation of nausea may result in increased salivation, including the morning sickness of pregnancy.

D. Smoking — Excessive smoking may cause increased salivary flow.

II. Pathologic Conditions

A. Oropharyngeal Lesions — Any oropharyngeal irritation, whether chemical or from infection, may cause increased salivation. In some of these disorders, pain or difficulty in swallowing results in drooling as well. The lesions include gingivostomatitis, aphthous ulcers, dental caries, tonsillar inflammation, peritonsillar and retropharyngeal abscesses, epiglottitis, supraglottitis, and foreign bodies.

B. Esophageal Obstruction — The appearance of increased salivation is mostly due to inability to swallow secretions. In newborns, esophageal atresia must be a primary consideration in an infant with increased secretions; in later infancy and childhood an esophageal foreign body is an important possibility.

C. Gastroesophageal Reflux

D. Systemic Afflictions

1. Central Nervous System and Muscular Disorders

Drooling due to defective swallowing coordination rather than increased salivation is common in neurologic diseases such as cerebral palsy and demyelinating disorders. Children with chorea and encephalitis as well as those with various myopathies and bulbar palsies also drool excessively.

2. Mental Retardation

Excessive drooling is not uncommon.

3. Rabies

4. Juvenile Rheumatoid Arthritis

Temporomandibular joint involvement may result in excessive drooling.

5. Allergies

Children with allergies may drool excessively.

6. Riley–Day Syndrome (Familial Dysautonomia)

Drooling is a minor symptom compared with dysphagia, recurrent pneumonitis, fevers, postural hypotension, insensitivity to pain, and various other signs.

III. Drugs and Chemicals

Various substances may enhance salivation including iodides, histamine, pilocarpine, acetylcholine, methacholine, nicotinic acid, sympathomimetics, mercurial compounds, and organophosphates. Poisoning with organophosphate compounds must always be considered in a child or adult with rather sudden onset of symptoms that include increased sweating, salivation, tearing, coughing, difficulty in breathing, vomiting, diarrhea, weakness, convulsions, coma, and others. The symptoms of acrodynia caused by mercury poisoning include irritability, muscle hypotonia, photophobia, a generalized pink rash, and painful extremities. Other poisonings causing increased salivation include mushrooms, arsenic, and thallium.

IV. Emotional Stress

Pleasurable excitation or, in some individuals, other forms of stress may result in increased salivation.

46

DECREASED SALIVATION

A reduction in the production of saliva results in dryness of the mouth (xerostomia). This is a relatively uncommon symptom in childhood and, when present, is most commonly caused by mouth-breathing or mild dehydration secondary to fever or exercise. Drug use and psychogenic disorders must also be considered.

I. Physiologic Causes
A. Exercise
B. Dehydration — The dryness of the mouth is usually more severe than would be expected with the degree of dehydration.
C. Fever
D. Mouth-Breathing — Mouth-breathing may be a habit but more often is a result of nasopharyngeal obstruction due to adenoidal hypertrophy, allergies, or upper respiratory infection.

II. Drugs
Xerostomia may be produced by the following: atropine, belladonna, antihistamines, amphetamines, phenothiazines, opiates, ergotamine, and phenylbutazone. Dryness of the mouth may be a clue to drug addiction with narcotics or amphetamines in adolescents or young adults.

III. Pathologic Disorders
A. Salivary Gland Inflammation — The inflammation may be secondary to mumps, sarcoidosis, or tuberculosis.
B. Central Nervous System Disorders — Multiple sclerosis is a rare cause of dry mouth in the pediatric age group.
C. Sjögren Syndrome — This condition is characterized by xerostomia and dry eyes (keratoconjunctivitis sicca) with or without manifestations of other autoimmune disorders, most commonly rheumatoid arthritis. The salivary glands may be enlarged.
D. Neoplasms — Primary tumors involving the salivary glands

as well as infiltrative neoplasms may disrupt the flow of saliva.

E. Obstruction of Salivary Ducts
A reduction in salivary flow may result from ductal obstruction by stones, tumors, inflammation, or scarring.

F. Miscellaneous Causes

1. Vitamin A Deficiency
Dryness of the eyes with loss of night vision and photophobia is more common than dry mouth.

2. Hypothyroidism

3. Uremia

4. Diabetes Insipidus
Xerostomia is probably secondary to fluid losses.

5. Botulism
Progressive weakness, ophthalmoplegias, and difficulty in swallowing are more prominent symptoms.

6. Mikulicz Syndrome
This refers to enlargement of salivary and lacrimal glands due to leukemic infiltration.

7. Acquired Postganglionic Cholinergic Dysautonomia
This rare disorder of unknown cause is characterized by bilateral internal ophthalmoplegia; lack of tears, saliva, and sweat; atony of the bowel and bladder and normal adrenergic function.

IV. Psychogenic Factors

Dryness of the mouth commonly occurs during acute stressful or anxiety-provoking situations. Chronic dryness suggests a hysterical trait or depression.

V. Congenital Disorders

A. Idiopathic Dry Mouth
This is a distinctly rare disorder in which the mucous membranes of the mouth become glazed, the mouth dry and filled with keratinaceous material.

B. Anhidrotic Ectodermal Dysplasia
Sparse hair, an inability to sweat, dryness of the nose, dental abnormalities, and thin depigmented skin are characteristic of this disorder.

SUGGESTED READINGS

Chudwin DS, Daniels TE, Wara DW et al: Spectrum of Sjögren syndrome in children. J Pediatr 98:213–217, 1981

Farb SN: Otorhinolaryngology, 2nd ed. Garden City, NY, Medical Examination Publishing Co, 1980

47

HOARSENESS

Hoarseness is the most important sign of laryngeal disease. The abnormal quality of the voice is usually the result of changes in the mass of the vocal cords or of disorders that interfere with the approximation of the edges of the cords. In infants, the cry may be hoarse because of anatomic abnormalities or cord paralysis. Larnygeal papillomas are an important cause of hoarseness in children between the ages of 1 and 4 years. In the immediate preschool and school-age groups, vocal cord nodules associated with voice misuse are by far the most common cause.

I. Infectious Causes

A. Acute Laryngitis	Laryngitis is often preceded by or associated with an upper respiratory tract infection. Hoarseness is the chief complaint and fairly sudden in onset. Cough and pain are also common symptoms.
B. Laryngotracheitis and Laryngotracheobronchitis	Children with croup commonly have hoarseness and a barking cough before the onset of stridor. Spasmodic croup is usually more acute in onset and is less likely to be preceded by signs of an upper respiratory tract infection.
C. Postnasal Drip	Children with acute or chronic postnasal drip caused by upper respiratory infection, sinusitis, or allergies often awaken with a hoarse voice.
D. Epiglottitis	The voice sounds muffled rather than hoarse. The symptoms of difficulty in swallowing, drooling, and sore throat come on rather quickly with progressive severity.
E. Laryngeal Diphtheria	The onset of laryngeal signs is usually preceded by a 3- or 4-day period of upper respiratory tract infection, often with a serosanguineous nasal discharge. A posterior pharyngeal membrane may be present.
F. Tuberculosis	The vocal cords may become distorted by tuberculous nodules.
G. Tetanus	

II. Trauma

A. Vocal Nodules

Misuse of the voice by excessive shouting or singing is relatively common in children. Tiny hemorrhages in the vocal cords are replaced by fibrous nodules. Hoarseness is the major complaint.

B. Sicca Syndrome

Children with disorders such as cystic fibrosis, ectodermal dysplasia, or collagen-vascular diseases in which mucous and salivary secretions are deficient or abnormal may become hoarse. This symptom is relieved by sips of water. Transient hoarseness may occur in very dry environments or during antihistamine or decongestant drug therapy.

C. Foreign Body

Hoarseness occurring after a sudden bout of choking suggests this possibility.

D. Hemorrhage in Vocal Cords

Occurrence is rare in coagulation disorders but has been reported following external or internal trauma, the latter during intubation attempts.

E. Laryngeal Fracture

Fracture may follow trauma from falls, auto accidents, clothes-line injuries, or strangulation attempts. Hoarseness and cough are present immediately after the trauma; Dyspnea and dysphagia are common.

F. Post-Intubation Hoarseness

A period of hoarseness and, in young children, stridor commonly follows endotracheal intubation.

G. Abnormal Arytenoid Cartilage

Displacement of the cartilage may be the result of trauma or may occur congenitally. Hoarseness and stridor are commonly present.

III. Tumors

A. Laryngeal Papillomas

These tumors are seen most frequently in children between 1 and 4 years of age. Hoarseness and loss of voice generally occur first, but difficulty in breathing may develop if the lesions enlarge and obstruct the airway. The papillomas are not malignant but can be life-threatening. This diagnosis must always be considered in young children with persistent hoarseness.

B. Vocal Cord Polyps

Polyps may develop following prolonged vocal abuse or trauma. The hoarseness may be intermittent.

C. Hemangioma — These tumors are most likely to appear in the first 2 years of life. Cutaneous hemangiomas may also be present.

D. Laryngeal Carcinoma — This lesion is distinctly uncommon in children, but any adult with hoarseness for more than 2 to 3 weeks should undergo laryngoscopic examination.

IV. Neurologic Disorders

A. Vocal Cord Paralysis — Stridor, respiratory distress, and feeding difficulties are the common symptoms of bilateral or unilateral cord paralysis in infants; the cry is usually hoarse. In older children, hoarseness tends to be a more prominent symptom. Some causes are listed below.

1. Central Nervous System Malformation — The Arnold–Chiari malformation may be associated with hoarseness.

2. Aberrant Great Vessels — A double aortic arch or abnormally placed subclavian artery may impinge on the recurrent laryngeal nerve.

3. Left Heart Failure — Hoarseness may be caused by pressure of an enlarged left pulmonary artery or left atrium on the recurrent laryngeal nerve.

4. Histoplasmosis — Enlarged hilar nodes may entrap the laryngeal nerve and produce hoarseness.

5. Cardiovocal Syndrome — Left recurrent laryngeal nerve paralysis associated with congenital heart disease. A weak cry and chronic hoarseness are presenting clues.

B. Bulbar Poliomyelitis — Other signs of pharyngeal dysfunction are also present.

C. Thiamine Deficiency (Beriberi) — Hyperesthesias and areflexia are early signs, as is hoarseness in infants. Edema and cardiac involvement with tachycardia and cardiomegaly are common.

V. Allergic Reaction

A. Angioneurotic Edema — Hoarseness associated with signs of oropharyngeal edema is a warning of possible impending airway obstruction.

VI. Anatomic Abnormalities

A. Laryngeal Web — Stridor and a weak cry are more common findings in this congenital abnormality.

B. Laryngomalacia — Congenital weakness of the cartilaginous structures of the larynx and trachea results in a partial collapse inward on inspiration. Stridor, more marked in the supine position, is the main symptom.

VII. Hysterical

This is an unusual cause in children. The cords are not adducted during speech but are during coughing. Onset is usually sudden.

VIII. Miscellaneous Causes

A. Hypothyroidism	The voice or cry may take on a hoarse quality in untreated infants.
B. Hypocalcemia	Infants with tetany secondary to hypocalcemia may have a hoarse cry and stridor.
C. Farber Disease	Hoarseness and stridor may appear at any time in the first few weeks of life. Palpable nodules develop in the skin, painful swellings occur in multiple joints, and hepatomegaly and central nervous system deterioration eventually occur.
D. Gaucher Disease	In the acute or infantile form, the presenting picture is that of pseudobulbar palsy with strabismus, swallowing problems, laryngeal spasm, developmental retardation, and hepatosplenomegaly.
E. Lipid Proteinosis	Marked hoarseness is a common early symptom that results from lipid deposition in the vocal cords. The tongue and lips become thickened, and papules develop on the skin along with areas of atrophic scarring.
F. Mucolipidosis II (I-Cell Disease)	Most patients have coarse facial features similar to those seen in Hurler syndrome, along with severe skeletal changes, psychomotor retardation, and frequent respiratory infections.
G. Amyloidosis	Deposition of amyloid in the vocal cords results in hoarseness.
H. De Lange Syndrome	The cry of infants with this striking syndrome is growling and coarse. The infants are hirsute, have a distinctive facies, and often have limb reduction defects.
I. Williams Syndrome	Children with this syndrome have an elf-like facies, failure to thrive, and a metallic-sounding voice.

J. Cricoarytenoid Arthritis — Rarely, a child with juvenile rheumatoid arthritis may have involvement of the cricoarytenoid. Symptoms also include stridor, a feeling of fullness in the throat on swallowing, and referred ear pain.

SUGGESTED READINGS

Bryce DP: Differential Diagnosis and Treatment of Hoarseness. Springfield Il, Charles C Thomas, 1974

Strome M: Differential Diagnosis in Pediatric Otolaryngology. Boston, Little, Brown & Co, 1975

48

PREMATURE LOSS OF TEETH

The deciduous or permanent teeth may become loose or may be lost for various reasons. Although trauma is the most common cause of tooth loss, this sign may be a prominent clue suggesting the presence of any of several disorders.

I. Trauma

During childhood, injury is the most common cause of premature loss or loosening of teeth. Child abuse must always be kept in mind if other suspicious signs and symptoms are present and the explanation of the injury is not commensurate with the findings.

II. Endocrine and Metabolic Causes

A. Juvenile Diabetes Mellitus

B. Hypoparathy-roidism — Tetany, hyperreflexia, and seizures are the result of hypocalcemia. The teeth may erupt late but are lost early.

C. Hypophospha-tasia — The clinical picture and radiographic findings are similar to those in rickets. The early loss of deciduous teeth is an important sign. The serum alkaline phosphatase is low, and phosphoethanolamine is found in the urine.

D. Hyperpituitarism — As the mandible grows excessively, the teeth may become separated and loose.

III. Hematologic Disorders

A. Leukemia — The gingiva may be swollen and infiltrated with leukemic cells, resulting in a loosening of the teeth.

B. Cyclic Neutrope-nia — Loosening of the teeth may occur after repeated episodes of oral ulceration associated with the neutropenia, which occurs at about 21-day intervals.

IV. Infection and Inflammation

A. Osteomyelitis — Mandibular or maxillary osteomyelitis may cause loosening of teeth in the involved area.

B. Juvenile Periodonitis — Chronic poor oral hygiene may result in alveolar bone destruction and loss of teeth, but this is uncommon in children.

C. Noma (Gangrenous Stomatitis) — This disorder is a rare, progressive infection of fusospirochetal origin that occurs in debilitated patients. Gangrenous ulcers develop and spread over the gums and buccal mucosa.

V. Poisonings

A. Acrodynia — This unusual syndrome is the result of mercury poisoning. Affected children are listless, irritable, and hypertonic; they sweat excessively and develop various rashes, often with erythema of the extremities and face. Photophobia and hair loss are common, but loss of teeth occurs only in severe cases.

B. Arsenic Poisoning — Symptoms of chronic arsenic poisoning include gradually increasing weakness, anorexia, intermittent vomiting, diarrhea or constipation, conjunctival congestion, and stomatitis.

VI. Dysmorphic Syndromes

A. Down Syndrome — The early loss of teeth is a result of peridontal disease, which is a common finding.

VII. Miscellaneous Disorders

A. Scurvy — The gums are swollen and fragile, the extremities are painful because of subperiosteal hemorrhage, and petechial hemorrhages occur in the skin.

B. Gaucher Disease — In the chronic or adult form, premature loss of teeth is overshadowed by splenomegaly, bone pain, joint swelling, and pathologic fractures.

C. Familial Dysautonomia — In this rare disorder, findings suggestive of autonomic nervous system dysfunction include abnormal temperature control, absent lacrimation, postural hypotension, indifference to pain, and recurrent pulmonary infection. Grinding of the teeth is responsible for early loss.

D. Histiocytosis X

Gingival swelling and tooth disruption is most common in Hand–Schüller–Christian disease but also occurs in Letterer–Siwe disease.

E. Papillon–Lefèvre Syndrome

The principal features of this uncommon disorder are hyperkeratosis of the palms and soles and destruction of the periodontal ligaments with early loss of teeth. The gingivae are red, swollen, and friable.

F. Acatalasemia

This rare disorder due to lack of catalase in the blood is seen most commonly in Japanese persons. The presenting symptom is painful ulcers around the teeth. Alveolar gangrene and atrophy ensue, with eventual loosening and loss of teeth.

G. Progeria

H. Hajdu–Cheney Syndrome

I. Werner Syndrome

J. Ehlers–Danlos Syndrome (Type VIII)

49

DELAYED DENTITION

The first primary teeth usually erupt between 6 and 7 months of age, and by 2 years of age, all 20 deciduous teeth have appeared. Various disorders may interfere with the normal sequence of dental development. Although failure of the dentition to appear by 1 year of age is considered to be a *bona fide* delay, this finding may be a normal variation in a small percentage of children.

I. Normal Variation

The appearance of the first tooth may be delayed until after the first birthday in some children.

II. Endocrine and Metabolic Causes

A. Hypothyroidism	In infants with congenital hypothyroidism, delayed eruption of teeth is one of the manifestations of the disorder. Other signs and symptoms predominate, however.
B. Hypopituitarism	Infants with congenital hypopituitarism have a delayed onset of teething and also retain their primary teeth longer than normal, sometimes throughout life.
C. Hypoparathyroidism	In primary hypoparathyroidism, delayed eruption of teeth and early loss may occur. Primary features include tetany, hyperreflexia, and convulsions from hypocalcemia. Other signs are diarrhea, dry scaly skin, brittle nails, alopecia, and recurrent candidal infections.
D. Pseudohypoparathyroidism	Hypocalcemia is also prominent in this disorder. Features of the unusual phenotype include short stature, moon-shaped facies, obesity, mental retardation, and short metacarpals and metatarsals. In pseudopseudohypoparathyroidism the serum calcium and phosphorus levels are normal.
E. Vitamin D Deficiency and Vitamin D-Resistant Rickets	Signs of florid rickets may not appear until late in the first year of life in deficiency rickets. Frontal bossing, thickening of the wrists and ankles, rachitic rosary (enlargement of the

costochondral junctions), and delayed closure of the anterior fontanel may be early signs. The signs in vitamin D-resistant rickets are more subtle, and tibial bowing may be the earliest sign.

III. Chromosomal Abnormality

A. Down Syndrome

The primary teeth may not appear until after the second birthday, and they are also retained longer than normal.

IV. Inherited Disorders

A. Achondroplasia

Although inheritance is autosomal dominant, most cases represent spontaneous mutation.

B. Cleidocranial Dysostosis

Features include macrocephaly with a large anterior fontanel, hypoplastic or aplastic clavicles, and delayed eruption of teeth. The inheritance is autosomal dominant.

C. Ectodermal Dysplasias

Various types of ectodermal dysplasia have been described. The hair and nails are affected as well as the skin, which tends to be thin and dry. There may be anodontia or hypodontia with abnormally shaped teeth.

D. Treacher Collins Syndrome

Delayed eruption of dentition occasionally occurs. The striking facial features of this condition, inherited as an autosomal-dominant trait, include malar hypoplasia, downslanting palpebral fissures, auricular deformities, and a hypoplastic mandible.

E. Osteopetrosis

In this rare inherited disorder, the development of dense, thick bone obliterates the cranial foramina, with resulting cranial nerve palsies. Pancytopenia results from bone marrow obliteration.

F. Amelogenesis Imperfecta

This hereditary defect of tooth structure is characterized by thin or absent enamel and brown teeth, which may wear down early in life.

G. Gardner Syndrome

Delayed eruption of teeth may be the only noticeable sign in the first decade of life. The other features—polyposis of the colon, epidermal and sebaceous cysts, and bony osteomas—do not appear until the second decade. The inheritance is autosomal dominant.

H. Fibromatosis Gingivae — Overgrowth of the gingiva may cover the dentition giving the appearance of later eruption.

I. Dubowitz Syndrome — Findings in this unusual disorder are small stature, mental retardation, mild microcephaly, short palpebral fissures, micrognathia, an eczema-like skin disorder, and a lag in eruption of teeth.

J. Ellis-van Creveld Syndrome (Chondroectodermal Dysplasia) — In this disorder inherited as an autosomal-recessive trait, small stature, short limbs, polydactyly, cardiac defects, and nail and teeth abnormalities are characteristic features.

K. Incontinentia Pigmenti — Verrucous or bullous lesions, often linear, are present in infancy; later, hyperpigmented patches or sworls appear as the initial lesions disappear. Defects of teeth, eyes, nails, hair, and central nervous system are common. It appears to be lethal *in utero* to males.

L. Osteogenesis Imperfecta — Late eruption of dentition is common in this disorder best known for its fragile bones.

M. Goltz Syndrome (Focal Dermal Hypoplasia Syndrome) — Areas of the skin may appear hypoplastic or sometimes bulging from the presence of lipomatous nodules. Syndactyly, dystrophic nails, strabismus, and dental abnormalities, including late eruption, are common.

N. Hunter Syndrome (Mucopolysaccharidosis II) — In this X-linked disorder, coarsening of features is more gradual than in Hurler syndrome.

O. Progeria — This is a most striking and unusual disorder characterized by premature degeneration of body tissues.

P. Hemifacial Atrophy

V. Infections

A. Congenital Rubella

B. Congenital Syphilis

VI. Other Causes

A. Serious Systemic Illness — Any serious illness may affect development and growth resulting in delayed dentition.

SUGGESTED READINGS

Smith DW: Recognizable Patterns of Human Malformation, 3rd ed. Philadelphia, WB Saunders, 1982

Stewart RE, Poole AE: The orofacial structures and their association with congenital abnormalities. Pediatr Clin N Am 29:572–573, 1982

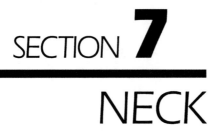

SECTION **7**

NECK

50

NUCHAL RIGIDITY

The sudden onset of a stiff neck with fever in an ill-appearing child usually indicates the presence of meningitis. In these cases, lumbar puncture should be performed immediately; the spinal fluid must be examined for cells, organisms, and protein and sugar content, as well as plated for culture. Nuchal rigidity is not, however, always the result of meningeal irritation secondary to infection; the history and other features of the physical examination may suggest other causes. A negative lumbar puncture should direct one's attention to other possibilities, because this symptom is too important to ignore.

The causes of nuchal rigidity have been divided into six categories: infections, vascular abnormalities, neoplasia, bony or muscular problems, metabolic disorders, and intoxications. Torticollis, a twisting of the neck, may also be associated with neck stiffness (see also Chap. 51, Torticollis).

I. Infections

A. Meningitis	Meningeal irritation may be the result of bacterial, viral, mycobacterial, fungal, or protozoal infections. Particularly in the latter three, the infection may be smoldering or chronic, whereas in others the onset of symptoms may be sudden and dramatic. Examination of the cerebrospinal fluid is essential. Special stains or cultures may be required in nonbacterial or nonviral cases.
B. Encephalitis	The pathogenetic organism may be any of those that cause meningitis. The onset may also be gradual or sudden. Fever, headache, ataxia, altered sensorium, convulsions, and coma are among the possible symptoms.
C. Cervical Adenitis	Acute adenitis secondary to pharyngitis or associated with other infections may result in nuchal rigidity. The swelling is tender, and the spinal fluid is normal. Posterior cervical adenitis is more likely than anterior to produce this symptom.
D. Pneumonia	Nuchal rigidity may be the presenting sign in upper-lobe pneumonia prior to auscultatory evidence.

E. Retropharyngeal Abscess

Other symptoms are prominent including dysphagia, drooling, and muffled voice. The neck is often held hyperextended. Subluxation of C1 and C2 vertebrae may occur.

F. Epiglottitis

The sudden onset of sore throat, dysphagia, drooling, and muffled voice, with a toxic appearance, is characteristic. Nuchal rigidity with the generalized illness may suggest meningitis, but a lumbar puncture could be catastrophic.

G. Guillain–Barré Syndrome

This condition is characterized by acute ascending motor paralysis, often with sensory changes and cranial nerve involvement. Deep tendon reflexes are usually decreased or absent; slight nuchal pain and rigidity are common.

H. Acute Cerebellar Ataxia

The onset of ataxia, especially involving the trunk, may be sudden, or signs may develop gradually. This disorder is most frequent in children between 1 and 4 years of age. Nuchal rigidity, if present, is mild.

I. Cervical Spine Osteomyelitis

Low-grade fever and slowly increasing pain on neck movement may be the only presenting signs.

J. Diskitis

These infections rarely cause rigidity.

K. Other Common Infections
1. Tonsillitis
2. Otitis Media
3. Pyelone-phritis
4. Mumps
5. Hepatitis
6. Shigellosis
7. Scarlet Fever
8. Infectious Mononucleosis
9. Cat-Scratch Disease
10. Roseola
11. Typhoid Fever
12. Herpes Zoster

L. Poliomyelitis

Poliomyelitis fortunately has become uncommon but was a scourge of the not-too-distant past. Affected children have rigidity of the back caused by muscle spasm.

M. Tetanus

Generalized muscle rigidity with muscle spasms occurs. Trismus (clenched jaw) is the classic sign; convulsions may also occur.

N. Brain Abscess

Signs and symptoms depend on the age of the child and the location and size of the lesion. Initially, headache, fever, and seizures may be present. Signs of increased intracranial pressure may be foremost.

O. Trichinosis

Periorbital edema, muscle pain, headache, fever, splinter hemorrhages of the nails, and eosinophilia are common signs.

P. Epidural Abscess

First symptoms are back pain with localized tenderness, and then nuchal rigidity, fever, and headache. Flaccid paralysis with loss of sensation below the level of the lesion then follows.

Q. Less Common Infections

1. Lymphocytic Choriomeningitis

There is abrupt onset of fever, headache, vomiting, photophobia, and abdominal pain, with cerebrospinal fluid pleocytosis in which the cells are almost all lymphocytes.

2. Chagas Disease

The findings of intermittent fever, nonpitting edema, lymphadenopathy, hepatosplenomegaly, urticaria, and behavioral problems suggest this disorder, although it is rare in the United States.

3. Cryptococcosis

India ink stain may be needed to demonstrate the organism.

4. Leptospirosis

Conjunctivitis, jaundice, albuminuria, and aseptic meningitis suggest this infection.

5. Malaria

6. Lyme Disease

Aseptic meningitis, encephalitis, and a host of other neurologic symptoms and signs may occur.

R. Dental Abscess
S. Postinfectious Encephalomyelitis

II. Vascular Abnormalities

A. Subarachnoid Hemorrhage	Meningeal irritation is present with irritability, severe headache, vomiting, loss of consciousness, and possibly coma.
B. Cerebral Aneurysms	If subarachnoid hemorrhage occurs, nuchal rigidity may develop. Affected children may have recurrent headaches and, rarely, episodes of nuchal rigidity prior to a massive hemorrhage.
C. Malformation of the Great Cerebral Vein (Vein of Galen)	Usual signs and symptoms occur after a subarachnoid bleed. Children with this anomaly may have cranial nerve palsies, nystagmus, ataxia, vertigo, and personality changes.
D. Primary Intracranial Venous Thrombosis	Thrombosis can be secondary to local infections, trauma, generalized sepsis, dehydration, and disorders causing a hypercoagulable state. Onset is often precipitous, with seizures, hemiparesis, lethargy and coma, and changing neurologic signs.

III. Neoplasms

A. Meningeal Leukemia	Invasion of the meninges usually occurs when the child is in hematologic remission. Progressive headache, nausea, vomiting, papilledema, and sixth nerve palsies may be present.
B. Posterior Fossa Tumors	Nuchal rigidity is more likely when the tumor extends through the foramen magnum into the upper spinal canal. A head tilt is common. Headache and vomiting may be present for long periods before clumsiness, strabismus, and ataxia occur.
C. Brain Stem Tumors	The triad of findings is characteristic: cranial nerve involvement, especially the seventh, ninth, and tenth nerves; pyramidal tract signs such as abnormal gait and posture and "handedness"; and signs of involvement of cerebellar pathways, such as ataxia, nystagmus, and occasionally, nuchal rigidity.
D. Tumors of the Third Ventricle	Pinealomas in particular may have ptosis as the first sign. Paralysis of upward gaze is the classical localizing sign. Nuchal rigidity, other signs of increased intracranial pressure, and ataxia also occur.
E. Osteoid Osteoma	This tumor may occur in cervical vertebrae. Pain is worse at night and may often be re-

lieved by aspirin. Roentgenograms show a small radiolucent area with surrounding sclerosis.

F. Eosinophilic Granuloma

This tumor may also occur in cervical vertebrae, giving rise to neck pain and rigidity. A punched-out lesion is seen on the roentgenogram.

IV. Bony or Muscular Disorders

A. Subluxations, Dislocations, and Fractures

Rigidity may be a presenting sign in these lesions of the cervical spine. The sudden onset of torticollis, even without a clear history of trauma, should suggest the possibility of these potentially dangerous lesions.

B. Myositis and Fibromyositis

A stiff neck may follow exposure to a cold draft or lying in an unusual posture. Neck muscles are tight and tender to palpation.

C. Vertebral Anomalies

Congenital block vertebrae may result in some lack of mobility. The condition is not painful, but is evident on roentgenograms.

D. Basilar Impression

Invagination of margins of the foramen magnum results in posterior displacement of the odontoid and compression of the spinal cord or brain stem. Other signs may include ataxia, nystagmus, head tilt, and cortical tract signs.

V. Metabolic Disorders

A. Infantile Gaucher Disease

This disease is almost always evident during the first 6 months of life. Hyperextension of the neck, strabismus, increased muscle tone, retardation, splenomegaly, laryngeal spasm, and seizures occur.

B. Maple Syrup Urine Disease

Rigidity and later opisthotonos occur in the first few days of life. Seizures and increased tone may suggest neonatal tetanus. Urine has the characteristic odor.

C. Kernicterus

Jaundice, irritability, and a shrill cry along with opisthotonos suggest this disorder.

VI. Intoxications

A. Phenothiazines

Dystonic manifestations from idiosyncratic reactions or overdose include nuchal rigidity, torticollis, opisthotonos, trismus, oculogyric crises, cogwheel rigidity, and other frightening signs. The child is usually awake.

B. Strychnine — Poisoning results in extreme rigidity of muscles, often intermittently simulating convulsions. Associated pain is intense. The child is awake.

C. Lead Poisoning

D. Methanol Poisoning

E. Hypervitaminosis A — Bone pain, headache, often associated with pseudotumor cerebri, hepatomegaly, and edema are more typical features.

VII. Miscellaneous Causes

A. Juvenile Rheumatoid Arthritis — Evidence of cervical spine involvement rarely may be a presenting sign. The presence of fever and leukocytosis may suggest infection. Other joint involvement may occur later.

B. Black Widow Spider Bite — Muscle spasm, particularly of the back, shoulders, and thighs, is apparent first. Abdominal pain may be exquisite.

C. Scorpion Sting

D. Kawasaki Disease

E. Paroxysmal Torticollis

F. Intussusception

REFERENCE

Stein MT, Trauner D: The child with a stiff neck. Clin Pediatr 21:559–563, 1982

51

TORTICOLLIS

Torticollis literally means "twisted neck." A head tilt is the primary physical sign, although some of the disorders listed below may be associated with neck stiffness as well.

The cause of torticollis may be as innocuous as exposure to a cold draft. A casual approach to the problem is to be condemned, however, because of the possibility of a vertebral subluxation or dislocation: In these conditions, manipulation of the neck or failure to recognize the injury may result in spinal cord compression with all of its serious consequences. For this reason, cervical spine films are suggested as part of the initial evaluation, particularly if pain or muscle spasm is associated with the torticollis. Information helpful in the differential diagnosis includes age of onset, a history of trauma or preceding infection, and associated systemic symptoms and signs.

I. Congenital Causes

A. Muscular Origin — The exact mechanism of production is unknown but may be a stretching of the sternocleidomastoid (SCM) muscle with resultant localized hematoma. Fibrosis of a portion of the SCM muscle develops with resultant shortening. The head is tilted toward the affected side; the chin is rotated to the opposite side. A "tumor" may be felt in the body of the SCM muscle within the first 10 days of life but disappears in 2 to 6 months. There is a higher incidence in breech and difficult forceps deliveries.

B. Vertebral Anomalies — Failure of segmentation of vertebrae, hemivertebrae, and the Klippel–Feil syndrome may be associated with torticollis. Cervical spine roentgenograms are diagnostic. In the Klippel–Feil syndrome, there is a reduction in the number of cervical vertebrae as well as fusion; the neck seems to ride on the shoulders. Sprengel deformity (elevation of the scapula) is often found in association with this anomaly.

C. Intrauterine Con-   During late fetal life the head may be fixed in
straint   position by the uterus. The head is oblique in
                        shape and the sternocleidomastoid may un-
                        dergo fibrosis. Most infants respond with pos-
                        tural manipulation for the restricted neck mo-
                        bility.

II. Trauma

A. Subluxation   Trauma may be described as minimal or may
                        not be remembered. Subluxation may occur
                        with sudden turning of the neck.
B. Dislocation   The C1–C2 instability common in various
                        dwarfism syndromes and bone dysplasias may
                        predispose to dislocation.
C. Fractures   Fracture of the clavicle as well as of vertebral
                        structures may result in torticollis.

III. Infection

A. Torticollis Fol-   A spontaneous subluxation may occur about 1
   lowing Upper   week after an upper respiratory infection.
   Respiratory In-   Children of 6 to 12 years of age are most fre-
   fection   quently affected.
B. Pharyngitis   Associated tissue swelling may be severe
                        enough to cause instability of the atlas (C1) on
                        the axis (C2).
C. Retropharyngeal   Fever, difficulty in swallowing, and drooling
   Abscess   are characteristic.
D. Cervical Adenop-   Localized irritation of the SCM muscle may
   athy   cause spasm.
E. Tuberculosis   Vertebrae or soft tissues may be affected.
F. Osteomyelitis   Pain is usually prominent.
G. Pneumonia   Characteristically the upper lobe is involved.
                        Cough, tachypnea, and fever are usual find-
                        ings.

IV. Tumors

A. Intraspinal Tu-   This tumor is commonly associated with mus-
   mor   cle spasm, back pain, and refusal to flex the
                        neck. Muscle weakness, abnormal reflexes,
                        and sensory losses may also occur.
B. Posterior Fossa   Headache, nausea, and vomiting are sugges-
   Tumor   tive findings.
C. Osteoid Osteoma   Pain at night, relieved by aspirin, is character-
                        istic.
D. Eosinophilic   Erosion of the vertebral structures may cause
   Granuloma   symptoms.

V. Neurogenic Torticollis

A. Poliomyelitis — Focal muscle weakness is responsible for the abnormal head posture.

B. Dystonia Musculorum Deformans — Affected children exhibit prolonged writhing and twisting motions.

C. Kernicterus — The neonatal history provides the key to diagnosis. Deafness or choreoathetosis may be present.

D. Huntington Chorea — Affected children have choreiform movements, but onset of symptoms is generally delayed until adulthood. The disorder is inherited as an autosomal-dominant trait.

E. Hepatolenticular Degeneration (Wilson Disease) — Other dystonic movements are present. Inspection of the irises may reveal the Kayser–Fleischer ring.

F. Neuritis of Spinal Accessory Nerve — The nerve is tender where it enters the neck, at the lateral border of the upper third of the SCM muscle.

VI. Ocular Torticollis

A. Superior Oblique Muscle Weakness — Children with fourth cranial nerve palsy may develop torticollis in an effort to prevent diplopia.

B. Congenital Nystagmus

VII. Miscellaneous Causes

A. Myositis or Fibromyositis — This is a fancy name for the common stiff neck following exposure to a cold draft. Neck muscles are tender and painful.

B. Fibrodysplasia Ossificans Progressiva — Onset of symptoms of this rare disorder is generally before 10 years of age. Lumpy, hard masses are palpable.

C. Juvenile Rheumatoid Arthritis — Cervical spine involvement may result in subluxation of C1 on C2.

D. Spasmus Nutans — Head nodding, tilt, and nystagmus are the characteristic findings; onset is before 6 months of age.

E. Paroxysmal Torticollis — Onset is between 2 and 8 months of age. Episodes last a few hours to 3 days; pallor, vomiting, and agitation may accompany the attacks. A relationship to migraine should be considered.

F. Reflux Esophagitis — The curious phenomenon of neck torsion without stiffness associated with hiatal hernia is known as Sandifer syndrome.

G. Drug-Induced | Phenothiazines may cause oculogyric crises, dystonia, opisthotonos, or trismus. Unless the overdose was large, the patient is awake and can obey commands. Dystonic reactions may occur with chlorpromazine (Thorazine), droperidol, fluphenazine, haloperidol, metoclopramide (Reglan), prochlorperazine (Compazine), thiethylperazine, thioridazine (Mellaril), thiothixene, trifluoperazine (Stelazine), and trimethobenzamide (Tigan).

H. Ligamentous Laxity | Laxity of the transverse ligament may be seen in patients on long-term oral steroid therapy. Subluxation or dislocation may occur with minimal or no trauma.

I. Functional Torticollis | This is rare in children.

J. Calcification of Intervertebral Disks | In this rare disorder of unknown etiology, the temperature may be mildly increased; there is local tenderness with muscle spasm. Fluffy calcification of the nucleus of the disk is noted on roentgenograms 1 to 2 weeks after onset.

SUGGESTED READINGS

Clark RN: Diagnosis and management of torticollis. Pediatr Ann 5:43, 1976

Jones MC: Unilateral epicanthal fold: Diagnostic significance. J Pediatr 108:702–704, 1986

Lipson EH, Robertson WC: Paroxysmal torticollis of infancy: Familial occurrence. Am J Dis Child 132:422, 1978

Murphy WJ, Gellis SS: Torticollis with hiatus hernia: Sandifer syndrome. Am J Dis Child 131:564, 1977

SECTION 8
CHEST

52

CHEST PAIN

The symptom of chest pain in children occurs considerably less frequently than abdominal or limb pain, but it may suggest an ominous underlying cause to the child or parent. In the study by Driscoll and colleagues[1] of chest pain in children seen as outpatients, 52% of the children or their parents thought that heart problems were the basis of the symptom, but none of the 43 patients had cardiac problems. Disorders affecting the chest wall accounted for 45% of the cases: costochondritis was the cause in 22.5% (a percentage slightly higher than that of most people's experience); coughing and bronchitis together, 12.5%; and muscle strain and trauma, 5% each. Curiously, chest pain in 45% of the patients in this study was labeled "idiopathic" after careful evaluation, including through history, physical, and laboratory examinations, failed to disclose evidence of a pathologic process. Selbst's study[2] attributed 28% as idiopathic, functional 17%, musculoskeletal 15%, and costochondral 10%. Although the chest pain in adults is a common manifestation of serious underlying problems, in children it infrequently is.

In the evaluation of chest pain, the presence or absence of other signs and symptoms should allow clear definition of the etiology of the problem or at least should limit the diagnostic possibilities to a few probable causes.

I. Chest Wall Lesions

A. Blunt Injury	The pain may be localized to an area of soft-tissue injury or rib fracture or may be located at costochondral junctions. The history is an important key to diagnosis, as is cutaneous evidence of trauma.
B. Muscle Strain	A careful history of preceding activities that may have resulted in muscle strain should be obtained. The strain may involve the pectoral, trapezius, latissimus dorsi, serratus anterior and shoulder muscles, and the coracoid process.
C. Trauma Secondary to Coughing	Protracted or severe coughing as with asthma or bronchitis may produce muscle strain and, occasionally, a rib fracture.

D. Costochondritis (Tietze Syndrome)

Swelling of one or two costochondral junctions, along with localized pain, is found. The cause is unknown, and the pain and swelling may last for months.

E. Herpes Zoster

Pain in a dermatome distribution may occur days before the appearance of cutaneous vesicles.

F. Tumors or Infiltrative Processes

Localized swelling or pain in the chest wall without obvious cause mandates a chest film.

G. Juvenile Rheumatoid Arthritis

Involvement of the costoclavicular joint rarely may be a presenting sign. Pleuritic chest pain is not uncommon.

H. Trichinosis

The combination of muscle pain, periorbital edema, and eosinophilia suggests this diagnosis.

I. Slipping Rib Syndrome

This sprain disorder is produced by trauma to the costal cartilages of the 8th, 9th, and 10th ribs. Pain on palpation is usually present. A hooking maneuver, inserting the fingers under the rib and pulling forward, will reproduce the pain.

J. Adolescent Breast Development

Girls and boys may have unilateral tenderness as the nubin of tissue develops.

K. Xipoid Process Syndrome

Pain may be increased by deep breathing.

L. Cervical Ribs

Symptoms often follow excessive exertion or trauma. Pain often radiates to the arms. Paresthesias are common.

M. Scalenus Anticus Syndrome

Pain is increased on abduction of the arm.

N. Costoclavicular Compression Syndrome

Pain is a result of distortion of the thoracic outlet causing compression of the brachial plexus. Paresthesias and signs of vascular compression are often present.

O. Juvenile Ankylosing Spondylitis

Costochondral and costovertebral pain may be present.

II. Cardiovascular Disorders

A. Pericarditis

The pain is usually precordial, dull, increased during inspiration, and sometimes referred to the left shoulder. Viruses are responsible for most cases, but collagen–vascular diseases, especially systemic lupus erythematosus and juvenile rheumatoid arthritis, are important causes.

B. Myocardial Ischemia — This is a distinctly uncommon cause of pain in children unless there is an underlying cardiac defect or coronary artery disease.

C. Chronic Pulmonary Hypertension — Pain may be present on exercise and relieved by rest. The pulmonic component of the second sound is accentuated. Congenital heart disease with increased pulmonary blood flow is the most common cause.

D. Mitral Valve Prolapse (Barlow Syndrome) — This possibility should be considered in children with an apical, late systolic murmur as well as chest pain. The disorder is much more common than previously thought.

E. Aortic Stenosis — Severe stenosis may result in decreased coronary artery blood flow and pain.

F. Pulmonary Stenosis — Severe stenosis may result in chest pain, especially during exercise.

G. Dissecting Aortic Aneurysm — In children the initial symptom may be either chest or back pain. This lesion may be associated with the congenital syndromes described below.

1. Marfan Syndrome — Arachnodactyly, dislocated lenses, pectus carinatum, scoliosis, and other features may be present.

2. Ehlers–Danlos Syndrome — Manifestations in affected children vary, ranging from hyperextensible joints to cutaneous laxity.

H. Pulmonary Vascular Obstruction — A pulmonary embolus or infarction produces sudden chest pain and anxiety.

I. Rheumatic Fever — Precordial pain may occur during the illness. The Jones criteria must be satisfied to make this diagnosis.

J. Sickle-cell Anemia — Chest pain probably is the result of vascular occlusion.

K. Dysrhythmias — Chest pain or discomfort may occur during supraventricular tachycardia, ventricular tachycardia, or any dysrhythmia affecting coronary artery flow.

L. Pericardial Defect — Herniation of the left atrial appendage through the defect produces sharp pain. Recurrent pleural effusions are common. Echocardiography will confirm the diagnosis.

M. Takayasu Arteri-
tis
The acute phase is characterized by fever, anorexia, weight loss, joint pain, and hypertension.

N. Pheochromo-
cytoma
Up to 40% of children with this tumor complain of chest or abdominal pain. Hypertension may be paroxysmal or sustained. Tachycardia, palpitations, headache, sweating, and pallor are other findings.

O. Pneumoperi-
cardium
A loud, metallic, splashing sound synchronous with the heart sounds may be heard on auscultation. A chest radiograph should confirm the diagnosis.

III. Pulmonary and Pleural Disorders

A. Pleurisy

1. Pneumonia
Inflammation of the pleural surface of the lung causes a "catching" chest pain during inspiration as the pleural surfaces rub together.

2. Primary Infec-
tion (Bacterial, Viral, or Tuberculous)
The pleural surface may be involved with little parenchymal disease. The pain is increased on inspiration.

3. Epidemic Pleurodynia (Devil's Grip)
The pain is sharp, stabbing, and accentuated on inspiration. Coxsackie B virus is the usual pathogenic organism.

4. Familial Mediterranean Fever
Although abdominal pain is more common, any serosal surface may be involved. The pain is sharp, usually lasts a few days, and is recurrent. The family history is important.

5. Familial Angioneurotic Edema
Chest pain may occur, but more frequent are recurrent episodes of swelling of the extremities and, occasionally, of the tongue and airway structures.

6. Systemic Lupus Erythematosus
The polyserositis may involve the pleura.

B. Pneumothorax
Chest pain may occur with a spontaneous pneumothorax or as a result of a pneumothorax associated with asthma or trauma.

C. Diaphragmatic Irritation
Shoulder pain usually results since the middle and anterior parts of the diaphragm are innervated by the phrenic nerve. A ruptured spleen is the classic cause of left shoulder pain, whereas the right hemidiaphragm may be irritated by a subphrenic abscess, a hepatic abscess, a tumor, or the perihepatitis of the

Fitz-Hugh–Curtis syndrome (associated with gonococcal infection).

D. Pneumome-diastinum

Crepitus may be noted at the suprasternal notch.

E. Asthma

The chest pain may be due to muscle strain, pneumothorax or pneumomediastinum, anxiety, or hypoxia.

F. Tracheitis

Irritation of the trachea may produce a substernal chest pain.

G. Precordial Catch (Stitch)

A sudden, brief catch of pain is common. The etiology is unclear.

H. Interstitial Pneumonitis

Dyspnea on exertion is the first symptom, followed by a dry, nonproductive cough. Anorexia and weight loss ensue. The chest pain may be pleuritic.

I. Mediastinitis

J. Mediastinal Tumor

A constant, boring, substernal pain is produced which may be associated with cough and dysphagia.

K. Sarcoidosis

Nonspecific chest pain, shortness of breath, a nonproductive cough, and occasionally hemoptysis may be the respiratory presentation of symptomatic patients with sarcoidosis. Hilar adenopathy can be found in 70% of these cases.

L. Pulmonary Tumors

IV. Esophageal Disorders

A. Foreign Body

The pain is usually increased on attempts at swallowing.

B. Achalasia

Achalasia produces an esophagitis with substernal burning, often worse in the recumbent position.

C. Ulceration and Strictures

Pain and difficulty in swallowing are primary symptoms.

D. Gastroesophageal Reflux

E. Esophageal Tear

This may follow pronounced vomiting.

V. Psychogenic Factors

A. Hyperventilation

Chest tightness or pain is a complaint along with lightheadedness, headache, acral paresthesias, and carpopedal spasm.

B. Conversion Reaction

Anxiety and stress may result in the complaint of chest pain, particularly if there is a family

member with chest pain related to cardiac
disease.

C. Malingering
D. Globus Hysteri-
cus

The complaint of inability to swallow because
of a lump or mass in the throat often has accompanying pain.

VI. Neurologic Disease

A. Spinal Cord
Compression

Pain in the chest may result from impingement on the cord or spinal roots by tumors or
abscesses or from compression following vertebral collapse.

VII. Extrathoracic and Referred Pain

A. Cholecystitis

Although uncommon in childhood, this inflammation is a notorious mimic of angina in
adults.

B. Pancreatitis

The pain is usually epigastric but may be substernal.

C. Hiatal Hernia

The substernal pain generally increases in a
recumbent position. Esophagitis is common.

D. Peptic Ulcer
E. Pancreatic
Pseudocyst
F. Pylorospasm

Pain is usually epigastric but may be over the
lower sternum.

G. Leukemia–Lym-
phoma

Pain is due to thoracic node involvement.

H. Nephrolithiasis

Pain may occur in the posterior left lower
chest as well as the back, groin, and genitalia.

REFERENCES

1. Driscoll DJ, Glicklich LB, Gallen WJ: Chest pain in children: A prospective study.
   Pediatrics 57:648–651, 1976
2. Selbst SM: Chest pain in children. Pediatrics 75:1068–1070, 1985

SUGGESTED READINGS

Brown LM: Mitral valve prolapse in children. In Barness LA (ed): Advances in Pediat-
rics, Vol 25, pp 327–348. Chicago, Year Book Medical Publishers, 1978
Pantell RH, Goodman BW Jr: Adolescent chest pain: A prospective study. Pediatrics
77:881–887, 1983
Porter GE: Slipping rib syndrome: An infrequently recognized entity in children.
Pediatrics 76:810–813,1985

53

GYNECOMASTIA

Enlargement of breast tissue in males is common in neonates and adolescents. In both age groups, regression of the enlargement is the rule. In neonates the gynecomastia invariably disappears, whereas in adolescents the persistence of the swelling, even though for less than 1 to 2 years in 90% of the cases, seems interminable to the young men. Occasionally, the breast enlargement may be so large or last so long that emotional difficulties arise. In some instances the breast tissue may require removal by an experienced surgeon.

In this chapter, causes of gynecomastia are divided into disorders of either pubertal or prepubertal onset. It is important to ascertain that the enlarged tissue is actually breast parenchyma; a third group of causes of breast enlargement mimicking gynecomastia is, therefore, included.

I. Onset During or After Puberty

A. Adolescence	Approximately 70% of boys develop some degree of gynecomastia during adolescence; the peak incidence is between 13 and 15 years of age. The enlargement may be unilateral or bilateral. Generally, the duration of gynecomastia is 1 to 2 years, but in up to 10% it may be as long as 3 to 4 years. Other disorders may cause gynecomastia, but they are uncommon.
B. Klinefelter Syndrome	About one third of boys with this chromosomal abnormality (XXY karyotype) develop gynecomastia during puberty. There is no known phenotypic picture in the preadolescent. Some children may have mental retardation. The small testes are not evident until puberty. Sparse facial hair and a feminine distribution of hair may be present.
C. Testicular Tumors	Interstitial cell tumors may cause feminization and gynecomastia. Choriocarcinomas of the testes may also cause gynecomastia and are characterized by the presence of large amounts of gonadotropins in the urine. Both kinds of tumors produce unilateral testicular enlargement.

D. Adrenal Tumors	In feminizing adrenal tumors and tumors producing early isosexual maturation with gynecomastia, there are advanced sexual maturation, elevated serum levels of estrogens, and increased urinary 17-ketosteroids. The testes, however, remain small.
E. Familial Gynecomastia	
1. Reifenstein Syndrome	This condition is characterized by testicular hypoplasia and sclerosis, gynecomastia, and variable degrees of hypospadias.
2. Kallman Syndrome	Gynecomastia with anosmia and testicular atrophy are findings in this rare disorder; transmission is through women who may have anosmia.
3. Gynecomastia with Hypogonadism and Small Penis	Hyperprolactinemia with galactorrhea is characteristic.
F. Chromophobe Adenoma of Pituitary	
G. Drugs	Several drugs have been implicated including digitalis, spironolactone, reserpine, phenothiazine, alpha-methyldopa, estrogen containing compounds, meprobamate, hydroxyzine, anabolic steroids, androgens, cimetidine, isoniazid, and human chorionic gonadotropin. Smoking marihuana may be associated with breast enlargement.
H. True Hermaphroditism	Gynecomastia in a boy with unilateral cryptorchidism may indicate true hermaphroditism.
I. Liver Disorders	Gynecomastia may occur in the presence of cirrhosis or liver carcinoma.

II. Prepubertal Onset

A. Neonatal Gynecomastia	Occurrence is common in newborns and is secondary to the transplacental passage of maternal estrogens.
B. Idiopathic Gynecomastia	This is a rare cause; diagnosis is made by exclusion of other disorders. The condition may be familial and often tends to regress within 1 year.
C. Testicular Tumors	Unilateral testicular enlargement is the primary clue.

D. Adrenal Tumors	Feminizing tumors accelerate growth and the bone age. Pubic hair may or may not be present. The testes and penis are normal in size for the child's age.
E. Congenital Adrenal Hyperplasia	Gynecomastia has been described with the 11-hydroxylase deficiency.
F. Precocious Puberty	Gynecomastia may occur as part of premature sexual development.
G. Exogenous Causes	Drugs such as those listed previously may be a cause.
H. Ectopic Gonadotropin-Secreting Tumor	
I. Liver Disorders	Cirrhosis and carcinomas may cause gynecomastia.
J. Testicular Feminization Syndrome	
K. Congenital Anorchia	
L. Secondary Testicular Failure	
M. Thyrotoxicosis	
N. Starvation	

III. Pseudogynecomastia
Breast enlargement may not be secondary to hyperplasia of true breast tissue. The following conditions may mimic gynecomastia.

A. Obesity	
B. Tumors	Lipoma, hemangioma, lymphangioma, neurofibroma, or carcinoma may involve the breast.
C. Infection	Cellulitis or abscess may cause enlargement.
D. Fat Necrosis	This condition may ensue following trauma to the breast area.

SUGGESTED READINGS

Latorre H, Kenny FM: Idiopathic gynecomastia in seven preadolescent boys. Am J Dis Child 126:771–773, 1973

Moore DC: Gynecomastia. In Kelley VC (ed): Practice of Pediatrics, Vol 7, Chap 41, pp 1–8. Hagerstown, Harper & Row, 1987

54

RESPIRATORY SYSTEM: COUGH

Cough is a common symptom in children. Acute infections, primarily upper respiratory ones, and allergic rhinnitis resulting in a postnasal drip are responsible for most coughs. Most causes listed in this chapter produce chronic cough, defined as that lasting more than a few weeks or as recurrent episodes.

Coughing is a reflex that renders an essential protective service: First, it serves to remove substances that may have been accidentally inhaled, and second, it removes excessive secretions or exudates that may accumulate in the airways. In some cases, cough is produced by extrinsic pressure on airway structures and serves neither of these purposes.

I. Infection

A. Upper Respiratory Infection
The common cold is caused by a variety of viruses. Coughing may be produced by pharyngeal irritation, postnasal drip, and other mechanisms.

B. Bronchitis
Inflammation of the bronchi is most commonly viral in origin, but mycoplasmal infection, pertussis, tuberculosis, and secondary bacterial infection may also be causative. In bronchitis, cough is the primary symptom and may initially be dry; later, it becomes loose and productive. Passive smoking may be a cause of chronic bronchitis.

C. Pneumonia
The majority of pneumonias are also viral in origin. In cases of bacterial origin, the course tends to be more acute and fulminant, sometimes without much cough. *Mycoplasma, Chlamydia,* and other organisms may be involved. Chlamydia pneumonia, which develops between 4 and 18 weeks of age, should be considered when the infant has an afebrile illness with congestion, wheezing, and a distinctive staccato cough. Cytomegalovirus may produce similar symptoms.

D. Bronchiolitis	Bronchiolitis is generally a disease of young infants primarily caused by viruses, especially respiratory syncytial virus. Tachypnea, wheezing, and cough are typical.
E. Croup	The croup syndrome has a variety of causes, some of which are infectious. Stridor is a predominant symptom, and the cough is barking in quality.
F. Sinusitis	Inflammation of the sinus cavities is often associated with a mucoid nasal discharge and postnasal drip, resulting in pooling of secretions in the hypopharynx with cough.
G. Pertussis	The paroxysmal, repetitive cough of pertussis may last for many weeks. The "whoop" may not be present in young children.
H. Pleuritis	Localized chest pain accentuated on inspiration is a more common symptom than cough.
I. Measles	The cough along with coryza, conjunctivitis, and fever followed by the rash completes the typical picture of rubeola. In atypical measles, pulmonary findings are more prominent than is the rash.
J. Tuberculosis	Most cases of tuberculosis are asymptomatic. Persistent fever and weight loss may be found. The "classic" bitonal cough and expiratory stridor are rare.
K. Fungal Infection	Histoplasmosis, coccidioidomycosis, and other fungal infections may involve the pulmonary structures, with resultant coughing often chronic in nature.
L. Parasitic Infestation	Cough and wheezing may be prominent during the lung migration phase in visceral larva migrans. In ascariasis, inhalation of the worms as they travel from the esophagus to the hypopharynx may produce coughing.
M. Psittacosis	Cough is not prominent. Fever, malaise, myalgia, and chills are nonspecific symptoms.
N. Q Fever	This is a rare disease in the United States.

II. Allergy

Allergy must be considered in the differential diagnosis when the cough is chronic.

A. Rhinitis	Acute or chronic nasal congestion and postnasal drip are common causes of cough. Clinical signs of allergy include allergic "shiners,"

	allergic salute, and Dennies lines (transverse creases on the lower lid).
B. Asthmatic Bronchitis	Cough is an integral part of the clinical picture of asthma. Prior to the development of expiratory wheezing, coughing may be the main clue.
C. Cough Variant Asthma	Cough may be the initial and occasionally the only presenting symptom of asthma. Most children who are affected will later have overt asthma. A clinical trial of bronchodilators will be helpful in this diagnosis.
D. Atelectasis	Recurrent atelectasis commonly develops in asthma owing to mucous plugs.
E. Hypersensitivity Pneumonitis	Various inhalants may trigger recurrent or chronic inflammatory responses with cough and other respiratory symptoms.
F. Allergic Bronchopulmonary Aspergillosis	This condition may be confused with chronic asthma. A low-grade fever, prolonged wheezing, a peripheral blood eosinophilia, and transient pulmonary infiltrates may be found.

III. Environmental Irritants

A. Dry Air	This is a common cause of coughing that is often overlooked in the differential diagnosis. Dryness of air passages may cause an irritative type cough or result in mucus production and pooling of secretions with a chronic cough, particularly during the winter months when the air in homes lacks proper humidity.
B. Fumes	Smoke from tobacco or fireplaces or fumes from chemicals, gases, or paints may trigger coughing following irritation of the airways.
C. Smoking	The airways may be irritated from tobacco smoke inhaled directly or passively from smoking in the household.

IV. Aspiration

A. Foreign Body	Most foreign bodies are associated with the sudden onset of coughing as they lodge in large airways. Small materials such as seeds or grasses may produce secondary irritation with the clinical picture of asthma or pneumonia. Other findings depend on size, position, and composition of the inhaled body.

B. Gastroesopha-
geal Reflux

In infants and young children, recurrent episodes of cough, wheezing, or pneumonitis
may be associated with aspiration of stomach
contents.

C. Neuromuscular
Disorders

Children with various neuromuscular disorders or cricopharyngeal incoordination may
experience recurrent episodes of aspiration,
particularly during feeding. The cough is wet
and often productive.

D. Other

Chalasia and achalasia are uncommon causes.

V. Congenital Anatomic Defects

A. Tracheoesopha-
geal Fistula

In most cases, the onset of symptoms is
shortly after birth, with coughing due to aspiration of saliva or feedings.

B. Lobar Emphy-
sema

Cough, wheezing, dyspnea, tachypnea, and
tachycardia are typical.

C. Bronchogenic
Cyst

These lesions usually are asymptomatic, although in some cases, the cyst may impinge
on the bronchi, producing cough.

D. Pulmonary Se-
questration

Recurrent episodes of pulmonary infection,
fever, and cough are the usual presenting
symptoms.

E. Anomalous
Blood Vessels
F. Tracheal Steno-
sis

Compression of the trachea or bronchi may
produce a cough, often brassy-sounding.

VI. Cystic Fibrosis

Cystic fibrosis should be included in the differential diagnosis in
every child with a chronic cough, particularly when gastrointestinal
symptoms are present.

VII. Airway Encroachment

A. Mediastinal
Tumors

Symptoms occur from airway compression.
Stridor or wheezing respiration may be
present. A brassy cough may occur if the tumor exerts pressure on the recurrent laryngeal
nerve.

B. Mediastinal
Adenopathy

Compression of airway structures by enlarged
nodes may occur in various infections and
inflammatory disorders.

C. Pulmonary Tu-
mors

These tumors are rare in childhood. Cough,
dyspnea, and signs of obstructive pneumonitis
are the most common symptoms.

D. Hemangiomas   There may also be cutaneous lesions.

E. Papilloma of Trachea and Bronchi   Dyspnea and stridor are the most common symptoms.

VIII. Psychogenic Origin: Habit Cough (Tics)

There is often a history of school phobia. The cough does not occur during sleep and remains unchanged with exertion, infection, and temperature changes. No systemic symptoms are present.

IX. Miscellaneous Causes

A. Auricular Nerve Stimulation   Stimulation of the auricular branch of the vagus nerve in the external auditory canal by cerumen or a foreign body is an uncommon cause of cough.

B. Congestive Heart Failure   Other signs and symptoms of failure predominate.

C. Enlongated Uvula   Rarely, the uvula may drag on the pharyngeal structures, precipitating a cough.

D. Tonsillar Concretions   Whitish balls of dried secretions may accumulate in the tonsillar crypts. They may be dislodged during swallowing and cause episodes of sudden coughing with the production of tiny amounts of this material.

E. Bronchiectasis   This disorder should be considered in the child with chronic cough, persistent atelectasis, and abnormalities on chest roentgenograms despite clinical resolution of infection. It may be associated with measles, pertussis, pneumonia, foreign bodies, cystic fibrosis, and immunodeficiency disorders.

F. Sarcoidosis   The cough is variable. Bilateral hilar adenopathy is typical on chest roentgenograms.

G. Pulmonary Emboli   Emboli are uncommon in the pediatric age group. Sudden coughing and dyspnea may occur at the time of embolization.

H. Exercise-Induced Airway Hyperreactivity   A relatively new concept as an important cause of chronic cough, this disorder does not appear to be mediated through allergic mechanisms. Pulmonary function testing appears to be the most appropriate means of confirming the problem.

I. Immotile Cilia Syndrome   The triad of a productive cough, sinusitis, and otitis has been present in all cases described;

in half, situs inversus was a finding. Infertility is common in affected boys.

J. Swyer–James Syndrome — This acquired condition follows bronchiolitis obliterans in infancy characterized by repeated bouts of pulmonary infections. A chronic cough may be present and bronchiectasis may occur.

K. Gilles de la Tourette Syndrome — Cough, with other verbal and motor tics, may support this diagnosis.

SUGGESTED READINGS

Cloutier MM, Loughlin GM: Chronic cough in children: A manifestation of airway hyperactivity. Pediatrics 67:6–12, 1981

Eigen H: The clinical evaluation of chronic cough. Pediatr Clin N Am 29:67–78, 1982

Hannaway PJ, Hopper GDK: Cough variant asthma in children. JAMA 247:206–208, 1982

Mellis CM: Evaluation and treatment of chronic cough in children. Pediatr Clin North Am 26:553–564, 1979

Williams HE, Phelan PD: Respiratory Illness in Children. London, Blackwell Scientific Publications, 1975

55

RESPIRATORY SYSTEM: DYSPNEA

Normally, breathing is accomplished without a conscious awareness of the effort involved. Dyspnea refers to that condition in which the patient is unpleasantly aware of the work of breathing or in which there is genuine discomfort or difficulty in breathing. Dyspnea is both a sign and a symptom: Difficulty in the respiratory effort may be obvious; older children may voice complaints about breathing difficulties.

The causes of dyspnea are too numerous to list individually. In this chapter, a few important examples are given for each major category; classification is based on the pathophysiologic mechanism involved. The cause of dyspnea does not always reside in the lung. When central nervous system irritation, particularly in meningitis or encephalitis, is the cause, early detection is essential to prevent serious consequences. Acidosis may also be mistaken for primary pulmonary disease.

It is also important to try to determine whether the respiratory effort is inspiratory or expiratory: The former suggests disease in the upper or large airways, whereas the latter is indicative of pathologic processes in the smaller airways or lower respiratory tract.

I. Interference with Gas Exchange

A. Pulmonary Infections	Gaseous exchange may be impaired in pneumonias of viral, bacterial, fungal, and mycobacterial origin. Air entry may also be compromised.
B. Aspiration	Gastroesophageal reflux, tracheoesophageal fistulae, near-drowning, and meconium aspiration may result in tissue reactions interfering with gaseous exchange.
C. Atelectasis	
D. Cystic Fibrosis	
E. Pulmonary Edema	Congestive heart failure, allergic pulmonary response, smoke inhalation, and chemical pneumonitis are some of the more common causes.
F. Pulmonary Fibrosis	Fibrosis resulting in alveolar-capillary block may develop with chronic lung irritation caused by inhalants or oxygen and respirator

therapy, or as a consequence of alpha-1-anti-trypsin deficiency.

G. Idiopathic Pulmonary Hemosiderosis

Recurrent episodes of alveolar hemorrhage may produce attacks of dyspnea, cyanosis, coughing, and hemoptysis.

H. Sarcoidosis

II. Interference with Air Entry

A. Bronchoconstriction
   1. Asthma
   2. Bronchiolitis

B. Upper Airway Obstruction
   1. Croup Syndrome

(See Chap. 58, Respiratory System: Stridor.)

   2. Foreign Body

There is usually an acute onset of dyspnea, cough, and other pulmonary symptoms.

   3. Epiglottitis
   4. Adenoidal or Tonsillar Hypertrophy

C. Compression of Lung
   1. Pneumothorax or Pneumomediastinum
   2. Tumors

If large enough, cysts, teratomas, or other mediastinal growths, including enlarged nodes secondary to malignancies, may compromise pulmonary reserve.

   3. Elevated Diaphragm

The lung may be compressed by elevation of the diaphragm caused by abdominal ascites or masses or secondary to a diaphragmatic hernia.

   4. Effusions

Lung expansion may be compromised by pleural effusions, empyema, hemothorax, or other fluid collections.

D. Emphysema

In infants, congenital lobar emphysema may produce early respiratory distress rather than the generalized emphysema seen in adults.

E. Thoracic Cage Disorders
   1. Flail Chest

Negative pressures cannot be generated to allow air entry.

2. Body Casts
3. Thoracic De-   Rarely, severe congenital constriction of the
   formities   thoracic cage occurs, with compromise of pul-
                     monary function.
F. Extreme Obesity
G. Painful Breath-
   ing
   1. Rib Fracture
   2. Pleurisy
   3. Peritonitis

III. Cardiovascular Problems

A. Congenital   Dyspnea is most prominent in disorders with
   Heart Disease   right-to-left shunts that create hypoxic states.
B. Congestive   Tachycardia, tachypnea, hepatomegaly, and
   Heart Failure   dyspnea are among the earliest signs.
C. Dysrhythmias   Circulation may be compromised as the car-
                     diac pump becomes inefficient. Paroxysmal
                     atrial tachycardia may produce intermittent
                     episodes of dyspnea.
D. Cardiac Com-
   promise
   1. Pericarditis   Dyspnea and chest pain may be the key
                     symptoms.
   2. Myocarditis   Compromise of circulation may occur with
                     viral myocarditis. Electrocardiogram changes
                     are usually prominent.
   3. Pneumoperi-   Symptoms are consistent with those of a peri-
      cardium   cardial effusion and pericarditis. A loud, me-
                     tallic, splashing sound synchronous with the
                     heart sounds may be heard on auscultation. A
                     chest radiograph is diagnostic.
E. Pulmonary Em-   Emboli are relatively uncommon in children.
   bolus   The sudden onset of dyspnea, apprehension,
                     cough, and in some cases, chest pain suggest
                     this diagnosis.
F. Mitral Valve
   Prolapse

IV. Insufficient Oxygen Supply to Tissues

A. Shock   Shock may follow trauma, sepsis, or hemor-
                     rhage.
B. Anemia
C. Exercise   Overexertion is a common nonpathologic
                     cause of dyspnea.

D. High Altitude
E. Carbon Monoxide Exposure
F. Methemoglobinemia   Various drugs and chemicals may reduce hemoglobin, decreasing its oxygen-carrying capacity.

V. Central Nervous System Disturbances

A. Acidosis   The respiratory center may be stimulated by changes in *p*H. In diabetic ketoacidosis, dehydration, inborn errors of metabolism, and salicylate poisoning, dyspnea may be a primary sign.

B. Central Nervous System Irritation
    1. Meningitis and Encephalitis   Children with central nervous system irritation from infection are often dyspneic. In some cases, investigation of pulmonary causes of the difficulty has delayed discovery of the primary cause.

    2. Tumors
    3. Hemorrhage

VI. Neuromuscular Problems

A. Muscular Dystrophy
B. Guillain–Barré Syndrome
C. Werdnig–Hoffman Disease
D. Poliomyelitis
E. Myasthenia Gravis
F. Hypokalemia
G. Organophosphate Poisoning
H. Diaphragmatic Paralysis
I. Botulism

VII. Psychogenic Causes

A. Fright
B. Pain
C. Hyperventilation Syndrome

VIII. Miscellaneous Causes
  A. Hyperthyroidism
  B. Fever

SUGGESTED READING

Holsclaw DS: Respiratory signs and symptoms. In Kaye R, Oski FA, Barness LA (eds): Core Textbook of Pediatrics, pp 248–274. Philadelphia, JB Lippincott, 1982

56

RESPIRATORY SYSTEM: HYPERPNEA

Hyperpnea is an increase in the depth of respirations. Many of the conditions listed in the classification below feature an increase both in depth and in rate of respiration. More than one pathophysiologic mechanism may be operative in the child with hyperpnea.

I. Hyperthermia
   A. Febrile States
   B. Warm Environment   The depth and rate of respirations are increased to assist in heat loss from the body.

II. Metabolic Acidosis
   A. Dehydration   Conditions producing dehydration such as severe diarrhea result in decreased renal perfusion and consequent retention of hydrogen ions.
   B. Starvation   Tissue catabolism results in increased hydrogen ion production.
   C. Diabetic Ketoacidosis   This is perhaps the best-recognized cause of tissue catabolism leading to metabolic acidosis and hyperpnea.
   D. Drugs and Toxins   Various substances may lead to metabolic acidosis.
       1. Salicylates   In acute salicylate intoxication, respiratory alkalosis is transient and metabolic acidosis soon ensues. Hyperpnea is an important clinical sign of toxicity during chronic salicylate therapy.
       2. Paraldehyde   The characteristic odor on the breath is readily apparent.
       3. Ammonium Salts
       4. Dinitrophenol
       5. Methanol
       6. Ethylene Glycol

7. Respiratory Stimulants — Aminophylline, epinephrine, and nikethamide are examples.

E. Chronic Renal Failure — Hydrogen ion retention occurs with inadequate renal function.

F. Renal Tubular Acidosis — In the distal form, the urine remains relatively alkaline despite systemic acidosis.

G. Intestinal Bicarbonate Loss — Intestinal fistulas may be the cause.

H. Inborn Errors of Metabolism

1. Glycogen Storage Disease, Type I — Marked hepatomegaly develops in young children. Recurrent episodes of lactic acidosis may result in death.

2. Galactosemia — Vomiting, diarrhea, jaundice, and hepatomegaly may occur in the neonatal period.

3. Ketotic Hyperglycinemia

4. Methylmalonic Acidemia

5. Isovaleric Acidemia — A "sweaty sock" odor is characteristic.

6. Lactic Acidemia — Children with this disorder may have intermittent ataxia, oculomotor nerve palsies, muscle weakness, and progressive motor deterioration.

7. Cystinosis — Signs of rickets are usually present.

III. Hypoxemia

A. Severe Anemia

B. Shock and Hypotension

C. Cardiac Failure

D. Cyanotic Congenital Heart Disease

E. Wilson–Mikity Syndrome — This condition is a form of pulmonary insufficiency that may occur in immature infants. Characteristic pulmonary changes are seen on roentgenograms. Hyperpnea and retractions resolve slowly.

IV. Neurogenic Hyperpnea

A. Hypoglycemia

B. Encephalitis — Respiratory alkalosis follows stimulation of the respiratory center.

C. Gram-Negative
   Sepsis
D. Cerebral Infarc-
   tion
E. Acute Salicylate   Stimulation of the respiratory center occurs
   Intoxication   before the metabolic acidosis.

V. Miscellaneous Causes

A. Psychogenic   Anxiety and hysteria are often associated with
   Causes   hyperventilation. Other symptoms include
                         headache, chest tightness, dizziness, and par-
                         esthesias of the extremities.
B. Reflex Hyperven-   Various stimuli may cause hyperpnea.
   tilation
   1. Pain
   2. Sudden Cool-
      ing of the Skin
   3. Urinary Blad-
      der Distension
   4. Pulmonary   For example, a pulmonary embolism may
      Vascular Oc-   cause occlusion.
      clusion
   5. Pneumothorax

SUGGESTED READING

Scarpelli EM, Auld PAM, Goldman HS: Pulmonary Disease of the Fetus, Newborn and Child. Philadelphia, Lea & Febiger, 1978

57

RESPIRATORY SYSTEM: HEMOPTYSIS

The coughing up of blood is a frightening symptom for the child, parents, and physician. In most cases, the origin of the blood is in the oropharynx, and a careful physical examination will disclose the site of bleeding. True hemoptysis of pulmonary origin has a variety of causes, the most common of which are bronchiectasis, cystic fibrosis, an aspirated foreign body, and pulmonary infections.

I. Infections

A. Bronchiectasis	A cough, productive of blood-tinged sputum, is usually present. Recurrent fever and signs of pneumonia are common. In chronic cases, clubbing of the fingers is found.
B. Cystic Fibrosis	Hemoptysis is rare but may occur in older patients with bronchiectasis. Hemoptysis is a poor prognostic sign since it indicates progressive pulmonary disease. Massive hemoptysis has been reported.
C. Pneumonia	A rusty sputum may occur in bacterial or viral pneumonias, but particularly in pneumococcal pneumonia.
D. Pulmonary Tuberculosis	A tuberculin skin test should be performed in all children with hemoptysis. Weight loss, night sweats, intermittent fever, and cough may be present.
E. Lung Abscess	Pus and sputum are often mixed with the blood.
F. Pertussis	Streaks of blood may be seen in the sputum produced after severe coughing episodes.
G. Influenza	In severe cases a hemorrhagic tracheobronchitis may develop.
H. Aspergillosis	An underlying pulmonary disorder predisposes to this condition. Fever and a necrotizing pneumonia with cavitation may develop. Hyphae may be found in the sputum.
I. Coccidioidomycosis	Most cases are asymptomatic, but mild respiratory symptoms develop in a small number

with fever, dry cough, malaise, anorexia, and myalgias. Rarely, if the cough is productive, the sputum may be blood-tinged.

J. Blastomycosis — In the pulmonary form, mild respiratory symptoms include a low-grade fever, chest pain, and a nonproductive cough. Progressive disease results in fever, weight loss, night sweats, and hemoptysis.

K. Hemorrhagic Fevers — This group of disorders, which is found in many parts of the world, is transmitted by arthropods. Some forms are associated with severe prostration, thrombocytopenia, and pneumonitis with hemoptysis.

L. Paragonimiasis — This infestation is also known as endemic hemoptysis in parts of Africa and Central and South America. A chronic pulmonary infection, caused by a trematode, is associated with cough and hemoptysis.

II. Trauma

A. Lung Contusion — Blunt or penetrating injuries of the chest wall may be associated with pulmonary injury and hemoptysis.

B. Foreign Body — Aspiration of a foreign object may cause hemoptysis following injury to the tracheobronchial tree such as laceration or chronic irritation.

C. Smoking Clove Cigarettes — Reaction to inhaled smoke may result in bronchospasm, pulmonary edema, and hemoptysis as well as lesser pulmonary symptoms.

III. Cardiovascular Causes

A. Pulmonary Embolus — Emboli may occur in subacute bacterial endocarditis or in peripheral venous thrombosis. Symptoms depend on the size of the embolus, the number of emboli, and the severity of the lesions. Dyspnea, pallor, cyanosis, and chest pain with a shock-like picture may be present.

B. Multiple Pulmonary Telangiectasis — This condition may be part of hereditary hemorrhagic telangiectasia (Rendu–Osler–Weber syndrome). The family history is important since the disorder is transmitted as an autosomal-dominant trait.

C. Ruptured Arteriovenous Fistula — The size of the fistula determines pre-rupture symptoms, which may include finger clubbing, polycythemia, and cyanosis. The lesion may be associated with the Rendu–Osler–Weber syndrome.

D. Mitral Stenosis — Hemoptysis may occur during paroxysmal dyspnea or pulmonary edema. Occasionally, the bleeding may be brisk when a bronchial or pleurohilar vein ruptures.

E. Endomyocardial Fibrosis — Hemoptysis is a late finding during left-sided heart failure.

F. Necrotic Pulmonary Arterial Lesions — Children with systemic lupus erythematosus and periarteritis nodosa may develop hemoptysis secondary to pulmonary vascular lesions.

IV. Tumors

A. Bronchogenic Cysts

B. Enterogenic Cysts — Duplications of the bowel may be present in the thoracic cavity. Symptoms depend on the size and position of the cyst and include recurrent pulmonary infections, chest pain, and hemoptysis.

C. Mediastinal Teratoma — The gastric mucosa of the teratoma may produce secretions that ulcerate into the lung parenchyma.

D. Bronchogenic Carcinoma — Occurrence in childhood is rare.

E. Bronchial Submucosal Gland Tumors — The two most common types are carcinoid tumors and adenoid cystic carcinomas. Cough is the most common presenting symptom, often with hemoptysis. Wheezing may confound the diagnosis.

F. Plasma Cell Granuloma of Lung — Additional findings may include clubbing, cough, chest pain, and weight loss.

V. Miscellaneous Disorders

A. Sickle-Cell Anemia — Pulmonary intravascular sickling resulting in infarction has been described.

B. Hemorrhagic Disorders

C. Primary Pulmonary Hemosiderosis — This uncommon disorder is characterized by chronic pulmonary symptoms including cough, dyspnea, wheezing, and hemoptysis, as well as changes seen on roentgenograms and iron-deficiency anemia.

D. Pulmonary Hemorrhage — Premature infants who have suffered hypoxic insults are most commonly affected.

E. Systemic Lupus Erythematosus (SLE)	A pulmonary hemosiderosis picture may appear long before other features of SLE occur.
F. Sarcoidosis	Patients with symptomatic respiratory presentations may occasionally have hemoptysis.
G. Swyer–James Syndrome	Unilateral hyperlucent lung acquired following bronchiolitis obliterans in infancy. Repeated bouts of pulmonary infection occur and may be followed by bronchiectasis.
H. Wegener Granulomatosis	Necrotizing granulomas of the upper and lower respiratory tract may result in hemoptysis. Evidence of renal vasculitis is usually present.

VI. Bleeding Without Pulmonary Involvement

The child must be examined carefully for evidence of upper-airway disorders associated with bleeding that may be mistaken for hemoptysis.
A. Epistaxis
B. Oral or Nasopharyngeal Trauma
C. Acute Tonsillitis
D. Gingivitis

58

RESPIRATORY SYSTEM: STRIDOR

Stridor is defined as a crowing sound heard usually during inspiration. The sound may be high-pitched or low-pitched and may also be present during expiration. Generally, stridor is indicative of obstruction somewhere along the respiratory tract, from the pharynx down to the major bronchi. This symptom demands immediate attention and thorough evaluation to uncover the precise cause.

It is important to determine whether the cause of the stridor is an acute or a chronic disorder. The following clues may be helpful in evaluating this sign: The presence of a weak cry, hoarseness, or aphonia strongly suggests a laryngeal problem. Inspiratory crowing is produced by partial obstruction of the upper airway, whereas expiratory stridor is the result of a lesion in the lower airway. If the child prefers to hold the neck in a hyperextended position, extrinsic pressure on the airway should be suspected.

In the classification that follows, the causes of stridor are divided into acute and chronic disorders. Associated signs and symptoms that may aid in the differential diagnosis are included.

I. Acute Causes of Stridor

A. Laryngotracheitis — Viral croup is the most common cause of acute stridor. There is usually a history of a preceding upper respiratory infection followed by the development, usually at night, of inspiratory stridor and a cough that sounds like a seal's bark. Hoarseness may be prominent. The term *laryngotracheobronchitis* should be reserved for lower tract infection, usually bacterial, secondary to viral croup.

B. Spasmodic Croup — Episodes of inspiratory stridor, not preceded by an upper respiratory infection, may occur without fever. Affected children are generally older than those in whom acute laryngotracheitis is found. The episodes may be recurrent.

C. Foreign Body Aspiration — Inspiratory stridor occurs if the foreign body is lodged in the subglottic area or above; both expiratory and inspiratory stridor are usually present if the obstruction is lower. A sudden choking episode followed by stridor and dyspnea suggests a foreign body.

D. Esophageal Foreign Body

Stridor may occur if the foreign body is lodged in the cervical esophagus. Drooling, dysphagia, and anorexia without signs of infection may be prominent.

E. Epiglottitis

Epiglottitis usually does not cause stridor. Onset of the infection is sudden, with fever, difficulty in swallowing, drooling, a muffled voice, and preference to sit upright. The child appears acutely ill.

F. Supraglottitis

The aryepiglottic folds rather than the epiglottis are inflamed. Group A β-streptococcus may be the cause. Symptoms are similar to epiglottitis.

G. Angioneurotic Edema

Acute swelling of the upper airway may cause alarming dyspnea and stridor; fever is uncommon. Swelling of the face, tongue, or pharynx may be present as well.

H. Ingestion of Corrosives

Stridor results from swelling of oral and pharyngeal structures. Drooling, mouth ulcers, and a history of ingestion are most important clues.

I. Trauma

Falls, auto accidents, clothes-line injuries, and violent blows may result in laryngeal fracture. Hoarseness and cough are presenting symptoms. Crepitation of the neck may be present, as well as dyspnea and dysphagia.

J. Peritonsillar Abscess

Stridor is a late sign as edema of the hypopharynx develops. Early signs are sore throat, dysphagia, drooling, and difficulty in opening the mouth. The uvula is shifted from the midline.

K. Retropharyngeal Abscess

Stridor develops as the pharyngeal wall becomes edematous. Drooling and dysphagia are present. Affected children hold the neck hyperextended.

L. Diphtheria

Stridor may be produced as the faucial membrane forms or drops into the glottic area. Fever, hoarseness or aphonia, a serous or serosanguineous nasal discharge, and cervical adenopathy may be prominent.

M. Hypocalcemic Tetany

This is a rare cause of stridor owing to the greatly reduced incidence of rickets. Other signs include carpopedal spasm, tremors, irritability, twitchings, and convulsions.

N. Laryngeal Aplasia In a newborn with marked inspiratory effort, cyanosis, and chest retractions, laryngeal aplasia or severe stenosis should be considered. Aplasia is not consistent with life unless a tracheostomy is performed immediately.

O. Psychogenic

P. Bacterial Tracheitis Acute serious upper-airway obstructive illness may be the result of this infection, usually due to *S. aureus.* Fever, toxicity, and stridor are clinical findings. Copious, thick, purulent tracheal secretions are found. It is critical to differentiate this infection from laryngotracheitis.

Q. Laryngeal Candidiasis

II. Chronic Causes of Stridor

A. Congenital Laryngeal Stridor This disorder, also called laryngomalacia, is thought to be caused by a relative immaturity of the laryngeal framework. On inspiration the loose tissues collapse inward, producing stridor that is more marked in the supine position. The stridor is more sonorous or stertuous in quality. The cry, however, is normal. The condition usually resolves with growth by 1 year of age. Direct laryngoscopy should be performed to confirm the diagnosis.

B. Floppy Epiglottis (Omega-Shaped Epiglottis) The epiglottis may fall back into the airway, causing partial obstruction. Stridor is more severe in the supine position.

C. Subglottic Stenosis Stridor is present from birth, but pronounced respiratory difficulty does not usually occur until an upper respiratory infection results in swelling or increased mucus production.

D. Laryngeal Paralysis The paralysis may be present at birth or develop later. The voice may take on a higher pitch with hoarseness and dyspnea in bilateral vocal cord paralysis, which usually signifies a brain stem injury or central nervous system malformation. Unilateral paralysis may follow recurrent laryngeal nerve entrapment by mediastinal tumor or aberrant great vessels or aortic arch. Onset of paralysis may be sudden in the Arnold–Chiari deformity. The cry is generally weak.

E. Laryngeal Web	A weak cry and stridor are evident. Direct laryngoscopy reveals failure of separation of the anterior portions of the vocal cords.
F. Vascular Ring/ Aberrant Vessels	In vascular ring anomalies such as a double aortic arch or abnormally placed subclavian artery, regurgitation of food with cyanotic attacks, and inspiratory or expiratory stridor may be the presenting signs. The infant may prefer to keep the neck hyperextended. An aberrant left pulmonary artery and aneurysmal dilation of the pulmonary arteries associated with absent pulmonary valve can produce dyspnea, stridor, and wheezing.
G. Micrognathia	In severe defects, as in the Pierre Robin syndrome, the tongue may fall back over the supraglottic aperature, producing stridor.
H. Abnormal Arytenoid Function	The arytenoid cartilage may be displaced congenitally or secondary to trauma. Hoarseness and stridor are present.
I. Laryngeal Papillomas	These lesions should be considered in any child who develops hoarseness and breathing difficulty without evidence of infection. Stridor may occasionally be present.
J. Chronic Laryngeal Stenosis	Stenosis is a frequent occurrence after tracheostomy owing to granuloma formation or cartilaginous overgrowth; it may also develop after infections, trauma, burns, or radiation.
K. Tracheal Stenosis	A congenitally small tracheal cartilaginous ring or absent cartilage may be associated with obstruction. If the defect is extrathoracic, the stridor is inspiratory; if intrathoracic, both inspiratory and expiratory crowing are present.
L. Hypertrophied Tonsils	Tonsillar tissue may be so large that the supraglottic airway becomes obstructed. Stridor is especially noticeable during sleep. Pulmonary hypertension and congestive heart failure may follow.
M. External Compression	Cystic masses, including lingual cysts, tonsillar teratomas, nasopharyngeal angiofibromas, and cystic hygromas, may obstruct the supraglottic area.
N. Aberrant Thyroid Tissue	A lingual thyroid or thyroglossal duct cyst may cause partial obstruction.
O. Mediastinal Cyst or Teratoma	Thoracic pain, a choking sensation, dyspnea, and stridor may be present.

P. Bronchial or Esophageal Cysts	Symptoms are suggestive of bronchial stenosis: cough, wheeze, progressive dyspnea, stridor, and cyanosis.
Q. Internal Laryngocele	The voice is muffled, and stridor is present. The mucosal pocket lies between the true and false cords.
R. Hemangiomas	Subglottic lesions gradually enlarge during the first few months of life. The stenosis produces a musical stridor similar to that of viral croup.
S. Macroglossia	The tongue may be enlarged enough to obstruct the hypopharynx.
T. Farber Disease	Hoarseness and stridor may appear at any time during the first few weeks of life. Palpable nodules develop in the skin, along with painful swelling of multiple joints. Hepatomegaly and central nervous system deterioration eventually occur.
U. Coccidioidomycosis	One case of subglottic infection has been reported.
V. Rheumatoid Arthritis	Involvement of the cricoarytenoid joint produces stridor and dyspnea.
W. Opitz–Frias Syndrome	Affected infants have feeding difficulties, often with recurrent aspiration, hypertelorism, and hypospadias. Stridor and a hoarse voice are often life-long findings.
X. Marshall–Smith Syndrome	A sporadic disorder with poor growth, advanced bone age, prominent eyes, low nasal bridge and upturned nose.
Y. Laryngotracheoesophageal Cleft	Partial clefts are the most common form of this rare anomaly. Respiratory distress, feeding difficulty and recurrent aspiration inevitably develop.

SUGGESTED READINGS

Hawkins DB, Udall JN: Juvenile laryngeal papillomas with cardiomegaly and polycythemia. Pediatrics 63:156–157, 1979

Quinn–Bogard AL, Potsic WP: Stridor in the first year of life: Clinical evaluation of the persistent or intermittent noisy breather. Clin Pediatr 16:913–919, 1977

Smith RJH, Catlin FI: Congenital anomalies of the larynx. Am J Dis Child 138:35–39, 1984

Tauscher JW: Esophageal foreign body: An uncommon cause of stridor. Pediatrics 61:657–658, 1978

59

RESPIRATORY SYSTEM: WHEEZING

The old adage "All that wheezes isn't asthma" is perhaps overdone; yet many physicians have been fooled by the apparently asthmatic child in whom elevated sweat chloride levels are later demonstrated or who is subsequently found to have a tracheal foreign body. Sometimes expiratory noises cannot be distinguished from inspiratory ones, and both may be present at one time. What may sound like wheezing may really be stridor, snoring, sighing, or just noisy breathing.

Wheezing is a musical sound caused by partial obstruction of the airway and is most often expiratory. Stridor is a coarser sound produced on inspiration. The following list of causes of wheezing has been divided into three primary categories: The first group represents the conditions that should be considered in the primary differential diagnosis; the second group represents much less likely causes of wheezing. In the third group are disorders in which wheezing is rarely found, or in which the respiratory noise may be mistaken for wheezing.

I. Common Causes of Wheezing

A. Asthma	Overall, asthma is the most common cause of wheezing in children. Repeated attacks of labored breathing, a tight cough, air trapping manifested by an increased antero-posterior diameter of the chest, and a "garden of sounds" heard on auscultation of the lungs (crackles, snaps, pops, rhonchi, whistles, and so forth) are characteristic. The family history is frequently positive for atopy. Attacks can be precipitated by exposure to various allergens, infection, exercise, ingestants, and, sometimes, emotions.
B. Bronchiolitis	Wheezing is frequently found in this viral infection of the lower airway, usually caused by respiratory syncytial virus. Fever may or may not be present; tachypnea and retractions are common. Bronchiolitis is most frequent in infants less than 6 months of age and unusual in those older than 18 months.

C. Aspiration

1. Foreign Body — There is usually a sudden onset of respiratory symptoms with cough, stridor, or wheezing. Symptoms depend on the type of foreign body, its size, where it is trapped, and the size of the patient. Signs may be unilateral on auscultation. Secondary infection may occur. Stridor is usually more prominent than wheezing. An esophageal foreign body may compress the trachea, producing a wheeze.

2. Gastroesophageal Reflux — Especially during infancy, reflux with aspiration into the lungs may produce recurrent episodes of wheezing mimicking asthma. There may not be a history of vomiting. Incidence is greater in the mentally retarded. Hiatal hernia or rarely esophageal stenosis may be demonstrated.

3. Defective Swallowing — Children with familial dysautonomia, bulbar palsy, and cleft palate may be predisposed to aspiration.

D. Cystic Fibrosis — Affected children may have associated wheezing and they sometimes have asthma. Other signs and symptoms of cystic fibrosis should be sought: chronic cough, repeated respiratory infections, persistent pulmonary changes on x-ray films, steatorrhea, and failure to thrive. A sweat test should be performed in equivocal cases.

E. Bronchitis and Pneumonitis — Infections (viral, bacterial, protozoal, or mycotic) may be associated with wheezing. Chest film changes, a clinical picture consistent with infection, and failure to respond to bronchodilators are findings that help in differentiation from asthma. Lower respiratory infections with wheezing in school-aged children in the fall are frequently related to M. pneumoniae.

F. Vascular Ring — This defect usually causes early onset of respiratory problems: brassy cough, dyspnea, stridor (much more common than wheeze), and repeated infections. Symptoms are often worse after feeding, and there may be some difficulty in swallowing. The neck may be held hyperextended. Double aortic arch and aberrant subclavian arteries are the most common anomalies.

G. Aberrant Vessels — In addition to vascular rings other vessels may impinge on the airway. An aberrant left pulmonary artery, absent pulmonary valve with aneurysmal dilation of the pulmonary arteries, and an aberrant innominate can also produce similar signs.

II. Less Common Causes of Wheezing

A. Congenital Obstructions

1. Tracheal or Bronchial Stenosis — Stridor is more common with tracheal stenosis; wheezing, with bronchial stenosis. Repeated lower respiratory infections are common.

2. Bronchomalacia — Bronchi may collapse on expiration, causing obstructive symptoms of cough, wheezing, and dyspnea with recurrent infections.

3. Tracheobronchomegaly — This disorder may be associated with cutis laxa. Redundancy of structures may result in recurrent infections and obstructive symptoms.

4. Lobar Emphysema — Tachypnea is a presenting sign in early infancy. Uncommonly, a wheeze may be heard over the affected lobe.

5. Sequestration — Recurrent infection, sometimes with hemoptysis, is a common manifestation.

B. Alpha$_1$-antitrypsin Deficiency — Adults are more likely than children to present with respiratory symptoms. Occasionally, cough and wheeze are findings.

C. Visceral Larva Migrans — *Toxocara* larvae may pass through the lung, producing an asthma-like picture. Affected children may have hepatomegaly, anorexia, and anemia; eosinophilia is usually pronounced.

D. Hypersensitivity Pneumonitis — Causes are numerous; it is more prevalent in adults.[1] Organic dust particles, chemicals, drugs (including aspirin), and fungi (*Aspergillus* and *Candida*) have been implicated.

E. Tumors

1. Tracheal and Bronchial Tumors — Symptoms depend on tumor location as well as its size. Cough, wheezing, and recurrent infection are prominent. Hemangiomas on neck and chest may be a clue but are not reliable indications of respiratory tract hemangiomas. External compression of the airway by

	cysts, lymphomas, and other mediastinal masses may produce dyspnea, chest pain, cough, and stridor as well as wheezing.
2. Carcinoid Tumors	These are very unusual in children. Wheezing, diarrhea, and sudden flushes of the skin may be present.
F. Heart Disease	Bronchial compression from cardiac enlargement may cause wheezing along with other symptoms. Congestive heart failure as a cause is usually obvious, with hepatomegaly, cardiomegaly, tachycardia, and tachypnea.
G. Miscellaneous Causes	
1. Tracheoesophageal Fistula	The H-type fistula is an uncommon cause of recurrent pneumonia or wheezing.
2. Pulmonary Vasculitis	Collagen–vascular diseases, especially systemic lupus erythematosus, may involve the pulmonary system. Pneumonitis, pleurisy, cough, hemoptysis, dyspnea, and sometimes wheezing may be found.
3. Idiopathic Pulmonary Hemosiderosis	Episodes of cough, wheezing, dyspnea, and hemoptysis are common. Anemia is always present.
4. Bronchopulmonary Dysplasia	This condition is seen in infants treated for hyaline membrane disease.
5. Immune Deficiency States	Affected children may have wheezing as a symptom in recurrent pulmonary infections.
6. Fibrous Mediastinitis	Involvement of the tracheobronchial tree may result in wheezing. There may be esophageal obstruction as well.
7. Immotile Cilia	The triad of cough, sinusitis, and otitis media have been present in all cases.

III. Conditions with Respiratory Noises Mimicking Wheezing

Other respiratory noises or symptoms may be mistaken for wheezing. Most discussions of the differential diagnosis of asthma or causes of wheezing include the disorders listed here. There should be no difficulty in distinguishing the associated dyspnea or stridor from wheezing.

A. Infections	
1. Laryngotracheobronchitis	Inspiratory stridor is the key feature. Rarely, wheezing may be a finding when involvement of the lower respiratory tract is extensive.

2. Other Causes of Croup Syndrome	Upper airway obstruction, as in spasmodic croup, epiglottitis, diphtheria, and retropharyngeal abscess, produces stridor rather than wheezing.
3. Pertussis	The repetitive cough should not be confused with wheezing.
B. Upper Airway Obstruction	Stridor or noisy respirations are produced. Causes include enlarged tonsils and adenoids, choanal stenosis or atresia, polyps, laryngeal papillomas, vocal cord paralysis, tetany, lingual thyroid, and allergic edema.
C. Congenital Malformations of Lungs 1. Hypoplasia 2. Cysts 3. Arteriovenous Malformation	Dyspnea, tachypnea, and cyanosis are symptoms.
D. Miscellaneous Causes 1. Neck Injury	Compression of the trachea produces stridor rather than wheezing.
2. Hysteria	Apparent respiratory difficulty in the hyperventilation syndrome should not be confused with wheezing.
3. Salicylate Intoxication	Deep, rapid respirations rather than an increased expiratory phase of respiration are found in salicylate toxicity.

REFERENCE

1. Bierman CW, Pierson WE, Massie FS: Nonasthmatic allergic pulmonary disease. In Kendig EL (ed): Disorders of the Respiratory Tract in Children, pp 670–696. Philadelphia, WB Saunders, 1977

SUGGESTED READINGS

Dees SC: Asthma. In Kendig EL (ed): Disorders of the Respiratory Tract in Children, pp 620–669. Philadelphia, WB Saunders, 1977
Leffert F: Asthma: A modern perspective. Pediatrics 62:1061–1069, 1978
Richards W: Differential diagnosis of childhood asthma. Current Probl Pediatr IV, No. 5, 1974

60

CARDIOVASCULAR SYSTEM: HYPERTENSION

Hypertension can be said to be a physical sign that has finally come of age. The last decade has seen a remarkable interest develop in the pathogenesis, etiology, and treatment of elevated blood pressure. As with so many other diseases, hypertension has been found to be amazingly frequent now that routine measurement has become commonplace.

There have been so many good reviews written—some of which are listed at the end of this chapter—that no attempt is made here to cover the many important considerations in obtaining and interpreting blood pressure readings. A few general points do require emphasis, however. The appropriate size of blood pressure cuff must be used. The rubber inflatable bladder should cover at least two thirds of the length of the upper arm and should be large enough to encircle the entire circumference of the extremity; a narrow cuff results in an elevated reading. If the pressure is taken in the sitting position, the arm should be supported at the level of the heart. Fear, agitation, apprehension, and other emotional factors, in addition to heat and exercise, may cause elevations in blood pressure. The importance of repeating measurements over time (if the elevations are not severe) cannot be overstated. If possible, a series of home readings should be attempted.

Rames and colleagues[1] found that 13.4% of school children 5 to 18 years of age had a blood pressure reading in excess of the 95th percentile on standard charts for age, or greater than 140/90 mm Hg, on the initial examination. Upon repeated screening, however, less than 1% of all children had a sustained high level. Furthermore, more than one half of these children had relative weights of 120% or more of the expected norm for height and body build. Obesity may be a much more common cause of high blood pressure in children than previously recognized. The implications for future health need further clarification, however.

The younger the child and the more severe the hypertension, the more likely a cause for the pressure elevation will be found. Generally, in private practice, the incidence of demonstrable causes of secondary hypertension, particularly renal, is not as high as that reported in studies of cases seen in referral centers. Essential hypertension was considered rare in the 1960s; by the late 1970s, however, essential hypertension was found to cause over half of blood pressure elevations in teenagers.

The following classification of causes of hypertension groups disorders by the organ system involved. Where possible, associated signs and symptoms are included to offer diagnostic clues. Most frequently, the elevation is "silent." Routine measurement of blood pressure is critical. Signs and symptoms that may be associated with hypertension are protean: headache, dizziness, nausea or vomiting, visual disturbances, facial nerve palsy, irritability, seizures, convulsions, personality changes, changes in conscious state, polyuria, polydipsia, weight loss, and so forth.

I. Miscellaneous Common Causes

A. Inappropriate Cuff Size	Overall, especially 5 to 10 years ago, this has been the most frequent cause of elevated blood pressure. The measurement must be repeated with use of the appropriate cuff.
B. Apprehension	The effects of the procedure and the milieu in which the pressure is obtained should not be underestimated. Repeated measurements over time (especially at home) are most helpful.
C. Obesity	Hypertension in obese children may be due in part to cuff size inaccuracy; however, do not ignore signs and symptoms of other disorders. Weight reduction is the key to therapy; lower readings following desired weight loss confirm the diagnosis.
D. Essential Hypertension	This form is asymptomatic, with no abnormal findings on physical examination. Often one or both parents also have essential hypertension. It is most commonly identified in teenagers, especially those who are obese.
E. Immobilization	Hypertension has only relatively recently been emphasized as a common accompaniment of immobilization following orthopedic or surgical procedures.[2] Children in body casts or cervical traction are particularly prone to develop hypertension.
F. Orthopedic Manipulation	

II. Renal Causes

A. Pyelonephritis	Renal parenchymal disease, especially pyelonephritis, acute as well as chronic, is the most common renal cause. Chronic pyelonephritis may be surprisingly asymptomatic.

B. Unilateral Renal Parenchymal Disease	In addition to pyelonephritis, parenchymal disease may result from obstructive uropathy, congenital defects, infarction, or trauma.
C. Renal Artery Abnormalities	Stenosis, aneurysms, arteritis, fistula, fibromuscular dysplasia, and thrombosis may all cause hypertension. Auscultation of the flanks may disclose bruits. If occlusion is severe, the onset is more abrupt. Headache, polyuria, polydipsia, and growth failure may be nonspecific symptoms. Café-au-lait spots of neurofibromatosis may be a clue. These abnormalities are second only to parenchymal disease as a cause of hypertension.
D. Acute Glomerulonephritis	This is a relatively common cause of hypertension of acute onset. Evidence of preceding streptococcal infection should be sought. Symptoms may be nonspecific such as malaise, headache, and anorexia, but edema, hematuria, and oliguria are common. Seizures and congestive heart failure may occur abruptly.
E. Other Nephritides	A host of other causes of glomerulonephritis must be considered. The presence of protein and cellular elements in the urine suggests this group of disorders; renal biopsy is usually required for differentiation. (See Chap. 77, Hematuria.)
F. Henoch–Schönlein Syndrome (Henoch–Schönlein Purpura)	A purpuric rash is characteristic. Abdominal pain, arthritis, and tissue swelling are also common.
G. Renal Trauma	Acute injury may have caused notable hematuria, gross or occult.
H. Hydronephrosis	The acute onset of hydronephrosis from obstruction may be associated with vomiting. A flank mass may be palpable.
I. Familial Nephritis	Recurrent episodes of hematuria, especially with intercurrent infections, are common; deafness may be a finding. Renal failure occurs in family members in the third and fourth decades.
J. Hemolytic-Uremic Syndrome	Persistent diarrhea, often bloody, and severe pallor draw attention to the hemolytic anemia and thrombocytopenia. Acute renal failure

may follow. Burr cells are seen on blood smear.

K. Renal Vein Thrombosis
Fever, hematuria, oliguria, and a flank mass are often present.

L. Renal Stones
There may be a history of renal colic with intermittent flank pain and hematuria. If stones obstruct the ureter, vomiting follows.

M. Nephrotic Syndrome
Edema, proteinuria, hypoalbuminemia, and hypercholesterolemia are present. The cause is most frequently idiopathic or nil disease.

N. Hypoplastic Kidney
There may be unilateral involvement of the entire kidney, or the defect may be segmental (Ask–Upmark), perhaps associated with vesicoureteric reflux.

O. Wilms Tumor
The usual presenting sign is an abdominal mass that is discovered by the parents. Abdominal pain and hematuria may also be present. Two thirds of affected children are under 3 years of age.

P. Neuroblastoma
Symptoms vary. Associated hypertension has been reported in from 10% to 50% of cases.

Q. Acute Renal Failure

R. Polycystic Disease
The infantile form results in renal failure in the first or second decade. The liver is cystic also, and abdominal masses are palpable. Inheritance pattern is autosomal recessive. In the adult form, hypertension begins in the second or third decade or later; renal insufficiency is prominent. Inheritance pattern is autosomal dominant.

S. Renal Tuberculosis
The finding of "sterile" pyuria is suggestive.

T. Radiation Nephritis

U. Retroperitoneal Fibrosis

V. Renin-Secreting Tumors
These lesions are a rare cause of severe hypertension. Symptoms may include polyuria, polydipsia, and enuresis. Hypokalemic alkalosis is usually present.

W. Liddle Syndrome
This is another cause of hypokalemic alkalosis with hypertension. Polyuria and polydipsia with an inability to concentrate urine are

present. Inheritance pattern is probably auto-somal dominant.

III. Endocrine Causes

A. Adrenogenital Syndrome

   1. 17-Hydroxy-lase Deficiency Syndrome — This rare deficiency results in hypogonadism with lack of secondary sex characteristics. Affected boys display pseudohermaphroditism; girls have amenorrhea.

   2. 11-β-Hydroxylase Deficiency — This defect results in rapid virilization with rapid somatic growth.

B. Cushing Syndrome — Obesity, moon facies, buffalo hump, arrested linear growth, acne, hirsutism, striae, malar flush, and elevated blood pressure are characteristic.

C. Pheochromocytoma — This tumor may produce episodic elevations in blood pressure with flushing, sweating, tachycardia, and headache. There may be a family history, or the lesion may be associated with neurofibromatosis or Sipple syndrome (multiple endocrinopathy).

D. Hyperthyroidism — Systolic pressure is elevated. Weight loss, irritability, tremor, tachycardia, sweating, and exophthalmos are strongly suggestive.

E. Primary Aldosteronism — The picture may include periodic muscular weakness, paresthesias, tetany, growth failure, polyuria, and polydipsia. Serum sodium levels are high, serum potassium low, and carbon dioxide high.

F. Primary Hyperparathyroidism — This is an unusual cause of hypertension. Symptoms are primarily those of hypercalcemia: muscle weakness, anorexia, nausea, vomiting, constipation, polyuria, polydipsia, weight loss, and fever. Calcium deposits in the kidney may result in renal damage and hypertension.

G. Diabetes Mellitus — Chronic nephropathy in childhood is unlikely unless the diabetes has been present for 10 or more years.

IV. Cardiovascular Causes

A. Coarctation of Aorta — Diminished or absent femoral pulses with hypertensive upper extremity pressures are characteristic.

B. Patent Ductus Arteriosus — Increased systolic pressure, wide pulse pressure, and a machinery-type murmur are findings.

C. Arteriovenous Fistula — Systolic pressure is increased; cardiac rate may also be increased.

D. Polycythemia

E. Anemia — In severe cases, systolic pressure may be elevated.

F. Subacute and Acute Bacterial Endocarditis

G. Leukemia

H. Pseudoxanthoma Elasticum — Yellowish papules on the neck, in the axillae, and around the umbilicus and groin become more apparent with age. There may be angioid streaks in the retina with hemorrhages.

Systemic vascular disease usually occurs later in life.

I. Takayasu Disease (Pulseless Disease) — Unequal pulses develop or are lost; large vessels are affected. The etiology is unknown.

V. Neurologic Causes

A. Increased Intracranial Pressure — Cerebral edema resulting from trauma, vascular accidents, pseudotumor cerebri, or infection (meningitis, encephalitis, abscesses) may cause hypertension.

B. Poliomyelitis

C. Guillain–Barré Syndrome (Acute Febrile Polyneuritis) — Progressive ascending paralysis is characteristic.

D. Familial Dysautonomia — Absent lacrimation and fungiform papillae on the tongue, diminished response to pain, recurrent episodes of vomiting, emotional lability, and paroxysmal hypertension are common.

VI. Drug-Induced Hypertension

A. Sympathomimetics — In particular, nose or eye drops and cough preparations have been implicated. Phenylephrine, ephedrine, isoproterenol, epinephrine, amphetamines, methylphenidate, and phenylpropanolamine are examples.

B. Corticosteroids

C. Oral Contraceptives

D. Methysergide

E. Phencyclidine

F. Excessive Ingestion of Licorice

G. Reserpine Overdose

VII. Miscellaneous Causes

A. Burns

B. Collagen–Vascular Diseases
1. Systemic Lupus Erythematosus
2. Scleroderma
3. Dermatomyositis
4. Polyarteritis

C. Heavy Metal Poisoning — Lead and mercury poisoning may cause hypertension.

D. Hypercalcemia — Hypercalcemia may be idiopathic or secondary to metastatic disease or sarcoidosis.

E. Stevens–Johnson Syndrome — This is a severe bullous form of erythema multiforme with mucous membrane involvement.

F. Hypernatremia

G. Sickle-cell Anemia

H. Malignancies — Rhabdomyosarcoma is an example.

I. Tuberous Sclerosis — Hypopigmented macules, café-au-lait spots, facial papules, and seizures are common. Inheritance pattern is autosomal dominant.

J. Acute Intermittent Porphyria

K. Fabry Disease (Angiokeratoma Corporis Diffusum) — Minute reddish blue or black lesions (angiokeratomas) are noted over the lower abdomen and scrotum late in the first decade of life. Paresthesias of extremities, recurrent fever, and proteinuria are other findings.

L. Amyloidosis

M. Neurofibromatosis — The hypertension is not always renovascular in origin.

N. Chronic Hypoxia

O. Malignant   The hypertension is associated with tachy-
    Hyperthermia   cardia, tachypnea and stiff muscles. Fever
                          develops and later a shock-like picture super-
                          venes.

REFERENCES

1. Rames LK, Clarke WR, Connor WE et al: Normal blood pressures and the evaluation in childhood: the Muscatine study. Pediatrics 61:245–251, 1978
2. Turner MC, Ruley EJ, Buckley KM et al: Blood pressure elevation in children with orthopedic immobilization. J Pediatr 95:989–992, 1979

SUGGESTED READINGS

Loggie JMH (ed): Hypertension in childhood and adolescence. Pediatr Clin North Am 25:1–188, 1978

Loggie, JMH, New MI, Robson AM: Hypertension in the pediatric patient: A reappraisal. J Pediatr 94:685–699, 1979

Makker SP, Moorthy B: Fibromuscular dysplasia of renal arteries: An important cause of renovascular hypertension in children. J Pediatr 95:940–945, 1979

National Heart, Lung and Blood Institute: Report of the Task Force on blood pressure control in children. Pediatrics 59:797–820, 1977

Saken R, Kates GL, Miller K: Drug-induced hypertension in infancy. J Pediatr 95:1077–1079, 1979

61

CARDIOVASCULAR SYSTEM: SYNCOPE

Syncope or fainting refers to the sudden and transient loss of consciousness, usually as a result of decreased cerebral perfusion and anoxia. Syncopal episodes are usually of short duration; however, if they last for over 20 seconds, a few clonic twitches may occur that may falsely suggest epilepsy.

The history is extremely important, particularly in attempting to define precipitating conditions that may be associated with the most common form of syncope, vasovagal. Recurrent episodes may suggest the need for further investigation to uncover cardiac or central nervous system causes. Hysterical fainting is characterized by its dramatic occurrence and seeming lack of concern on the part of the child.

I. Vasovagal (Vasodepressor) Syncope
The most common cause of sudden fainting is termed vasovagal syncope. A family history of syncope can often be obtained. Occurrence is most common in adolescence; a single incident rarely suggests emotional maladjustment. Episodes are usually provoked by factors such as pain, sudden emotional upset, hunger, fatigue, prolonged standing, heat, or the loss of or sight of blood. A prodrome of lightheadedness, dizziness, cold sweat, and pallor is common.

II. Hysterical Fainting
Fainting may be an attention-getting device. The situation tends to be dramatic, often is repeated, and has no prodrome; usually the child shows little concern for the episode. The period of unresponsiveness is generally much longer in duration than with vasovagal syncope.

III. Cardiovascular Causes
Overall these account for a small percentage of actual syncopal episodes.

A. Cardiac Anomalies	Syncopal episodes may occur with a number of cardiac defects, particularly after exercise.
1. Severe Aortic Stenosis	

    2. Severe Pulmonic Stenosis

    3. Tetralogy of Fallot

    4. Truncus Arteriosus

    5. Transposition of the Great Vessels

B. Dysrhythmias

    1. Paroxysmal Atrial Tachycardia

    2. Stokes–Adams Syncope — Complete atrioventricular block causes loss of consciousness.

    3. Familial Paroxysmal Ventricular Fibrillation

    4. Mitral Valve Prolapse — Usually, children or adults with prolapse of a mitral leaflet are asymptomatic. In some, dysrhythmias may occur, or precordial chest pain may be a presenting symptom. The presence of an apical late systolic murmur or a midsystolic click suggests this disorder. Prolapse may coexist with Marfan syndrome, the straight back syndrome, idiopathic hypertrophic subaortic stenosis, or ostium secundum defect of the atrial septum.

    5. Cardioauditory Syndrome (Jervell and Lange–Nielsen Syndrome) — Fainting attacks may begin in infancy or childhood, usually precipitated by emotions or physical exertion. The attacks may be mild, severe, or even fatal and are probably secondary to ventricular fibrillation. The electrocardiogram is useful in demonstrating large T waves and a prolonged Q-T interval. Perceptive, profound, and symmetric deafness is part of this disorder inherited as an autosomal-recessive trait and is congenital or very early in onset.

    6. Long Q-T Syndrome Without Deafness — Syncopal episodes commonly begin in early childhood and may be mild and transient or severe, leading to several minutes of unconsciousness or even sudden death. As many as

	half of those affected by this autosomal-dominant disorder die before adolescence. Attacks are most commonly precipitated by violent emotions or physical exercise.
7. Sinus Node Dysfunction	Dysfunction may occur with or without structural heart disease. Irregular cardiac rhythms or abnormally slow rates are clues. Other symptoms include chest pain with exercise, palpitations, and dizzy spells.
8. Emery–Dreifuss Muscular Dystrophy	Initial features include toe walking, partial flexion of the elbows, and inability to fully flex the neck and spine. A distinct pattern of contractures in the absence of major weakness is the earliest clue to diagnosis. In early adulthood atrial conduction abnormalities occur with exertional chest pain and recurrent syncope. If rhythm disturbances are untreated, the disorder proves fatal by mid-adulthood. There is an X-linked inheritance.
C. Primary Pulmonary Hypertension	
D. Carotid Sinus Syncope	Attacks appear to be related to a hyperactive carotid sinus reflex with slowing of the heart and hypotension.
E. Postural Hypotension	Assuming a standing position suddenly after recumbency may be associated with light-headedness or syncope.
F. Left Atrial Myxoma	A pedunculated myxoma may suddenly block left atrial outflow. A changing murmur may be a clue. This lesion may occur in tuberous sclerosis.
G. Myocardial Infarction	

IV. Breath-Holding

Some young children may have recurrent episodes of breath-holding and sometimes syncope. The breath-holding occurs during crying precipitated by injury or a deliberate attention-getting device during anger or frustration. During the syncopal episode there may be a few muscular twitches that may be mistaken for seizures by the parents. Two types of breath-holding spells have been described: (1) a cyanotic spell following crying and (2) a pallid one with the sudden onset of pallor and collapse without prior crying.

V. Hyperventilation

Prolonged deep breathing, either intentional or unrecognized during emotional stress, may lead to lightheadedness, generalized weakness, carpopedal spasm, and chest tightness. Occasionally, if the $PaCO_2$ is reduced far enough, syncope may occur. A dangerous form of intentional hyperventilation has been reported in swimmers prior to races, who may subsequently become unconscious while underwater and drown.

VI. Epilepsy

Convulsive episodes, particularly akinetic or drop seizures, may mimic syncopal episodes; there is no postictal phase, and they are not associated with jerking movements. Affected older children do not report lightheadedness or other symptoms prior to the collapse.

VII. Miscellaneous Causes

A. Cough	Prolonged coughing episodes may raise intra-thoracic pressure, decrease venous return to the heart, and lower cardiac output, resulting in syncope.
B. Micturition	This unusual form of syncope occurs during urination.
C. Paracentesis	Syncope may occur after the sudden removal of fluid from the pleural space, peritoneal cavity, or bladder.
D. Cerebellar or Brain Stem Tumors	Syncopal episodes may occur in children with these tumors after coughing or straining.
E. Adrenal Insufficiency	Weakness, lightheadedness, and fainting may occur in adrenocortical insufficiency, most commonly after the withdrawal of oral steroids.
F. Severe Anemia	
G. Drugs	Some antihypertensive agents may cause postural hypotension and fainting. Antihistamines often cause dizziness and sometimes syncope.
H. Anterior Mediastinal Tumors	Stridor, orthopnea, cough, and edema of the head and neck should suggest this possibility.
I. Acquired Postganglionic Cholinergic Dysautonomia	This is a rare disorder of unknown cause characterized by strabismus, lack of tears, saliva and sweat and atony of the bowel and bladder. Orthostatic hypotension may lead to syncope.
J. Swallowing	An unusual cause in children related to increased vagal tone with second-degree heart block.

K. Migraine
L. Pregnancy

SUGGESTED READING

Ruckman RN: Cardiac Causes of Syncope. Pediatrics in Rev 9:101–108, 1987

SECTION **9**

ABDOMEN

62

ABDOMINAL DISTENSION

A distended or protuberant abdomen may result from a wide variety of disorders. The diagnostic possibilities may be rapidly narrowed by information supplied by the history and a careful physical examination.

If the enlargement occurs suddenly and is associated with vomiting and abdominal pain, intestinal obstruction or peritonitis must be considered. An abdominal mass or visceromegaly is easily distinguishable from other less well-defined causes. The presence of ascites opens another list of diagnostic possibilities.

I. General Considerations

A. Poor Posture — An excessive lordosis either from poor posture or as the normal curve seen in the toddler may make the abdomen seem protuberant.

B. Excessive Feeding — This is most commonly seen in infants, but older children may voluntarily ingest large enough quantities of food or drink to distend the abdomen.

C. Aerophagia (Air Swallowing) — The excessive swallowing of air may result from improper feeding techniques, with pacifiers, from gum chewing, and during times of excitement or stress. The abdomen tends to be tympanitic; excessive gas passage, from both above and below, is a helpful clue.

D. Chilaiditi Syndrome — This is a rarely discussed entity in recent times; it refers to the presence of pain in the right upper quadrant associated with excessive air swallowing.

E. Malnutrition — Wasted extremities contrast with the pot-bellied appearance.

F. Muscle Weakness — Disorders causing muscle weakness may be associated with an increased lumbar lordosis and consequent abdominal protuberance.

G. Chronic Constipation — A careful history of elimination patterns is helpful. If the stool is hard, left lower quadrant masses may be palpable. A rectal examination is mandatory. Occasionally, an abdominal roentgenogram may reveal massive fecal retention not apparent on palpation.

II. Intestinal Obstruction

In most instances obstruction produces an acute onset of symptoms. Vomiting, pain, and failure to pass stools along with the abdominal distension should direct attention to this group of disorders.

A. Neonatal Disorders

1. Duodenal Atresia — Vomiting develops shortly after the first feeding or prior to it as a result of amniotic fluid ingestion. The vomitus may be bile-tinged; the epigastric area is distended.

2. Gastrointestinal Atresia or Stenosis — The time of onset of symptoms depends on the level of obstruction, but in most, symptoms begin in the first day or two. Meconium may be passed despite obstructive lesions.

3. Imperforate Anus

4. Tracheoesophageal Fistula — Generally, coughing and regurgitation of saliva are more common than the abdominal distension that may occur with some types.

5. Meconium Ileus — Up to 25% of children with cystic fibrosis have been reported to present in the neonatal period with obstructive symptoms secondary to meconium ileus.

6. Meconium Peritonitis — Most frequently the peritonitis is the result of an intestinal atresia or meconium ileus. Generally, affected infants appear quite ill, with a hugely dilated abdomen, flank and genital edema, and distended abdominal wall veins.

7. Necrotizing Enterocolitis — Infants particularly at risk are those who may have had a neonatal insult. Early signs are vomiting, lethargy, temperature instability, apnea, and abdominal distension.

8. Hirschsprung Disease (Congenital Megacolon) — Vomiting, distension, and constipation are the usual presenting signs, but symptoms may not appear until later.

9. Gastric Perforation — Vomiting, refusal to feed, respiratory distress, and cyanosis are followed quickly by abdominal distension.

B. Disorders with Later Onset

1. Incarcerated Hernias — Inguinal hernia incarceration is most common.

2. Intussuscep-
   tion

This disorder is usually characterized by episodic crampy abdominal pain; distension occurs later.

3. Malrotation
   with Volvu-
   lus

The sudden onset of vomiting followed by the
rapid development of abdominal distension
should suggest this possibility. Shock follows
rapidly.

4. Bezoar

Hair, vegetable matter, or casein from formu-
las may agglutinate to form an obstructive
mass. Distension may not be as evident as is
the epigastric mass.

5. Intestinal
   Tumors

These are relatively rare causes of obstruction
in children.

III. Abdominal Masses

A. Neoplasia

1. Wilms Tumor

Generally, parents note abdominal enlargement during bathing of the child.

2. Neuroblas-
   toma

In young infants, hepatic metastases may produce the enlargement.

3. Hepatic Tu-
   mors

Hepatomas, hemangiomas, or abscesses may
be large enough to distend the abdomen.

4. Lymphoma

5. Ovarian Tu-
   mors

There may be abdominal pain as well owing
to torsion of the ovarian pedicle.

B. Storage Diseases

Hepatic and splenic enlargement may produce
abdominal distension (see Chaps. 65 and 66,
Hepatomegaly and Splenomegaly).

1. Tay–Sachs
   Disease

2. Gaucher Dis-
   ease

3. Glycogen
   Storage Dis-
   eases

4. Mucopolysac-
   charidoses

C. Pancreatic Cyst

Fullness in the left upper quadrant and epigastrium may be present, sometimes associated with ascites. There may be a history of
abdominal trauma.

D. Gallbladder
   Disease

1. Choledochal
   Cyst

The triad of abdominal pain, mass in the right
upper quadrant, and jaundice is often present.

2. Hydrops	Acute swelling of the gallbladder is usually associated with abdominal pain and swelling of the right upper quadrant in an acutely ill child.
E. Peritoneal, Mesenteric, or Omental Cysts	Usually, progressive abdominal enlargement is the only symptom.
F. Amyloidosis	Primary or secondary amyloidosis may be associated with significant hepatic enlargement.
G. Genitourinary Disorders	
1. Hydronephrosis	
2. Bladder Distension	
3. Polycystic Kidneys	In the infantile form, abdominal enlargement may be the only presenting sign.
4. Pregnancy	In the postpubertal girl with lower abdominal distension, pregnancy must always be considered.
5. Hydrometrocolpos	An imperforate hymen or vaginal atresia may result in massive distension of the uterus owing to retained secretions.
H. Anterior Meningocele	

IV. Ascites
Flank fullness, generalized dullness to percussion, and demonstration of a fluid wave indicate the presence of ascitic fluid. See Chapter 63, Ascites, for diagnostic possibilities.

V. Infection and Inflammation

A. Peritonitis	
1. Bacterial Peritonitis	Abdominal pain is usually intense. Bowel sounds are decreased or absent.
2. Bile Peritonitis	The leakage of bile produces a sudden, severe illness with distension, abdominal pain, fever, and shock.
3. Tuberculous Peritonitis	Onset may be insidious without much pain or tenderness.
B. Abdominal Abscess	
C. Botulism	Symptoms may begin several hours or days after toxin ingestion. Nausea, vomiting,

	blurred vision, diplopia, and abdominal fullness are followed by weakness and dysphagia.
D. Amebiasis	A large hepatic abscess may produce distension of the right upper quadrant. General abdominal distension may also be part of the picture, as well as diarrhea, abdominal pain, and growth failure.
E. Malaria	Splenic and hepatic enlargement may result in abdominal distension.
F. Regional Enteritis	Distension may be part of the clinical presentation along with weight loss, recurrent or persistent fevers, anorexia, and intermittent diarrhea.
G. Ulcerative Colitis	Diarrhea and abdominal pain are the most common presenting symptoms. Abdominal distension may also occur, but it is most pronounced during the complication of toxic megacolon in which there are stasis and marked bowel dilatation.
H. Congenital Cytomegalic Inclusion Disease	

VI. Endocrine and Metabolic Disorders

| A. Hypothyroidism | The abdomen is often protuberant with an umbilical hernia. |
| B. Rickets | A pot-belly appearance may be part of the picture of developing rickets, along with poor muscle tone, lordosis, and difficulty in walking. |

VII. Malabsorption

A. Celiac Disease	The symptoms of full-blown gluten enteropathy include failure to thrive, chronic diarrhea, muscle wasting, irritability, and anorexia, along with the abdominal distension.
B. Cystic Fibrosis	Abdominal distension may be present in the child with steatorrhea and failure to thrive or as part of the meconium ileus equivalent with recurrent abdominal pain and intermittent obstruction from fecal impactions.
C. Abetalipoproteinemia	Growth failure during the first few months of life is followed by the development of steatorrhea and abdominal distension during the first year. Ataxia and weakness develop later.

VIII. Miscellaneous Causes

A. Hypokalemia	This condition may produce an ileus with vomiting and abdominal distension.
B. β-Thalassemia	During the second half of the first year of life, pallor, irritability, anorexia, fever, and an enlarging abdomen owing to hepatosplenomegaly become part of the picture.
C. Carbohydrate Intolerance	Abdominal bloating may be noticeable along with crampy abdominal pain and loose bowel movements.
D. Scurvy	Distension is a late manifestation of vitamin C deficiency.
E. Beriberi	Thiamine deficiency is usually manifested by a peripheral neuritis, encephalopathy, and cardiac failure.
F. Absence of Abdominal Wall Musculature	The prune-belly syndrome is associated with renal abnormalities.
G. Pneumoperitoneum	Perforation of the bowel or stomach may result in the accumulation of free abdominal air. Peritonitis usually accompanies or quickly follows this emergent condition.
H. Beckwith–Wiedemann Syndrome	Macroglossia, visceromegaly, and omphalocele or umbilical hernia should suggest this syndrome.
I. Chloramphenicol Toxicity	The "gray baby syndrome" may occur in infants treated with chloramphenicol. Toxic accumulations result in a shock-like picture with abdominal distension.
J. Necrotizing Enterocolitis	Although primarily seen in low-birth-weight infants, older infants and children may be affected. Bloody stools and pneumatosis intestinalis are usually present.

63

ASCITES

Ascites is the intraperitoneal collection of fluid. In general there are three underlying mechanisms for the production of this fluid: (1) a reduction in the oncotic pressure of the plasma; (2) an obstruction to venous or lymphatic drainage; and (3) irritation of the peritoneum by infection, trauma, or neoplasia. In diseases that are associated with ascites, combinations of these mechanisms may often be operative.

In this chapter, disorders that may be associated with the production of ascitic fluid have been divided into four groups, among which there may be some overlap. It seems especially worthwhile to separate the neonatal period from other age groups, particularly for enumeration of diseases that may produce a hydrops-like picture. The other three groups reflect an attempt to categorize disorders associated with ascites by their mode of onset and associated symptoms: sudden onset in an ill-appearing child; subacute onset, with other symptoms; and insidious onset.

I. Neonatal Period
A. Genitourinary
   Causes
   1. Urinary Tract Obstruction With Perforation — Urine is the most commonly found ascitic fluid in the neonate. In some cases the actual leakage site may be difficult to locate; posterior urethral valves, unilateral ureteral stenosis, and urethral atresia must be considered as possible causes of obstruction.
   2. Hydrometrocolpos — The clinical picture may falsely suggest ascites when the uterus is grossly distended with retained secretions. These secretions may spill into the peritoneal cavity, producing ascites.
   3. Ruptured Perinephric Cyst
   4. Congenital Nephrosis — Nephrosis is usually not present at birth, but edema and ascites may be noticeable in the neonatal period.
   5. Renal Vein Thrombosis — Ascites is a late finding. Flank mass, oliguria, and hematuria occur first.

B. Peritonitis

1. Meconium
   Peritonitis

Most infants with prenatal perforation of the bowel are acutely ill, with tachypnea, grunting, and cyanosis. The abdominal wall is distended with prominent superficial veins. In some infants, mild-to-moderate distension and hydroceles may be the only presenting signs. Bowel perforation occurring suddenly after birth causes acute illness. Air as well as fluid may be identified on abdominal roentgenograms.

2. Bile Peritonitis

Newborns are rarely affected; they may not be as acutely ill as older children with peritoneal irritation from bile. Fluctuating jaundice and acholic stools, inguinal hernias, and abdominal distension are diagnostic clues.

3. Acute Bacterial
   Peritonitis

Affected infants are acutely ill. Underlying causes include acute appendicitis, perforation of a hollow viscus, gangrenous bowel, trauma, and septicemia.

C. Chylous Ascites

The etiology usually cannot be determined. Generally, these infants do not appear ill. The ascitic fluid is milky owing to a high fat content. The onset is insidious and may be associated with pleural effusions and lymphedema of the extremities.

D. Disorders That
   May Produce a
   Hydrops-like
   Picture

1. Erythroblasto-
   sis Fetalis

Infants with severe isoimmune disease, most commonly a result of Rh incompatibility, may present with ascites and anasarca. ABO incompatibility is a rare cause.

2. Congestive
   Heart Failure

In utero causes include premature closure of the foramen ovale and supraventricular tachycardia.

3. Circulatory
   Abnormalities

Arteriovenous malformations, hemangioendothelioma, umbilical or chorionic vein thrombosis, twin-to-twin transfusions, and fetal–maternal hemorrhage may be causes.

4. Fetal Infections

Cytomegalovirus, toxoplasmosis, congenital hepatitis, congenital syphilis, leptospirosis, and Chagas disease have all been implicated.

5. Neoplasia	Placental chorioangioma, choriocarcinoma *in situ,* and fetal neuroblastomatosis may be causes.
6. Miscellaneous Causes	
a. α-Thalassemia (Bart's Hemoglobin)	
b. Maternal Diabetes	
c. Achondroplasia	
d. Pulmonary Lymphangiectasia	
e. Ruptured Ovarian Cyst	
f. Cystic Adenomatoid Malformation of the Lung	
g. Lysosomal Storage Diseases	Congenital ascites may be a presenting sign of these disorders which include infantile sialidosis, Salla disease, GM_1 gangliosidosis, and Gaucher disease.

II. Sudden Onset in an Ill-Appearing Child

A. Acute Bacterial Peritonitis	Severe, sudden onset of abdominal pain with fever and distension is characteristic. Some ascitic fluid or exudate may form. Children with nephrosis are particularly predisposed to bacterial peritonitis.
B. Bile Peritonitis	Escape of bile into the peritoneal cavity results in a sudden, severe illness with abdominal distension, tenderness, fever, and shock.
C. Acute Hemorrhagic Pancreatitis	Clues include a bluish discoloration around the umbilicus or in the flanks. There may be a hemorrhagic pleural effusion.
D. Hepatic Vein Occlusion (Budd–Chiari Syndrome)	There is usually an abrupt onset of abdominal enlargement. Abdominal pain, hepatomegaly, and less commonly splenomegaly and jaun-

dice may be present. This syndrome may be secondary to a number of underlying disorders including hepatomas, hypernephromas, leukemia, sickle-cell disease, inflammatory bowel disease, and allergic vasculitis.

E. Acute Glomeru-
lonephritis

Ascites is uncommon and usually overshadowed by other signs and symptoms.

III. Subacute Onset with Other Symptoms

Ascites develops during the course of some diseases that have other more prominent signs and symptoms.

A. Cirrhosis

A large variety of disease processes may cause cirrhosis, the leading cause of ascites after the neonatal period. Although the first manifestations of cirrhosis may be those of portal hypertension (splenomegaly and esophageal varices, with hematemesis and ascites), there are often other clues in the past history or on physical examination that may suggest a specific cause. The development of ascites may be insidious or acute.

1. Obstructive
Biliary Disease
   a. Biliary Atre-
      sia

In the neonate, the initial picture is that of obstructive jaundice, followed by liver and spleen enlargement. Growth failure and, later, ascites become evident.

   b. Choledochal
      Cyst

Early signs are the triad of abdominal pain, jaundice, and a mass in the right upper quadrant.

   c. Cystic Fi-
      brosis

Biliary cirrhosis may occur late in the course.

   d. Ascending
      Cholangitis

Stones and tumors are rare causes of obstruction of the biliary tree that may produce cirrhosis if long-standing.

2. Infection and
Inflammation
   a. Hepatitis

A, B, and non-A and non-B forms have been implicated.

   b. Rubella;
      Coxsackie
      Virus Infec-
      tion; Cyto-
      megalovirus

Infection;
Herpes
Simplex

c. Toxoplas-
mosis

d. Syphilis

e. Neonatal   A catch-all group of diseases, not caused by a.
Hepatitis   through d.

f. Ascending
Cholangitis

g. Chronic   Persistent jaundice, of 4 weeks' duration or
Active Hep- longer, or relapsing episodes may be clues.
atitis   Other symptoms include arthritis, fever, ery-
             thema nodosum, lethargy, and hepatospleno-
             megaly.

h. Ulcerative
Colitis and
Regional
Enteritis

3. Vascular
Causes

a. Constrictive   Signs of heart disease may or may not be
Pericarditis   present. Hepatomegaly and dyspnea on exer-
                  tion precede the ascites. The liver may be ten-
                  der to palpation.

b. Cardiac   Ascites is seen only in children with chronic
Failure   right heart failure, as in pulmonic stenosis,
                  tricuspid atresia, and pulmonary hyperten-
                  sion.

c. Hereditary   Cutaneous telangiectasia may suggest liver
Hemor-   involvement. Cirrhosis develops as a result of
rhagic Tel-   hepatic cell fibrosis that follows shunting of
angiectasia   blood.

4. Genetic and   Some of the more common causes are listed
Metabolic Dis-   below.
orders

a. Wilson Dis-   There may be neurologic, hematologic, or gas-
ease (Hepa-   trointestinal signs. Cirrhosis with ascites or
tolenticular   hematemesis may be the initial symptom.
Degenera-
tion)

b. Alpha$_1$-   Affected children may present in the neonatal
antitrypsin   period with jaundice or later in life with cir-
Deficiency   rhotic manifestations.

c. Galactos-emia	Vomiting, jaundice, hepatosplenomegaly, failure to thrive, and corneal clouding may precede the signs associated with cirrhosis.
d. Glycogen Storage Disease, Type IV	Hepatomegaly and poor muscle tone precede signs of cirrhosis.
e. Tyrosinemia	Infants with the acute form present in the first 6 months of life with vomiting, diarrhea, hepatosplenomegaly, edema, ascites, and failure to thrive. Jaundice is present in half of the cases. In the chronic form, cirrhosis may be a later presenting sign.
f. GM_1 Gan-gliosidosis	Congenital ascites and hepatosplenomegaly may be the initial clues.

5. Drugs

a. Veno-occlu-sive Disease	Cirrhosis, splenomegaly, and ascites may occur following ingestion of toxins such as "bush tea" in the Caribbean islands.
b. Hepatotoxic Drugs	Methotrexate and similar preparations may produce ascites.
6. Hypervitamin-osis A	Although uncommon, ascites has been described along with headache, bone pain, and scaly dermatitis.

B. Renal Disorders

1. Nephrosis	Edema, proteinuria, hypoproteinemia, and hypercholesterolemia characterize nephrosis. Ascites may be a prominent finding.
2. Chronic Renal Failure	

C. Malignancy

1. Leukemia	
2. Hodgkin Disease	
3. Granulosa Cell Tumor of Ovary	Ascites occasionally is part of the symptom complex in young girls, as well as early breast development, advanced height for age, pubic hair, and intermittent vaginal bleeding.

D. Systemic Lupus Erythematosus	Serosal involvement may uncommonly result in ascites.
E. Kwashiorkor	
F. Hypersensitivity Peritonitis	Abdominal distension and pain, nausea, vomiting, diarrhea, and weight loss appear gradually. Hypersensitivity angiitis probably represents an allergic reaction.

IV. Insidious Onset

A. Pancreatitis	Abdominal pain is the most constant symptom, but it may be mild and ascitic fluid formation gradual. Inapparent or intentional abdominal trauma (as in a battered child) may result in chronic pancreatic fluid leakage.
B. Protein-Losing Enteropathies	A wide variety of disorders may be causative. Abdominal symptoms, such as diarrhea and cramping, may be chronic.
C. Intraperitoneal Tumors	These tumors may cause occlusion of inferior vena cava or hepatic veins, or they may seed the peritoneal cavity or metastasize to the liver, resulting in fluid formation.
D. Tuberculous Peritonitis	Presentation may be vague, with low-grade fever and few localizing symptoms.
E. Chylous Ascites	Affected children rarely have symptoms other than abdominal swelling. This form is usually the result of an injury to, obstruction of, or anomaly of the thoracic duct.
F. Portal Vein Obstruction	

V. Mimics of Ascites

A. Omental or Mesenteric Cysts
B. Celiac Disease
C. Severe Megacolon

SUGGESTED READINGS

Avery ME, Taeusch HW (eds): Diseases of the Newborn, 5th ed. Philadelphia, WB Saunders, 1984

Forfar JO, Arneil GC: Textbook of Pediatrics, 2nd ed., Edinburgh, Churchill Livingstone, 1978

Giacoia GP: Hydrops fetalis (fetal edema). Clin Pediatr 19:334–339, 1980

Roy CC, Silverman A: Pediatric Clinical Gastroenterology, 3rd ed. St. Louis, CV Mosby, 1983

Vaughan VC, McKay RJ, Behrman RE (eds): Nelson Textbook of Pediatrics, 11th ed. Philadelphia, WB Saunders, 1979

Wyllie R, Arasu TS, Fitzgerald JF: Ascites: Pathophysiology and management. J Pediatr 97:167–176, 1980

64

ABDOMINAL PAIN

Abdominal pain is a common pediatric problem with such a variety of causes that a listing of all the diagnostic possibilities would read like a pediatrics textbook index. In the classification that follows, abdominal pain has been divided into two general categories— recurrent and acute. However, there may be a great deal of overlap between these two groups: Separate instances of recurrent pain may appear to be acute; conversely, disorders with acute presentations often may become recurrent.

For both recurrent and acute abdominal pain, common causes, less common ones, and then unusual causes are listed. An additional category of trauma-induced causes has been included for acute abdominal pain.

The history is important in the evaluation of this symptom and should include information about the site of the pain, its pattern of radiation, duration and events surrounding onset of pain, and systemic symptoms, as well as past medical history, social history, and family history. The physical examination obviously is also critically important. There are extraabdominal causes of abdominal pain as well.

I. Recurrent Abdominal Pain
A. Common Causes

1. Chronic Non-specific Abdominal Pain of Childhood	Up to 10% of all children, particularly those between 5 and 12 years of age, may have chronic "bellyaches." This disorder, despite its undetermined pathogenetic mechanism, is so common that whole books have been written about it.[1] Characteristics of the pain may vary, but generally, the pain is poorly localized— most children vaguely refer to the periumbical area; the episodes are generally less than an hour's duration and frequently only minutes long. The children prefer to lie down and may look pale; upon cessation of the pain they are up and about as if nothing had happened. Appetite and growth are unaffected. A family history of abdominal pain may be elicited.
2. Lactose Intolerance	Liebman found lactose intolerance in about one third of children with chronic nonspecific

abdominal pain.[2] Bloating and cramping after lactose ingestion is common in populations at high risk (*e.g.*, blacks, Orientals, and Indians).

3. Psychogenic Pain

The subjective complaint of pain in a child has special meaning: It may represent a wish to avoid school or a cry for attention or help, as in abuse or molestation; it is also a common familial response to stress, among other causes. The difficult but important task for the physician is to uncover, if possible, the situational forces being experienced by the child.

4. Allergic-Tension Fatigue Syndrome

Abdominal pain may be a primary complaint in this poorly understood complex of symptoms attributed to food allergy. Headaches, irritability, lethargy, and leg pains may accompany the pain. Elimination diets should be tried in suspected cases.[3]

5. Constipation

Chronic stool withholding may be associated with vague, recurrent abdominal pain resulting from colonic spasm. The etiology of constipation may be varied. History of elimination habits and rectal examination are essential for diagnosis.

6. Irritable Colon

The crampy episodes of abdominal pain may be especially increased at times of stress.
There may be a family history of the disorder. Stools are usually pellet-like and frequent but occasionally may be loose.

7. Dysmenorrhea

This poorly understood disorder is common in adolescents and young adults. The discomfort does not begin until regular ovulation is established and seems to be related to endometrial prostaglandin release.

8. Mittelschmerz

Ovulatory pain midway through the menstrual cycle often occurs only on one side, especially the right. Affected girls usually have some abdominal tenderness; guarding and even an increased white blood cell count may also be found.

B. Less Common Disorders
   1. Peptic Ulcer

This may perhaps be more common than has been recognized. Only half of children with a peptic ulcer manifest the classic picture of burning epigastric pain increased on fasting and relieved by foods or antacids. Vomiting and gastrointestinal blood loss are prominent symptoms.

2. Parasites
Most children harboring intestinal parasites have no symptoms, although these organisms are frequently suggested as a cause of abdominal pain. Ascariasis, infestation by the large roundworm, rarely causes symptoms. Large numbers of parasites may cause some cramping, but other symptoms such as lethargy, flatulence, bloating, diarrhea, and anorexia usually accompany the cramps. When eosinophilia occurs in association with peptic ulcer symptoms, strongyloidiasis should be suspected.

3. Air Swallowing (Aerophagia)
This may be a more common cause of crampy abdominal pain than has been allowed. The child may have increased belching and flatulence as well. Excessive gum chewing has been considered as a cause. Pain in the right upper quadrant associated with air swallowing, called *Chilaiditi's* syndrome in the past, is thought to be caused by interposition of the colon between the liver and the diaphragm.

4. Inflammatory Bowel Disease
Regional enteritis and ulcerative colitis may have few symptoms early in their development. Diarrhea, blood loss, weight loss, unexplained fever, anemia, growth failure, and a host of other symptoms may occur during the course of the illness.

5. Sickle-cell Anemia
Abdominal crises may be seen along with other vaso-occlusive syndromes.

6. Urinary Tract Disorders
Chronic pyelonephritis, hydronephrosis, ureteroceles, and other urinary tract disorders may be associated with recurrent abdominal pain.

7. Masses and Tumors
Vague symptoms or recurrent pain may be seen with any intra-abdominal mass or tumor, including splenomegaly, hepatomegaly, ovarian cysts, teratomas, bezoars, Wilms tumor, and neuroblastomas. Careful palpation of the abdomen is mandatory in every child with this symptom.

8. Hiatus Hernia
Epigastric or substernal discomfort is common. Associated reflux of gastric contents into the

distal esophagus may also result in "heart-burn" symptoms that may increase during recumbency. Torsion spasms of neck (Sandifer syndrome) is another clue to the presence of a hiatus hernia.

9. Drug Therapy — The diagnosis is usually obvious, especially with aspirin, but effects of antibiotics, anticonvulsants, and bronchodilators should also be considered.

10. Collagen–Vascular Diseases — Abdominal pain is not uncommon in juvenile rheumatoid arthritis and systemic lupus erythematosus.

C. Uncommon and Unusual Causes

1. Migraine — Controversy exists whether recurrent pains are a manifestation of a migraine variant or precede the classic picture. Cyclic vomiting is sometimes present.

2. Abdominal Epilepsy — Even greater controversy abounds here than with migraine. Some researchers feel these episodes are migrainous; others have described children whose pain has ceased during anticonvulsant therapy.

3. Familial Mediterranean Fever — This disease is characterized by febrile attacks of peritonitis, pleuritis, or synovitis, usually brief in duration. Inheritance pattern is autosomal recessive.

4. Hereditary Angioneurotic Edema — Recurrent attacks of abdominal pain are often accompanied by swelling of the extremities and occasionally life-threatening laryngeal edema.

5. Diskitis — Abdominal pain may be a presenting symptom of inflammation of an intervertebral disk space. Back pain or decreased movement becomes apparent over time.

6. Endometriosis

7. Recurrent Pancreatitis — This condition may be hereditary as well as associated with cystic fibrosis, hyperparathyroidism, and hyperlipoproteinemia. Pancreatic calcifications on plain films of the abdomen are a later finding.

8. Brain Tumor — Other signs and symptoms of increased intracranial pressure predominate.

9. Hyperthyroidism — Irritability, weight loss, heat intolerance, and tachycardia are usually present.

10. Addison Disease	Anorexia, weight loss, lethargy, and muscular weakness are common symptoms.
11. Porphyria	Moderate or severe pain, often colicky, is characteristic. Constipation is usually marked. Onset before puberty is rare.
12. Heavy Metal Poisoning	Abdominal pain may be an early sign of lead, arsenic, or mercury poisoning.
13. Duplication of Bowel	Affected children usually present with symptoms of obstruction but may have ectopic gastric mucosa resulting in ulceration.
14. Tuberculosis of Spine	
15. Choledochal cyst	A mass in the right upper quadrant, jaundice, and abdominal pain point to this lesion.
16. Superior Mesenteric Artery Syndrome	This syndrome may be seen in teenagers who have recently lost weight or have been in body casts. Vomiting, nausea, bloating, and early satiety on eating are common.
17. Abdominal Angina	Colicky abdominal pain occurs after meals; weight loss usually follows. A bruit is frequently heard over the epigastrium.
18. Dysrhthymias	Particularly, paroxysmal supraventricular tachycardia may cause pain.
19. Hyperlipoproteinemia	Familial type I is characterized by eruptive xanthomatosis, lipemia retinalis, recurrent abdominal pain, pancreatitis, and hepatosplenomegaly. Type IV may be associated with pancreatitis when serum triglyceride levels are very high.
20. Linea Alba Hernia	In some cases, pain may not be localized to the palpable nodule, which is most often near the umbilicus.
21. Hematocolpos	A bulging imperforate hymen may be seen on pelvic examination. A lower abdominal mass is usually palpable.
22. Mesenteric Cysts	
23. Coarctation of the Aorta	Hypertension with weak femoral pulses is characteristic.
24. Familial Dysautonomia	
25. Cystic Fibrosis	Pain may be a manifestation of the meconium ileus–equivalent syndrome seen in older children with cystic fibrosis.

26. Transient Protein-Losing Enteropathy	This disorder is ushered in by the onset of anorexia, emesis, or abdominal pain followed by generalized edema.
27. Spinal Cord Tumors	Leg weakness or pain, back pain, and bowel or bladder problems are much more common.
28. Slipping Rib Syndrome	Pain is often localized to the upper quadrants. Palpation of the chest wall over the costal cartilages 8 to 10 will often localize the pain.
29. Meconium Ileus Equivalent	As many as 10% of children with cystic fibrosis may develop severe constipation and abdominal pain.
30. Wegener Granulomatosis	Recurrent abdominal pain may be seen in this rare disorder primarily characterized by renal vasculitis and upper and lower respiratory tract necrotizing granulomas.

II. Acute Abdominal Pain

Any cause of recurrent abdominal pain may produce acute symptoms.
A. Common Causes

1. Acute Appendicitis	The variations in appendiceal position may result in "atypical" pictures. Fever, anorexia, and vomiting are helpful clues.
2. Mesenteric Adenitis	Enlargement of lymph nodes in the terminal ileum, probably caused by a viral infection, mimics acute appendicitis, but the pain is less localized.
3. Gastroenteritis	Viral origin is most common. Diarrhea is usually a more prominent symptom than in appendicitis. There is no rebound tenderness; bowel sounds are hyperactive. Pain tends to be diffuse.
4. Bacterial Gastroenteritis	Infection by *Shigella, Yersinia, Campylobacter,* and occasionally *Salmonella* organisms may produce abdominal pain.
5. Pharyngitis	Especially when streptococcal, pharyngitis may be associated with abdominal pain and vomiting, simulating an acute intestinal process.
6. Pneumonia	Children with pneumonia of the right lower lobe may present with abdominal pain. Careful auscultation of the chest and timing of respiratory rate are required.
7. Acute Pyelonephritis	Presenting symptoms may be gastrointestinal—vomiting, abdominal pain, and diar-

	rhea with none of the classic urinary tract signs.
8. Dietary Indiscretion	The amount and type of food or fluid intake prior to onset of the pain should be ascertained.
9. Food Poisoning	Vomiting and diarrhea are frequent accompaniments. Other family members may be ill.
B. Less Frequent Causes	
1. Pelvic Inflammatory Disease	Pain is most frequent during the menstrual period. Pain in the right upper quadrant may result from gonorrheal perihepatitis (Fitz–Hugh–Curtis syndrome).
2. Hypoglycemia	
3. Diabetes Mellitus	Abdominal pain is an often overlooked presentation of diabetic ketoacidosis. Polyuria persists even though the child may appear dehydrated. Respirations are heavy and deep.
4. Hepatitis	In both infectious and serum hepatitis, vomiting and anorexia are common. Pain is usually not well localized.
5. Infectious Mononucleosis	
6. Iliac Adenitis	There may be a history of lower extremity injury or infection days to weeks before onset of abdominal pain. Hip pain may also be present.
7. Henoch–Schönlein Syndrome (Henoch–Schönlein Purpura)	Hemorrhagic rash, especially on the lower extremities, is the most consistent finding. Arthritis, nephritis, and areas of skin edema are common.
8. Herpes Zoster	Acute abdominal pain may precede the appearance of the vesicles over the abdominal wall.
9. Intussusception	The sudden onset of acute severe recurring episodes of pain may be accompanied by vomiting; there may be an unusual degree of lethargy. Dark blood-tinged mucousy stools occur later.
10. Meckel Diverticulum	Profuse, painless rectal bleeding is a more common presentation than pain. Pain symptoms may mimic appendicitis. Perforation may

	lead to peritonitis. Diverticulum may be the lead site of intussusception.
11. Peritonitis	A rigid, tender abdomen with rebound tenderness is typical, with diminished or absent bowel sounds. Affected children appear acutely ill.
12. Obstruction Secondary to Adhesions	There is usually a prior history of surgery or peritonitis. Bowel sounds are high-pitched, with rushes; vomiting is common.
13. Volvulus	There may be a history of intermittent pain prior to midgut volvulus. Shock may quickly ensue.
14. Cholecystitis; Cholelithiasis; Acute Hydrops of Gallbladder	Gallstones may be a finding in disorders with hemolysis. A hydroptic gallbladder is generally palpable.
15. Acute Glomerulonephritis	
16. Leukemia, Lymphoma	
17. Acute Rheumatic Fever	
18. Acute Pancreatitis	Pain is initially epigastric. As symptoms progress, vomiting of bile occurs.
19. Electrolyte disturbances	Ileus and pain are associated with hypokalemia.
20. Hernias	Pain is severe if the hernia is strangulated or incarcerated.
21. Abdominal Abscesses	Abscesses may be perinephric, psoas, subdiaphragmatic, and so forth.
C. Uncommon and Unusual Causes	
1. Mesenteric Artery Occlusion	Abdominal distension, nausea, and vomiting develop, followed rapidly by shock.
2. Testicular Torsion or Neoplasm	Pain is usually scrotal or lower abdominal, allowing separation from other abdominal processes.
3. Nephrotic Syndrome	
4. Ascites	
5. Renal Colic	Stone formation may occur because of urinary infection or obstruction, with immobilization,

or in genetic and metabolic defects. Gross hematuria is present as well as the colicky abdominal or flank pain.

6. Hemolytic Crisis

Children with hereditary spherocytosis may present with acute abdominal pain and anemia associated with infections. The spleen is usually palpable.

7. Black Widow Spider Bite

8. Serositis

Connective tissue disorders, especially systemic lupus erythematosus, may be associated with episodes of serositis and chest or abdominal pain.

9. Vasculitis

Vasculitis from numerous causes may be associated with abdominal pain. Periarteritis nodosa and mucocutaneous lymph node syndrome are best known in children.

10. Pericarditis

Epigastric as well as chest pain may be present.

11. Spinal Cord Tumors

12. Erythromycin-Induced Cholestasis

The estolate ester may induce cholestasis, particularly in children over age 12 years. The abdominal pain may be acute or the picture may resemble one of obstructive jaundice.

13. Eosinophilic Gastroenteritis

Nausea, vomiting, and diarrhea with recurrent abdominal pain and peripheral blood eosinophilia are found in this unusual disorder.

D. Trauma Induced

1. Abdominal Wall Muscle Bruise or Strain

This is the most common by far of the traumatic causes of acute pain. Tenderness is superficial. There may be a history of a blow to the abdomen or of new or excessive exercise activity such as sit-ups.

2. Splenic Rupture or Hematoma

Left shoulder pain may be an early clue.

3. Liver Laceration or Hematoma

Injury is usually the result of blunt trauma and should be suspected if the hematocrit continues to drop following abdominal trauma.

4. Pancreatic Pseudocyst

Symptoms of pain, fever, and vomiting, with a palpable epigastric mass, usually begin some time after trauma. Serum amylase levels are usually elevated. Ascites and pleural effusions may be present.

5. Perforated Viscus	Signs of peritonitis develop. Free air may be seen on upright films of the abdomen.
6. Intraperitoneal Blood	The presence of blood in the peritoneum from any cause produces abdominal pain.

REFERENCES

1. Apley J: The Child with Abdominal Pains, 2nd ed. Oxford, Blackwell Scientific Publications, 1975
2. Liebman WM: Recurrent abdominal pain in children: Lactose and sucrose intolerance, a prospective study. Pediatrics 64:43–45, 1979
3. Crook WG: Food allergy—the great masquerader. Pediatr Clin North Am 22:227–238, 1975

SUGGESTED READINGS

Bugenstein RH, Phibbs CM: Abdominal pain in children caused by linea alba hernias. Pediatrics 56:1073–1074, 1975
Burrington JD: Superior mesenteric artery syndrome in children. Am J Dis Child 130:1367–1370, 1976
Stickler GB, Murphy DB: Recurrent abdominal pain. Am J Dis Child 133:486–489, 1979

65

HEPATOMEGALY

Hepatomegaly, or the presence of an enlarged liver, is a relatively common finding in the pediatric age group. Diseases that may be associated with hepatomegaly are numerous; pathophysiologic mechanisms of enlargement include congestion, hyperplasia of Kupffer cells, cellular infiltrates, storage products, inflammation, fatty infiltration, and intrinsic tumors.

The amount of extension of the liver below the right costal margin at the midclavicular line must not be used as the sole criterion for enlargement. The diagnosis of hepatomegaly is best based on liver span measurements. A discussion of the technique of measurement and graphs of the normal range for children can be found in the article by Walker and Mathis.[1]

In this chapter, causes of hepatomegaly have been divided into groups by age of onset and by the presence or absence of systemic signs or illness. The largest group contains disorders that may appear at any age.

I. Appearance in Neonatal Period

A. Intrauterine and Neonatal Hepatitis

A diffuse array of infections, both congenital and acquired, may be associated with hepatomegaly. Fulminant intrauterine infections may be recognized during the first few days of life. Jaundice is common. Microcephaly, petechiae, and splenomegaly may also be present. Infections that should be considered include cytomegalovirus infection, rubella, toxoplasmosis, herpes simplex, syphilis, and varicella. Bacterial sepsis and acquired viral infections, including infectious hepatitis and Coxsackie virus infections, may also be causes.

B. Maternal Diabetes

Infants are generally large for gestational age and appear plethoric, hypotonic, and lethargic.

C. Isoimmunization Disorders

Infants with erythroblastosis fetalis, most commonly as a result of Rh or ABO sensitization, may have marked hepatomegaly.

D. Congestive Heart Failure

Cardiac failure, especially right-sided, produces significant hepatomegaly.

E. Hemolytic Anemias

Children with disorders associated with hemolytic anemia, such as congenital spherocytosis, may have liver enlargement.

F. Biliary Atresia

In extrahepatic atresia, infants appear normal at birth. Jaundice appears after the first week of life. Intrahepatic atresia must also be considered in any unexplained obstructive jaundice. The liver becomes slightly enlarged and smooth.

G. Inspissated Bile Syndrome

This syndrome usually follows a moderately severe hemolytic disease. Persistent low-grade hyperbilirubinemia and hepatomegaly are found. Stools are pale to dark yellow in color.

H. Hemangioma of Liver

The development of congestive heart failure of obscure origin in a child with hepatomegaly may be the presenting sign. Occasionally, cutaneous hemangiomata may be found.

I. Metastatic Neuroblastoma

Cutaneous as well as hepatic tumor involvement may be present.

J. Hemorrhage into the Liver

Birth trauma may result in bleeding into the liver with hepatic enlargement and anemia.

K. Galactosemia

Affected infants appear normal at birth but then develop vomiting, diarrhea, hepatosplenomegaly, and jaundice. They often die of early fulminant sepsis; failure to thrive and cataracts are often present in survivors.

L. Beckwith–Wiedemann Syndrome

Macroglossia, omphalocele or umbilical hernia, and postnatal gigantism are suggestive findings.

M. Zellweger Syndrome

Hypotonia with a high forehead, flat and narrow facies, redundant skin folds of the neck, and hepatomegaly are characteristic findings.

N. Disorders of the Urea Cycle

Citrullinemia, argininosuccinicaciduria, or argininemia should be considered in infants with vomiting, lethargy, coma, and seizures.

O. Tyrosinemia

Earliest signs appear in the first 2 months of life. Hypoglycemia, hypoproteinemia, and a hemorrhagic diathesis are attributed to acute hepatic necrosis.

P. Alpha$_1$-antitrypsin Deficiency

Signs of cholestatic disease such as jaundice and hepatosplenomegaly may occasionally be present in the neonate. More commonly, the deficiency produces an anicteric hepatitis progressing to cirrhosis later in life.

Q. Achondrogenesis Affected infants usually die shortly after birth. Very small stature is obvious.

R. Methylmalonic Acidemia Infants with the vitamin B_{12}-responsive form present with early nursing difficulties, vomiting, episodes of metabolic acidosis during infections or following increased protein intake, failure to thrive, and microcephaly or macrocephaly.

S. Infantile Sialidosis This is a rare, primary neuraminidase deficiency characterized by dwarfism, failure to thrive, congenital ascites, pericardial effusions, skeletal abnormalities, and early death.

II. Appearance in Infancy with Prominent Systemic Findings

A. Neuroblastoma Liver enlargement occurs with hepatic metastases. The abdominal mass associated with an abdominal primary tumor may also be mistaken for liver enlargement.

B. β-Thalassemia First symptoms usually begin after 6 months of age. Hepatosplenomegaly is striking; pallor, irritability, fever, anorexia, and frontal bossing are other findings.

C. Mucopolysaccharidoses

  1. Mucopolysaccharidosis I (Hurler Syndrome) Coarse features gradually appear; macrocephaly, claw hands, hirsutism, hepatosplenomegaly, and mental deterioration become prominent.

  2. Mucopolysaccharidosis II (Hunter Syndrome) Features are less coarse than in Hurler syndrome, but stiff joints, dwarfism, and hepatosplenomegaly occur.

  3. Mucopolysaccharidosis III (Sanfilippo Syndrome) Onset is between 1 and 3 years of age. Splenomegaly is minimal, but mental retardation is severe. Features are coarse.

  4. Mucopolysaccharidosis VI (Maroteaux–Lamy Syndrome) Affected children have coarse features as well as stiff joints, cloudy corneas, and hepatosplenomegaly.

D. Histiocytosis X (Letterer–Siwe Disease) Onset of symptoms is generally in infancy, with scaly, crusted skin lesions, enlargement of liver and spleen, lymphadenopathy, fever, anemia, thrombocytopenia, and leukopenia.

E. Sickle-Cell Disease | Splenomegaly is common during infancy. Hepatomegaly is present in almost all affected infants and children and becomes more severe during crises.

F. Glycogen Storage Diseases

1. Type I (Von Gierke Disease) | The abdomen is protuberant; the enlarged, firm, smooth liver may extend to the iliac crest. Splenomegaly and cardiomegaly are absent. Profound hypoglycemia and acidosis may be present in early infancy. Short stature and a doll-like facies are other features.

2. Type II (Pompe Disease) | Signs including profound hypotonia with decreased reflexes develop in the first few weeks of life. Cardiac failure is common and probably the cause of hepatomegaly.

3. Type III (Forbes Disease) | Hepatomegaly and failure to thrive may be the only symptoms. Fasting hypoglycemia and hyperlipidemia may be present.

4. Type IV (Andersen Disease) | Infants present at approximately 1 year of age with enlarged nodular liver and splenomegaly. Cirrhosis develops, and death eventually occurs as a result of portal hypertension.

5. Type V (Hers Disease) | An enlarged liver and growth retardation may be prominent.

G. Hereditary Fructose Intolerance | Affected infants are normal at birth. Clinical manifestations appear after dietary introduction of fructose and sucrose. Vomiting and diarrhea occur early; hepatomegaly develops after continued ingestion of fructose; bleeding, jaundice, and renal tubular acidosis may follow.

H. Generalized Gangliosidosis (Type 1) | Accumulation of the ganglioside GM_1 results in hepatosplenomegaly and an appearance resembling that of Hurler syndrome. Foam cells are present in the bone marrow.

I. Fucosidosis | Moderate hepatosplenomegaly, dementia, spasticity, and cardiomyopathy are characteristic.

J. Gaucher Disease | The malignant infantile form can develop at any time in the first few months of life. Feeding problems, vomiting, hepatosplenomegaly, muscular hypertonia, and developmental deterioration are characteristic. Cough and respiratory difficulty are common.

K. Niemann–Pick Disease

The infantile form is characterized by hepato-splenomegaly and developmental retardation. A cherry-red retinal spot develops early in the course.

L. Farber Disease

Hoarseness and stridor may appear in the first few weeks of life. Painful nodules develop in the skin and subcutaneous tissues, particularly over joints. Hepatomegaly and central nervous system deterioration occur later.

M. Wolman Disease

Failure to thrive with vomiting and diarrhea may be present from birth; massive hepato-splenomegaly occurs. A key finding is enlarged, calcified adrenal glands on abdominal roentgenograms.

N. Crigler–Najjar Syndrome

This disorder is characterized by a severe, persistent hyperbilirubinemia with the un-conjugated form, often with early kernic-terus.

O. Mannosidosis

Coarse facies, opacities of lens, and psycho-motor retardation are present.

P. Familial Intrahe-patic Cholestasis

Jaundice, pruritus, and abdominal distension with hepatosplenomegaly are found. Some types are familial with phenotypic characteristics.

Q. Albers–Schön-berg Syndrome

Severe osteopetrosis. The bones are thick, dense and fragile. Macrocephaly, frontal bossing, pancytopenia, and cranial nerve palsies occur.

R. Mucolipidosis I

Myoclonus, mental retardation, cherry-red spots of the retina, skeletal dysplasia, small stature, coarse features, and hepatospleno-megaly are findings.

S. Mucolipidosis II (I-cell Disease)

Alveolar ridge hypertrophy with limited joint mobility is found. Liver enlargement is min-imal.

T. Aase Syndrome

Triphalangeal thumb and hypoplastic anemia are the major features.

U. Klippel–Trenau-nay–Weber Syn-drome

There is hypertrophy of one or more limbs, with hemangiomas, varicosities, and arterio-venous fistulae.

V. Systemic Carni-tine Deficiency

This disorder is characterized by acute epi-sodes of encephalopathy associated with he-patic dysfunction and progressive muscle weakness. Symptoms may mimic Reye syn-drome.

W. Familial Erythro-phagocytic Lymphohistiocytosis — This is a rapidly fatal illness with fever, pancytopenia, central nervous system involvement, and hepatosplenomegaly.

X. Lysinuric Protein Intolerance — This rare autosomal recessive disorder also features splenomegaly, muscle weakness, and osteoporosis.

Y. Multiple Sulfatase Deficiency — An autosomal recessive disorder characterized by an initial period of normal development followed by the onset of motor and mental difficulties during the first or second year. In later stages most patients have coarse facial features, ichthyosis, hepatosplenomegaly, and skeletal abnormalities. Appearance may be confused with mucopolysaccharidoses.

III. Appearance in First Decade Without Apparent Chronic Illness

A. Iron Deficiency — Hepatomegaly may occur in iron-deficiency anemia, especially in young children.

B. Hepatoblastoma — Asymptomatic abdominal enlargement is the most frequent sign. This tumor is most likely to appear before 3 years of age; as it progresses, other symptoms such as poor appetite, failure to gain weight, and pallor are common.

C. Congenital Lipodystrophy — There is a striking absence of subcutaneous fat. Hepatomegaly eventually develops.

D. Type I Hyperlipoproteinemia — Hepatosplenomegaly develops early in the first decade. Episodes of abdominal pain may occur; xanthomata can occur early. Serum chylomicrons and cholesterol levels are increased.

E. Homocystinuria — Arachnodactyly, subluxation of lenses, malar flush, and mental retardation with minimal hepatomegaly may be found. Vascular thromboses frequently occur, especially as these children age.

F. Moore–Federmann Syndrome — Hepatomegaly may be found in this familial syndrome characterized by short stature that becomes evident during childhood.

G. Chronic Active Hepatitis — Infants with chronic viral hepatitis B may have hepatomegaly without other overt signs of illness. Liver enzymes are elevated.

H. Acquired Immune Deficiency Syndrome — Other common features include generalized lymphadenopathy, recurrent opportunistic infections, splenomegaly, and failure to thrive.

IV. Appearance in First Decade with Apparent Illness

A. Visceral Larva Migrans (Toxocariasis) — This infestation should be considered in any child with recurrent fever, cough, and wheezing in the presence of hepatomegaly, especially if a marked eosinophilia is found.

B. Hemolytic Anemias — Various types of hemolytic anemia, such as congenital spherocytosis, may be associated with hepatomegaly.

C. Hand–Schüller–Christian Disease — The classic triad of exophthalmos, diabetes insipidus, and punched-out lesions of the skull seen on roentgenograms suggests this form of histiocytosis.

D. Chédiak–Higashi Syndrome — Affected children usually have problems with recurrent infections. Partial albinism, variable hepatosplenomegaly, neutropenia, anemia, and thrombocytopenia are found. Large cytoplasmic inclusions are seen in the white blood cells.

E. Chronic Granulomatous Disease — Recurrent infections, suppurative lymphadenopathy, dermatitis, osteomyelitis, chronic enteritis, and malabsorption are prominent symptoms.

F. Metastatic Tumors

V. Appearance at Any Age—Relatively Asymptomatic

A. Cirrhosis — Several disorders producing cirrhosis are associated with liver enlargement early in the course (see Chap. 63, Ascites). Many of these disorders may be silent in their progression.

B. Hepatic Tumors — Most tumors produce asymmetric liver enlargement.

   1. Hepatocarcinoma — This tumor is uncommon before 3 years of age. There may be some abdominal discomfort as the tumor enlarges. Hemihypertrophy, macroglossia, and absence of a kidney have been described in some cases.

   2. Hemangioendotheliomas — Associated cutaneous lesions are common.

and Cavernous
Hemangiomas
3. Hamartomas
4. Solitary Cysts

C. Ascariasis — Hepatomegaly may occur during the extraintestinal migration of the worm. If the child is symptomatic, colicky abdominal pain is the most common complaint.

D. Inflammatory Bowel Disease — Although there may have been symptoms of inflammatory bowel disease, hepatomegaly may be insidious during an asymptomatic period.

E. Benign Hepatomegaly — Slight liver enlargement may frequently be associated with a mild, self-limited illness, often viral, with some gastrointestinal involvement.

F. Polycystic Disease of the Liver — This disease is often discovered incidentally. The hepatic enlargement is asymptomatic.

G. Hemochromatosis — Hepatomegaly, increased skin pigmentation, and diabetes mellitus are the classic features.

H. Tangier Disease — Striking, enlarged orangish yellow tonsils may be the initial clue. The liver is occasionally enlarged.

I. Echinococcosis (Hydatid Disease) — Liver enlargement is localized, distinct, smooth, and round.

J. Amyloidosis — In primary amyloidosis many organs are involved. Hepatic function is rarely disturbed. Secondary amyloidosis is occasionally seen in children with chronic illnesses, but again the liver involvement is usually asymptomatic.

K. Rendu–Osler–Weber Syndrome (Hereditary Hemorrhagic Telangiectasia) — Cutaneous telangiectatic lesions suggest this possibility.

L. Mulibrey Nanism — The early onset of growth failure, a triangular facies, prominent forehead, and hepatomegaly with pericardial constriction characterize this disorder.

VI. Appearance at Any Age—Generally Appearing Ill

A. Sepsis — Hepatomegaly may occur during acute viral and bacterial infections.

B. Starvation

C. Hepatitis	Several viruses may cause hepatitis. Mononucleosis affects the liver in most cases. A granulomatous hepatitis may be seen in tuberculosis and sarcoidosis.
D. Drugs and Toxins	Hepatocellular injury or cholestasis may occur during treatment with a number of drugs or on exposure to toxic materials. Phenobarbital, hydantoins, sulfonamides, acetaminophen, tetracyclines, and corticosteroids are commonly used drugs that may produce hepatomegaly.
E. Leukemia and Lymphoma	Generally, children with these diseases manifest other signs and symptoms
F. Cystic Fibrosis	Signs of pulmonary and pancreatic involvement are the usual presenting symptoms. Abdominal distension, ascites, or esophageal varices with bleeding may be the first sign of the cirrhosis.
G. Congestive Heart Failure	Liver enlargement is more common in right heart failure.
H. Constrictive Pericarditis	This disorder may be chronic, with an insidious onset of fatigue, dyspnea, abdominal swelling, and hepatosplenomegaly.
I. Diabetes Mellitus	Hepatomegaly may be an acute phenomenon during ketoacidosis or may be chronic with poor disease control.
J. Chronic Active Hepatitis	Persistent or relapsing jaundice is the earliest finding. Hepatosplenomegaly is present in most children. Arthritis, arthralgias, fever, erythema nodosum, or colitis may be present.
K. Juvenile Rheumatoid Arthritis	Hepatomegaly may be a finding, particularly in the systemic form.
L. Systemic Lupus Erythematosus	
M. Alpha$_1$-antitrypsin Deficiency	The first symptoms may be those of an acute hepatitis or an anicteric hepatitis progressing to cirrhosis. Chronic lung disease occurs in some children.
N. Wilson Disease	The presentation of this inherited disorder is varied. Children may present with an acute hepatitis, asymptomatic cirrhosis with portal hypertension and bleeding from varices, acute hemolysis, renal disturbances, or neurologic symptoms.

O. Liver Abscess	Incidence is greater in children receiving anti-inflammatory or antineoplastic drugs. Pain in the right upper quadrant is an early symptom, with tenderness over the liver. Weight loss, anorexia, fever, and jaundice may be present.
P. Parasitic Disorders	
1. Amebiasis	This is most commonly seen in the tropics or subtropics. Hepatic involvement is characterized by high fever, profuse sweating, hepatic tenderness, and occasionally, right shoulder pain.
2. Schistosomiasis	Fever, urticaria, malaise, weight loss, and anorexia with eosinophilia are the most prominent symptoms.
3. Liver Flukes	Fever, dyspnea, and hepatomegaly with eosinophilia are common. Pain in the upper quadrant, urticaria, and jaundice may also be found.
Q. Leptospirosis	Symptomatic disease is characterized by an abrupt onset of fever, myalgia, headache, and vomiting. The associated vasculitis may affect any organ system.
R. Reye Syndrome	Vomiting follows a prodromal illness such as an upper respiratory infection or chickenpox. Irrational behavior, lethargy, and coma may follow.
S. Brucellosis	Brucellosis is often associated with a remittent type of fever; fatigability and vague muscle pains may be the only symptoms.
T. Malaria	
U. Rocky Mountain Spotted Fever	
V. Histoplasmosis	
W. Rickets	
X. Budd–Chiari Syndrome	This syndrome must be considered in children with the abrupt onset of ascites in the absence of known liver disease.
Y. Veno-occlusive Disease	This disorder occurs in certain endemic areas such as Jamaica and India. Ascites, hepatomegaly, and jaundice develop rapidly, usually after exposure to a toxin.
Z. Hyperlipoproteinemia	Onset of symptoms in types IV and V is after the first decade. Xanthomata and premature

		arteriosclerotic heart disease in family members are clues.
AA.	Infantile Pyknocytosis	Hepatosplenomegaly with pallor and jaundice is found, as well as characteristic burr cells on peripheral blood smear.
BB.	Hypervitaminosis A	Leg and forearm pain, anorexia, and irritability are other symptoms.
CC.	Tuberculosis	The declining incidence of this disease may catch us off guard in considering this diagnosis.
DD.	Primary Sclerosing Cholangitis	This rare disorder is occasionally associated with ulcerative colitis. Progressive liver failure, cholestatic jaundice, weight loss, and steatorrhea are other features.
EE.	Babesiosis	This protozoal illness has been reported with increasing frequency in the United States. Fever, chills, hepatomegaly, and signs of hemolysis may be present.
FF.	Generalized Histiocytic Proliferation Syndromes	Several of these syndromes show erythrophagocytosis and have been reported under various names. Clinical findings are similar and include organomegaly and pyrexia. One group is precipitated by viral infections, usually in immunosuppressed patients.

REFERENCE

1. Walker WA, Mathis RK: Hepatomegaly: An approach to differential diagnosis. Pediatr Clin North Am 22:929–942, 1975

SUGGESTED READINGS

Fanaroff AA, Martin RJ (eds): Behrman's Neonatal-Perinatal Medicine, 3rd ed. St. Louis, CV Mosby, 1983

Mowat AP: Liver Disorders in Childhood. Scarborough, Ont, Butterworth & Co, 1979

Risdall RJ, McKenna RW, Nesbit ME et al: Virus associated hemophagocytic syndrome. Cancer 44:993–1002, 1979

66

SPLENOMEGALY

The spleen serves two primary functions: (1) filtration of particulate matter and formed elements from the blood and (2) assistance in protection from infection by means of the production of humoral factors needed for opsonization. During the first 5 or 6 fetal months, it also serves as a site of blood formation.

Although it has been stated that the spleen is not palpable until enlargement to 3 or 4 times its normal size occurs, this is not always the case. As outlined under the section on Normal Variants, as many as 1% of all children, and a higher percentage of children under 1 year of age, have palpable but normal spleens. Whereas the normal palpable spleen is soft and just barely felt, the pathologically enlarged spleen is usually more easily palpated; it often has an abnormal surface or consistency; and it is generally associated with other signs and symptoms.

I. Normal Variants

The spleen is usually palpable in most premature infants and in as many as 30% of term infants. By 1 year of age, 10% of healthy infants still have a palpable spleen, and even after 10 years of age approximately 1% of children and adolescents have palpable spleens. In the older infants and children the spleen tip is just barely palpable in the left midclavicular line and is soft; it can often only be palpated on deep inspiration. Most of these children have visceroptosis of the spleen—that is, the spleen hangs in a slightly lower position than normal.

II. Infection

The most common cause of splenomegaly overall is infection. In most cases the enlargement subsides over a few weeks.

A. Acute Infections

1. Bacterial Infections   Many bacterial infections are accompanied by splenic enlargement: severe pneumonia, septicemia, bacterial endocarditis, typhoid fever, brucellosis, tularemia, plague, and others. A splenic abscess must also be considered. Usually the splenomegaly is only one part of a systemic illness.

2. Viral Infections	A number of viral infections may cause splenic enlargement, particularly infectious mononucleosis and cytomegalovirus infection.
3. Rickettsial Infection	Rocky Mountain spotted fever and typhus are examples.
4. Protozoal Infection	Malaria and trypanosomiasis may be causes. Babesiosis seems to be increasing in the United States. Fever, chills, signs of hemolysis, and hepatosplenomegaly may be present. The peripheral blood smear should be examined for parasitized erythrocytes.
5. Spirochetal Infection	Leptospirosis may be associated with splenomegaly.
B. Chronic Infections	
1. Bacterial Infection	Subacute bacterial endocarditis, brucellosis, and staphylococcal infection involving ventriculojugular shunts are examples.
2. Viral Infection	Splenomegaly may especially accompany congenital infections such as rubella, herpes, and cytomegalovirus infection.
3. Protozoal Infection	Toxoplasmosis, malaria, schistosomiasis, and visceral larva migrans may cause splenic enlargement.
4. Fungal Infection	Histoplasmosis and coccidioidomycosis are examples.
5. Mycobacterial Infection	Splenomegaly may be a finding in tuberculosis.
6. Spirochetal Infection	Syphilis may be a cause.
C. Altered Host Defense	
1. Immunodeficiency Disorders	The spleen may be greatly increased in size, especially after repeated infections
2. Chédiak–Higashi Syndrome	Features include recurrent infections, partial albinism, variable degrees of hepatosplenomegaly, neutropenia, anemia, and thrombocytopenia.
3. Familial Lipochrome Histiocytosis	This rare disorder is similar to chronic granulomatous disease. Splenomegaly, pulmonary infiltration, and arthritis, with increased susceptibility to bacterial infections, are prominent features.

4. Chronic Granulomatous Disease	This disorder is characterized by recurrent infections, significant adenopathy, and furunculosis with onset at an early age. Hepatic and splenic enlargement may signify abscesses.
5. Acquired Immune Deficiency Syndrome	More prominent features include recurrent opportunistic infections, hepatomegaly, generalized lymphadenopathy, and failure to thrive.

III. Hematologic Disorders

A. Iron Deficiency	If splenomegaly is present, it is mild.
B. Hemolytic Disorders	Altered red blood cell properties, either surface immunoglobins or loss of deformability, may result in their trapping and removal by the spleen, with consequent splenic enlargement.
1. Isoimmunization Disorders	Rh and ABO incompatibilities in infants are the best known of these disorders.
2. Hereditary Spherocytosis	Jaundice may be present in infancy. Later, affected children present with pallor and splenomegaly, occasionally with aplastic crises. Spleen size increases with age.
3. Sickle-cell Anemia	As the child ages the spleen usually shrinks owing to repeated infection. Acute, life-threatening enlargement of the spleen is seen in sequestration crises, most commonly occurring during the second 6 months of life and less frequently after age 2 years.
4. Thalassemia Major	Hepatosplenomegaly and pallor are prominent in affected children over 6 months of age.
5. Other Red Cell Disorders	Hemoglobin C disease, SC disease, elliptocytosis, stomatocytosis, pyruvate kinase deficiency, glucose-6-phosphate dehydrogenase deficiency, and other enzyme disorders may be associated with splenomegaly.
6. Autoimmune Hemolytic Anemias	
7. Congenital Erythropoietic Porphyria	Prominent features include cutaneous lesions (vesicles, bullae, and scarring) upon sun exposure, red urine, hypertrichosis, and splenomegaly.

8. Extramedullary Hematopoiesis
Osteopetrosis and myelofibrosis may be associated with splenomegaly as fetal sites of blood formation again become active.

9. Idiopathic Myelofibrosis
Fibrosis of the bone marrow usually begins before 3 years of age. Anemia, thrombocytopenia, leukoerythroblastosis, splenomegaly, and occasionally hepatomegaly are found.

IV. Storage Diseases
A. Lipid Storage Diseases

1. Gaucher Disease
Splenic enlargement occurs in both acute and chronic forms. In early-onset types progressive developmental deterioration is generally seen; in the chronic or adult form, onset is insidious, with splenomegaly followed by hepatomegaly, patchy brown or yellow skin discoloration, and bony lesions.

2. Niemann–Pick Disease
Various types have been described, with onset ranging from 6 months to 5 years of age. Hepatosplenomegaly and progressive mental deterioration are common. Cherry-red spots are commonly found on funduscopic examination, and foam cells abound in the bone marrow.

3. Gangliosidoses
An increasing number of forms of this storage disorder are being described. Coarse features, often resembling those seen in Hurler syndrome, are characteristic of the forms involving gangliosides GM_1 and GM_3. Progressive deterioration is common.

4. Mucolipodoses
Affected children also have coarse features like those of Hurler syndrome, progressive deterioration, and progressive hepatosplenomegaly. Mucolipidoses I and II, mannosidosis, and fucosidosis may all be associated with splenomegaly.

5. Metachromatic Leukodystrophy
Mild visceromegaly may be present with the progressive neurologic deterioration.

6. Wolman Disease
Failure to thrive and diarrhea are present from birth. Calcified adrenal glands seen on abdominal roentgenograms are pathognomonic.

7. Lactosyl Ceramidosis	Onset of symptoms is by 1 year of age, with failure to thrive, mental deterioration, and hepatosplenomegaly.
8. Cholesterol Ester Storage Disease	Hepatomegaly is a constant feature; splenomegaly occurs less frequently. Affected children may have advanced atherosclerosis. Hyperlipemia is usually present.
9. Analphalipoproteinemia (Tangier Disease)	A red orange coloration of the tonsils is characteristic; splenomegaly is common. A peripheral neuropathy is the most serious complication.
10. Hyperchylomicronemia (Type 1 Hyperlipoproteinemia)	The spleen and liver are occasionally enlarged; hyperlipemia is typical. Attacks of abdominal pain and crops of eruptive xanthomata are found.
B. Mucopolysaccharides	The syndromes of Hurler, Hunter, Sanfilippo, and Maroteaux–Lamy may be associated with splenomegaly. Dysmorphogenic features of these disorders overshadow the splenomegaly.
C. Glycogen Storage Disease	In type IV (Andersen disease), the liver is enlarged and nodular with early onset of cirrhosis. Splenomegaly may be a later finding.
D. Other Storage Diseases	
1. Amyloidosis	Proteinuria with hepatosplenomegaly in a child with a chronic inflammatory disease suggests this diagnosis.
2. Sea Blue Histiocyte Disease	Reticuloendothelial cells contain large blue cytoplasmic granules. Splenomegaly is common. The clinical course may be mild, with purpura caused by thrombocytopenia, or may be characterized by progressive hepatic cirrhosis.

V. Vascular Congestion

A. Portal Hypertension with Congestive Splenomegaly	
1. Cirrhosis	This is the most common cause of portal hypertension. Various infectious and hereditary disorders may be responsible (see Chap. 65, Hepatomegaly).

    a. Hepatitis   Both infectious and serum types have been
                        implicated.
    b. Chronic
       Active
       Hepatitis
    c. Biliary
       Atresia
    d. Cystic Fi-
       brosis
    e. Wilson
       Disease
    f. Galactos-
       emia
    g. Alpha$_1$-
       antitrypsin
       Deficiency
    h. Cystinosis
    i. Hemosid-
       erosis
    j. Tyrosinosis
    k. Fructose
       Intolerance
 2. Extrahepatic
    Lesions
    a. Cavernous   This lesion may be a sequela of umbilical vein
       Transfor-   catheterization in the neonatal period.
       mation of
       Portal Vein
    b. Splenic
       Vein
       Thrombosis
    c. Splenic
       Artery
       Aneurysm
    d. Congenital
       Portal Vein
       Stenosis or
       Atresia
    e. Chronic
       Congestive
       Heart Fail-
       ure
 3. Constrictive   Hepatomegaly appears before splenomegaly.
    Pericarditis

4. Splenic Trauma A splenic hematoma may follow abdominal injury.

VI. Tumors and Infiltrations

A. Leukemia Over half of children with acute lymphocytic leukemia will have splenomegaly sometime during their disease.

B. Lymphomas Splenomegaly may be an isolated finding in some cases of both Hodgkin disease and other forms of lymphoma.

C. Cysts Cysts may be congenital or follow trauma. An asymptomatic smooth mass is typical.

D. Splenic Hemangioma Cutaneous hemangiomas are sometimes present.

E. Splenic Hamartoma This rare disorder is characterized by failure to thrive, recurrent infections, and pancytopenia.

F. Histiocytosis X Both Letterer–Siwe disease and Hand–Schüller–Christian disease may be associated with splenomegaly. Other signs and symptoms predominate.

G. Generalized Histiocytic Proliferation Syndromes Several of these disorders show erythrophagocytosis and have been reported under various names. Clinical findings are similar and include organomegaly and pyrexia.

H. Metastatic Disease Neuroblastoma is most common.

VII. Miscellaneous Causes

A. Serum Sickness

B. Connective Tissue Disorders
  1. Juvenile Rheumatoid Arthritis
  2. Systemic Lupus Erythematosus

C. Beckwith–Wiedemann Syndrome Splenomegaly may be part of the generalized visceromegaly.

D. Hemihypertrophy Splenic enlargement may be found if the left side of the body is hypertrophied.

E. Sarcoidosis

F. Hyperparathy-   In neonatal disease early symptoms include
roidism   failure to thrive, constipation, hepatosplenomegaly, anemia, seizures, polyuria, polydipsia, and hypotonia.

G. Cockayne Syn-   Hepatosplenomegaly has been reported in
drome   affected children, who have short stature,
pinched facies, microcephaly, and progressive
deterioration.

H. Gingival Fibro-   Absent or dysplastic nails, clubbed digits, gin-
matosis and Dig-   gival overgrowth, and soft, bulky nose and
ital Anomalies   ear cartilage are prominent signs. One half of
cases have hepatosplenomegaly.

I. Hyperdibasic   Splenomegaly is occasionally found in affected
Aminoaciduria   children, whose protein intolerance causes
failure to thrive, diarrhea, vomiting, and aver-
sion to protein-rich foods.

J. Miller–Dieker   This disorder is characterized by severe failure
Syndrome (Lis-   to thrive, microcephaly, high and narrow fore-
sencephaly)   head, prominent occiput, anteverted nares,
and micrognathia. Cyanotic attacks are frequent in the neonatal period.

K. Infantile Pykno-   Pallor, jaundice, hepatosplenomegaly, and the
cytosis   presence of burr cells on the peripheral smear
are characteristic findings.

L. Dyskeratosis   This rare genetic disorder is characterized by
Congenita   atrophy and a reticular pigmentation of the
skin, dystrophic nails, and leukoplakia. Some
patients have developed a severe hematologic
disease resembling Fanconi anemia.

M. Lysinuric Protein   This rare autosomal recessive disorder also
Intolerance   features hepatomegaly, muscle weakness, and
osteoporosis.

67

ABDOMINAL MASSES

In differential diagnosis of abdominal masses in childhood, the age group of the affected child should be considered: In newborn infants over half of all abdominal masses are renal in origin, and of these, most are caused by multicystic kidney disease or congenital hydronephrosis. In older infants and children, most abdominal masses are due to enlargement of the liver and spleen, often from diseases such as leukemia or lymphoma or as a result of portal hypertension. However, retroperitoneal tumors, especially Wilms tumors and neuroblastomas, make up a sizeable percentage of masses found in children over 1 year of age.

In this chapter, masses that are the result of hepatomegaly (Chap. 65) or splenomegaly (Chap. 66) are not included. Abdominal masses from other causes generally lie in the area of the organ of origin, which aids in the selection of diagnostic studies. Before extensive laboratory investigations are undertaken, it is important to rule out the presence of large amounts of stool in the large intestine or of urine in the bladder as the cause of the distension.

I. Genitourinary Disorders
  A. Renal Disease
    1. Hydrone-
      phrosis
    2. Polycystic or
      Multicystic
      Kidney Disease
    3. Solidary Cysts
    4. Renal Vein   This lesion is more likely to occur in newborn
      Thrombosis   infants, especially in those of diabetic mothers, or rarely, during severe dehydration. Hematuria is common.

    5. Ectopic or
      Horseshoe
      Kidney
    6. Ureterocele
    7. Perinephric
      Abscess
  B. Bladder Disten-   The mass is globular and located in the mid-
     sion   line, usually below the umbilicus. In the newborn, obstruction of urine outflow—for in-

stance, as a consequence of posterior urethral valves—should be considered. In older infants and children, causes of bladder distension include anticholinergic drugs, spinal cord tumors, spinal cord abnormalities, and bladder irritation from inflammatory conditions in the pelvis or infection within the bladder. Urethral irritation may also cause urinary retention.

C. Urachal Cyst

The cyst may be palpated as a midline swelling below the umbilicus attached to the abdominal wall.

D. Bladder Diverticulum

E. Uterine Enlargement

    1. Pregnancy

Pregnancy must always be considered in adolescents with midline, lower abdominal masses.

    2. Hydrometrocolpos

In early infancy, a suprapubic mass and vomiting as a result of hydronephrosis from obstruction of the ureters may be signs. Adolescents with an imperforate hymen may have uterine distension from retained secretions and menses.

F. Ovarian Disorders

    1. Ovarian Cyst

Occasionally, the ovary may twist on its pedicle, producing symptoms similar to those of acute appendicitis.

    2. Ovarian Tumors

These tumors are uncommon in childhood.

II. Neoplasia

A. Wilms Tumor

The mass is often discovered by parents while bathing the child. In over 60% of the cases, the tumor is found before 5 years of age. The mass may extend to the midline and into the iliac fossa.

B. Neuroblastoma

About half of these tumors arise in the abdomen. The mass frequently crosses in the midline. The tumor may produce excessive catecholamines, resulting in tachycardia, diarrhea, hypertension, skin flushing, and perspiration. Almost 50% occur within the first 2 years of life.

C. Lymphoma — Enlargement of the liver and spleen is generally found, but abdominal lymph nodes are frequently enlarged as well.

D. Teratoma — An abdominal mass, high in the retroperitoneal region, usually becomes evident in the first 2 years of life. Roentgenograms of the tumor often reveal spotty calcifications.

E. Retroperitoneal Lymphangioma — This tumor is palpable as an ill-defined cystic mass.

F. Congenital Mesoblastic Nephroma — This rare embryonic tumor is usually present at birth.

G. Embryonal Rhabdomyosarcoma

III. Intestinal Disorders

A. Fecal Material — Masses of stool are frequently palpable in the left lower quadrant. Generally they are mobile and disappear after a cleansing enema.

B. Intussusception — Other symptoms such as pain and vomiting, are much more prominent than the mass, which is palpable in the right lower or upper quadrant.

C. Intestinal Duplication — In addition to the mass, abdominal pain, vomiting, or gastrointestinal hemorrhage may be present.

D. Incarcerated Hernia

E. Malrotation with Volvulus — The sudden onset of abdominal pain and vomiting heralds this catastrophic event.

F. Bezoar — In premature infants fed milk with a high casein content, lactobezoars may form. Hair ingestion may also result in gastric masses.

G. Intestinal Tumors — Leiomyosarcomas and other solid tumors are uncommon. Peritoneal, mesenteric, or omental cysts may occur.

H. Regional Enteritis — Palpable masses may be caused occasionally by mesenteric node inflammation or by fistula or abscess formation.

I. Pyloric Stenosis — Projectile vomiting in a hungry young infant is usually the first clue.

IV. Biliary Disorders

A. Choledochal Cyst — Symptoms include a mass in the right upper quadrant with jaundice or pain.

B. Hydrops

Infants with acute hydrops of the gallbladder present with poorly localized, continuous abdominal pain, and a mass in the right upper quadrant.

C. Distended Gall-
   bladder

Distension occurs occasionally in cystic fibrosis.

V. Miscellaneous Causes

A. Pancreatic Cyst

Blunt injury to the abdomen may be the cause. The mass is palpable in the epigastrium and left upper quadrant. Ascites may accompany the cyst.

B. Anterior Menin-
   gocele

C. Adrenal Hemor-
   rhage

D. Abscesses

Abdominal abscesses are generally associated with fever, abdominal discomfort, anorexia, and frequently, vomiting and diarrhea.

E. Aortic Aneurysm

The occurrence of aortic aneurysm is rare in children. The mass is pulsatile.

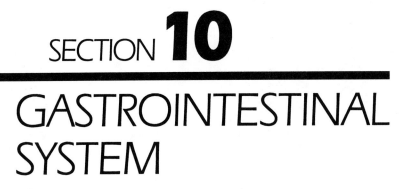

SECTION **10**

GASTROINTESTINAL SYSTEM

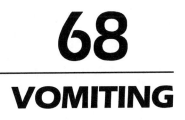

68

VOMITING

Vomiting is such a common symptom in childhood that it is difficult to present a nice, neat, clear classification of possible causes. Fortunately, in most cases, vomiting is merely part of a relatively benign gastrointestinal infection; the problem ceases in a day or two. Vomiting is a worrisome symptom when it persists, develops in the neonatal period, is associated with abdominal distension or severe abdominal pain, or is projectile (see Chap. 69); when the vomitus contains blood or bile; or when there are other significant systemic signs and symptoms or other warning signals.

The acute onset of vomiting suggests different disorders from those associated with chronic or recurrent vomiting; however, there may be some overlap between these groups. The various other clues obtained from the history and physical examination should quickly narrow the diagnostic possibilities to a few likely causes.

It is important to ascertain that the symptom complaint *is* vomiting and not regurgitation or spitting up. This differentiation is particularly important in infancy: Is the infant bringing up stomach contents forcefully, or is there a nondramatic flow of small amounts of fluids or food from the mouth? Is the vomiting preceded by a cough or choking that in turn precipitates the vomiting? In this latter case, disorders involving areas other than the gastrointestinal tract should be considered.

The following classification of causes of vomiting begins with some general possibilities and then groups disorders by the organ system involved.

I. General Considerations
    A. Poor Feeding Technique

1. Overfeeding	This is usually seen in infants but may occur in youngsters with poor dietary discretion.
2. Improper Formula Preparation	The formula may contain excessive amounts of protein or solutes, or mistaken ingredients—such as salt for sugar—may be added.
3. Excessive Air Swallowing	The nipple opening may be too small. A propped bottle may also cause excessive air swallowing with consequent vomiting.
4. Inappropriate Handling After Feeding	Bouncing the infant on the knee after feeding may bring up what just went down.

B. The Active Child   Spitting up and occasional vomiting may be found in the infant who is constantly moving.

C. Coughing   Coughing episodes may trigger vomiting. Pertussis is a classic example.

D. Postnasal Drip   Excessive mucous production may cause pharyngeal gagging with vomiting; the presence of large amounts of mucus in the stomach may induce vomiting in some children.

E. Emotional Deprivation   Vomiting may be a nonspecific symptom of the altered maternal–infant relationship.

F. Psychogenic Vomiting   Vomiting may be self-induced or may be caused by anxiety or stress, or it may be brought on by sights, smells, or occasionally sounds.

G. Cyclic Vomiting   Cyclic vomiting may be psychogenic[1] or in some cases related to migraine.

H. Immobilization   Occasionally, young children or infants who are immobilized by casts may vomit for unexplained reasons.

II. Gastrointestinal Disorders

A. Pharyngeal and Esophageal Disorders

   1. Gastroesophageal Reflux   Recurrent coughing spells, choking, wheezing episodes, and pneumonia may be prominent features.

   2. Hiatus Hernia   Recurrent episodes of vomiting begin at an early age. Affected children may develop failure to thrive, anemia secondary to blood loss from esophagitis, and torsion spasms of the neck (Sandifer syndrome).

   3. Chalasia   Chalasia is a common cause of regurgitation in neonates. The lower esophageal sphincter fails to close fully, allowing reflux of gastric contents. Rarely, the condition may persist, giving rise to recurrent episodes of regurgitation, often with pneumonitis and esophagitis.

   4. Achalasia   The occurrence of achalasia is uncommon in childhood; usually older children are affected. The lower esophagus fails to relax with swallowing.

   5. Tracheoesophageal Fistula   Choking and coughing may be associated with vomiting.

6. Esophageal Stenosis or Web — Infants with congenital lesions present with early onset of vomiting and dysphagia.

7. Esophageal Tumors

8. Esophageal Duplication — Compression by the duplication causes stenosis. Dyspnea owing to tracheal compression may be present.

9. Cricopharyngeal Incoordination — The inability to swallow liquids and secretions results in recurrent aspiration, choking, and occasionally vomiting.

10. Congenital Short Esophagus

B. Gastric Disorders

1. Gastritis — Irritation of the gastric mucosa may result from aspirin and other drugs or toxic ingestants including corrosives.

2. Gastric Bezoars — Bezoars may be composed of hair, vegetable fibers, or, in small infants, coagulated milk protein.

3. Pyloric Stenosis

4. Pylorospasm

5. Gastric Mucosal Diaphragm — The egress of contents from the stomach may be blocked.

6. Pyloric Atresia

7. Peptic Ulcer — Vomiting, intestinal blood loss, and abdominal pain are more common after 6 years of age; the abdominal pain is uncommon under 6 years and is often atypical after age 6.

8. Gastric Volvulus — Onset may be acute, with epigastric pain and vomiting, or the condition may be chronic, with recurrent postprandial discomfort, vomiting, belching, and upper gastrointestinal bleeding.

9. Gastric Tumors — Large tumors or those close to the pylorus may cause obstruction.

10. Gastric Duplication — Intestinal blood loss is typical.

11. Microgastria — A congenital small stomach results in an inability to take normal-sized feedings.

12. Chronic Granulomatous Disease (CGD) — Gastric outlet obstruction resulting from granulomatous inflammation of the antral wall may be the first manifestation of CGD. Blood in the stool, anorexia, and poor weight gain are other features.

C. Intestinal Disorders

1. Obstruction — A host of congenital or acquired obstructive lesions may result in vomiting. Whether the distension is epigastric or abdominal depends on the site of the obstruction. Bilious vomitus indicates obstruction unless proven otherwise.

   a. Duodenal Web
   b. Intestinal Atresia or Stenosis
   c. Meconium Ileus or Equivalent Syndrome — A meconium plug may occur in small or sick infants.
   d. Malrotation
   e. Volvulus
   f. Incarcerated Hernias
   g. Congenital Adhesions or Bands
   h. Intestinal Duplication
   i. Imperforate Anus
   j. Hirschsprung Disease
   k. Intussusception — Episodic crampy abdominal pain with vomiting should suggest this disorder. Lethargy is often a prominent feature.
   l. Foreign Body
   m. Superior Mesenteric Artery — Duodenal compression is most likely to be seen in children in body casts or during prolonged recumbency and is associated with rapid weight loss.

n. Tumors

o. Mesenteric Cysts — Vomiting occurs if the cyst becomes infected or filled with blood.

p. Duodenal or Intestinal Hematomas — If there is no clear history of a traumatic episode, child abuse should be considered.

q. Adhesions

r. Paralytic Ileus — A number of conditions including infections (*e.g.,* pneumonia), hypokalemia, perforation, pancreatitis, diabetic ketoacidosis, and others may produce an ileus with resultant vomiting.

s. Omental Infarction — Increasing abdominal pain and nausea, sometimes with vomiting, may be seen. Abdominal tenderness is usually diffuse.

2. Inflammation and Irritation

   a. Appendicitis — Anorexia and vomiting are often early manifestations.

   b. Regional Enteritis — Crohn disease uncommonly causes vomiting unless there are complications or unless inflammation involves the stomach or duodenum, resulting in symptoms of obstruction.

   c. Peritonitis

   d. Food Poisoning — Abdominal pain, vomiting, and diarrhea develop within the first 12 hours following ingestion of the contaminated food. Enterotoxins are responsible.

   e. Ulcerative Colitis — Diarrhea, rectal bleeding, and weight loss are the most frequent symptoms. Vomiting may occur later, particularly with toxic dilatation of the colon.

   f. Necrotizing Enterocolitis

   g. Ileocecal Inflammation in Leukemia (Typhlitis) — Right lower quadrant pain, abdominal distension, diarrhea, and vomiting in a child with leukemia should alert the physician to this diagnosis.

3. Infection — Almost any systemic infection may result in vomiting. A few intestinal infections and infestations are listed.

   a. Gastroenteritis — Viral infections affecting the gastrointestinal tract, such as those caused by the rotavirus group, commonly produce vomiting and diarrhea.

b. Streptococcal Infection — Acute streptococcal infections may produce symptoms of fever and vomiting, particularly in young children.

c. Shigellosis — Onset of symptoms may be abrupt, with fever, abdominal pain, anorexia, and vomiting. Diarrhea, crampy abdominal pain, tenesmus, and occasionally meningismus may follow.

d. Toxogenic E. coli Infection — Vomiting may be an early manifestation before onset of diarrhea or may accompany it.

e. Yersinia enterocolitica — This disease may begin as an upper respiratory tract infection and progress to a prolonged illness with vomiting, diarrhea, fever, and abdominal pain.

f. Cholera — Vomiting may be severe. Profuse, watery diarrhea without fecal characteristics is the primary symptom.

g. Giardiasis — Symptomatic infestations usually result in diarrhea and abdominal distension. Uncommonly the infestation may mimic peptic ulcer disease, with epigastric pain and vomiting.

h. Strongyloidiasis — Upper gastrointestinal involvement may be associated with abdominal pain and vomiting. Migration of the larvae to the lung results in cough, dyspnea, and pneumonia.

i. Hookworm
j. Amebiasis
k. Ascariasis

4. Other Intestinal Disorders

a. Gastrointestinal Allergy — Abdominal pain, diarrhea, and occasionally vomiting may be related to the ingestion of certain foods.

b. Lactose Intolerance — Familial forms may be associated with prominent vomiting. Acquired forms are generally characterized by diarrhea.

c. Gluten Enteropathy — Diarrhea and growth failure are the most common symptoms, but vomiting and abdominal pain may be prominent.

III. Extraintestinal Abdominal Disorders

A. Hepatitis — Nausea and vomiting may appear early. Lethargy, right upper quadrant tenderness, and jaundice strongly suggest hepatitis.

B. Acute Cholecys-
titis

This is an uncommon cause of vomiting in children. Abdominal pain is right-sided, with tenderness to palpation. Nausea and vomiting are found in most cases.

C. Cholelithiasis

Intermittent colicky pain is characteristic. There may be vomiting and fatty food intolerance.

D. Choledochal Cyst

Typical symptoms are abdominal pain, jaundice, and a right upper quadrant mass. Vomiting, fever, and alcoholic stools are occasionally present.

E. Liver Abscess

F. Hepatoma

G. Pancreatitis

Children with the hereditary form have episodes of recurrent abdominal pain progressing to nausea and vomiting lasting 4 to 6 days. In acute pancreatitis, epigastric abdominal pain predominates.

IV. Genitourinary Tract Disorders

A. Pyelonephritis

Symptoms of fever, chills, and abdominal and back pain with vomiting may falsely suggest an acute gastroenteritis.

B. Hydronephrosis

C. Urinary Tract
Obstruction

Any acute obstruction of the urinary tract with proximal distension may cause vomiting.

D. Renal Stones

E. Pregnancy

"Morning sickness" may be the cause in the sexually active adolescent.

F. Hydrometro-
colpos

Uterine distension from retained products may produce vomiting that may be projectile in young infants.

V. Metabolic and Endocrine Disorders

A. Diabetic Ketoaci-
dosis

Abdominal pain and vomiting may be prominent as an initial presentation of diabetes or in the known diabetic whose disease is poorly controlled.

B. Uremia

C. Renal Tubular
Acidosis

D. Hypercalcemia

E. Congenital Adre-
nal Hyperplasia
(Adrenogenital
Syndrome)

Vomiting progressing to shock in the infant with ambiguous genitalia demands investigation for this disorder.

F. Withdrawal of
Corticosteroids

G. Diabetes Insip-
idus

H. Galactosemia   Onset of vomiting, diarrhea, and jaundice
coincides with the introduction of milk to the
diet.

I. Fructose Intoler-
ance

J. Fructose 1, 6-Di-
phosphate Defi-
ciency

K. Lysosomal Acid
Phosphate Defi-
ciency

L. Gangliosidoses

M. Wolman Disease

N. Niemann–Pick
Disease

O. Glycogen Stor-
age Disease,
Type I

P. Amino Acid and   Many of the inborn errors of amino acid and
Organic Acid   organic acid metabolism or transport may be
Disorders   associated with vomiting, particularly after
feedings are begun in the neonatal period.
Ketoacidosis, changes in sensorium, seizures,
and abnormal odors should suggest the possibility of any of the following: phenylketonuria,
methylmalonic acidemia, maple syrup urine
disease, hypervalinemia; hyperlysinemia; ketotic hyperglycinemia, propionicacidemia, bu-
tyric or hexanoic acidemia, isovaleric-acidemia,
or argininosuccinicaciduria.

Q. Hypoparathy-   Vomiting may be the result of increased intra-
roidism   cranial pressure associated with the hypocalcemia. Seizures, cataracts, tetany, headaches,
and mucocutaneous candidiasis may be findings.

VI. Disorders of the Central Nervous System

Any of the large number of diseases causing central nervous system
irritation or increased intracranial pressure may produce vomiting.

A. Infections   Meningitis, encephalitis, or brain abscess may
be a cause. Some infections may be subacute;

	in tuberculous meningoencephalitis, for example, presenting symptoms may suggest a gastroenteritis.
B. Trauma	Vomiting frequently follows head injury. Collections of blood (acute or chronic) may also be associated with vomiting: subdural hematoma, subarachnoid hemorrhage, or epidural hematoma.
C. Brain Tumors	Morning vomiting and headache should suggest the presence of central nervous system tumors. Other signs include cranial nerve palsies, ataxia, increasing head size, and a bulging fontanel.
D. Hydrocephalus	
E. Other Causes of Increased Intracranial Pressure	Lead poisoning and pseudotumor cerebri may be causes.
F. Migraine	Vomiting is a common symptom, especially early in the onset of the attack. In young infants who cannot relay the symptom of headache, recurrent vomiting attacks may be the primary symptom. A history of motion sickness is found in up to half of the children.
G. Epilepsy	Episodes of vomiting may accompany convulsive attacks.

VII. Other Systemic Disorders

A. Parenteral Infections	Any systemic infection may cause vomiting. The neonate with septicemia may have bile-stained vomitus, suggesting obstruction.
B. Reye Syndrome	Recurrent vomiting ushers in the encephalopathy.
C. Vestibular Injury or Inflammation	Middle ear disorders associated with vertigo may stimulate intense vomiting upon movement.
D. Familial Dysautonomia	Affected children may have recurrent aspiration, postural hypotension, absent lacrimation, absent deep tendon reflexes, and episodic fevers, among other signs and symptoms.
E. Acrodermatitis Enteropathica	Other symptoms such as a malabsorptive diarrhea, skin lesions, alopecia, and irritability overshadow the occasional vomiting.
F. Black Widow Spider Bite	

REFERENCE

1. Reinhart JB, Evans SL, McFadden DL: Cyclic vomiting in children: Seen through the psychiatrist's eye. Pediatrics 59:371–377, 1977

SUGGESTED READINGS

Gryboski J: Gastrointestinal Problems in the Infant. Philadelphia, WB Saunders, 1975
Roy CC, Silverman A: Pediatric Clinical Gastroenterology, 3rd ed. St. Louis, CV Mosby, 1983

69

PROJECTILE VOMITING

Forceful or projectile vomiting in an infant usually brings immediately to mind the diagnosis of pyloric stenosis. However, a knowledge of other possible causes is important, particularly in cases where other findings make this diagnosis unlikely: For example, the child may be beyond the usual age for presentation, or the symptoms may be abrupt in onset.

In this short chapter are listed some disorders that may be associated with projectile vomiting; many of the others cited in Chapter 68, Vomiting, may also produce occasional projectile episodes. However, the disorders listed here are somewhat more notorious.

I. Gastrointestinal Disorders

A. Pyloric Stenosis	Vomiting usually begins within the first few weeks of life and becomes progressively more severe and projectile. Visible gastric peristalsis may be noted. Affected infants feed avidly, even after vomiting.
B. Pylorospasm	Some researchers have questioned the existence of this disorder; perhaps it represents one end of the spectrum of which pyloric muscle hypertrophy is the other. Most cases respond nicely to conservative treatment.
C. Gastric Mucosal Diaphragm	Folds of mucosa may intermittently block the egress of stomach contents.
D. Pyloric Atresia	Signs are obvious at the first feeding.
E. Gastric Volvulus	Onset may be acute, with epigastric pain and vomiting, or the disorder may be chronic, with recurrent postprandial discomfort, vomiting, belching, and upper gastrointestinal tract bleeding.
F. Hiatal Hernia	In severe cases in which symptoms begin in the first few weeks of life, the vomiting may be projectile, mimicking pyloric stenosis.
G. Peptic Ulcer	Channel or antral ulcers may produce colicky symptoms with episodes of forceful vomiting.
H. Duodenal Obstruction	Atresia, stenosis, or webs commonly produce projectile vomiting. The epigastrium may ap-

pear distended, and the vomitus usually contains bile.

II. Infection

A. Sepsis

Systemic infections, particularly in neonates, may be associated with projectile vomiting. The vomitus may be bile-stained. Affected infants appear sick, and the onset is acute.

B. Pyelonephritis

An unsuspected pyelonephritis is a notorious mimic of pyloric stenosis, especially in young infants.

III. Genitourinary Tract Disorders

A. Urinary Tract Obstruction

Marked dilatation of any part of the urinary tract from obstruction, such as renal stones, ureteral kinking, or tumor, may result in forceful emesis.

B. Hydrometro-colpos

Children with imperforate hymen or vaginal atresia resulting in uterine distension from retained secretions may present with projectile vomiting along with a lower abdominal mass.

IV. Central Nervous System Disorders

Vomiting may occur in several central nervous system disorders, although projectile vomiting is infrequent. Infection, irritation, and increased intracranial pressure must be considered. Usually, changes in sensorium and other central nervous system signs indicate a central lesion.

A. Meningitis and Encephalitis

B. Acute Intracranial Hemorrhage

Intraventricular, epidural, or subarachnoid bleeding should be considered.

C. Hydrocephalus

Sudden blockage of cerebrospinal fluid flow is a much more likely cause than gradual ventricular enlargement.

D. Brain Tumors

E. Lead Encephalop-athy

V. Other Disorders

A. Congenital Adrenal Hyperplasia (Adrenogenital Syndrome)

Hypoadrenalism in young infants may be associated with forceful vomiting. Virilization and ambiguous genitalia are important clues.

B. Hypercalcemia   Associated symptoms include anorexia, constipation, polydipsia, and polyuria, along with nausea and vomiting.

C. Wolman Disease   In this rare disorder of cholesterol storage, diarrhea, weight loss, and hepatosplenomegaly occur in the first few weeks of life. Calcifications in enlarged adrenal glands are characteristic on abdominal roentgenograms. Forceful vomiting occasionally occurs.

D. Phenylketonuria   Vomiting (sometimes projectile) and irritability may be seen in the first few months of life.

70

DIARRHEA

Diarrhea denotes the passage of an increased number of stools of variable nonsolid consistency. The passage of an excessive amount of fluid with the stool is the primary manifestation of diarrhea. The basic pathophysiologic mechanisms responsible for this fluid loss are multiple; more than one of these malfunctions may be present at the same time. (For discussion of these mechanisms, see the Suggested Reading list at the end of this chapter.)

Fortunately, most of the common causes of diarrhea either are not life-threatening or are disorders that can be managed fairly easily. Of the many possible causes, only a few are commonly seen: dietary indiscretions, viral and bacterial infections, extraintestinal infections, carbohydrate intolerance, and the irritable bowel syndrome.

Causes of diarrhea have been divided into those seen in the newborn infant, in the well-appearing child, and finally, in the ill-appearing child. The more common disorders are listed first; the less common ones follow.

I. Diarrhea in the Newborn

A. Overfeeding — Excessive caloric or fluid intake may result in loose stools.

B. Viral Infections

C. Bacterial Infections — *E. coli* and *Salmonella* infections are most common, but other organisms may also cause infections.

D. Cow's Milk Allergy — This is an uncommon cause of diarrhea but should not be overlooked.

E. Necrotizing Enterocolitis — Abdominal distension, lethargy, temperature irregularities, and vomiting are findings.

F. Congenital Lactase Deficiency — Occurrence is rare. Stools are frothy and contain sugar.

G. Glucose or Galactose Malabsorption

H. Familial Chloride Diarrhea — Profuse watery diarrhea may begin even *in utero*. The stools resemble urine. Abdominal distension and ileus develop as part of hypokalemic hypochloremic alkalosis.

I. Enterokinase Deficiency	Intermittent diarrhea may be present from birth. Vomiting, irritability, and failure to thrive become prominent features.
J. Hypoadrenalism	The adrenogenital syndrome is the most likely cause of this problem.
K. Maternal Ulcerative Colitis	Infants born to affected mothers may have transient diarrhea for the first few days of life.

II. Diarrhea in a Well-Appearing Child

A. Overfeeding	Excessive food or liquid intake may result in frequent loose stools.
B. Irritable Colon Syndrome or Chronic Nonspecific Diarrhea of Childhood	These two disorders may be related. Chronic nonspecific diarrhea, seen in healthy thriving children from 6 months to 3 years of age, is characterized by frequent loose stools, most prevalent in the morning, and more frequent after ingestion of cold liquids. In the irritable colon syndrome, seen in older children, the stools are frequent and small, often passed with gas and sometimes preceded by mild cramping.
C. Inadequate Dietary Fat	The deficiency may result in bulky, frequent stools.
D. Other Dietary Peculiarities	A careful history may reveal excessive intake of a number of foodstuffs that may result in diarrhea. Dietetic candies and gums, apple juice, and salad dressing are among the culprits.
E. Allergic–Tension–Fatigue Syndrome	Some children, particularly those with an atopic background, may manifest a host of signs and symptoms including headache, abdominal pain, lethargy, irritability, and diarrhea secondary to intolerance of various foods, particularly milk, chocolate, and eggs.
F. Constipation with Encopresis	Children with fecal impactions may present with the complaint of diarrhea due to leakage of loose stool around the bolus of hard stool.
G. Antibiotics	Diarrhea may be associated with or follow a course of antibiotics. Causes include the vehicle for the antibiotic and a change in bacterial flora; other mechanisms, as yet unidentified, are suspected.
H. Parasites	Often children with infestation by any of a variety of parasites may not appear ill. Giardiasis, amebiasis, and ascariasis are possibilities.

I. Carbohydrate Intolerance	The defect may be primary or follow gastrointestinal infections. Lactose intolerance is most common. The stools are frothy, smell like vinegar, and contain sugar.
J. Milk Protein Allergy	A true allergic reaction to cow's milk protein may occur with diarrhea and mild abdominal cramps. Soy protein may also produce an allergic gastrointestinal picture. Heiner syndrome, caused by severe milk allergy, is characterized by bloody diarrhea and shock after ingestion of small amounts of cow's milk protein.
K. Familial Polyposis	Although diarrhea is not a common manifestation, its presence may lead to a rectal examination and discovery of the diagnosis.
L. Medications	Ingestion of various medications, such as decongestants and theophylline preparations, may be associated with the passage of frequent loose stools.
M. Well Water	The high mineral content of some well water may result in diarrhea.

III. Diarrhea in an Ill-Appearing Child

A. Infectious Gastroenteritis	
1. Viral Infection	A host of viruses have been found to cause diarrhea. Rotavirus is the most important cause of vomiting and diarrhea in the United States during the winter months, particularly in children 6 months to 2 years of age; in most cases, a disaccharidase depression follows this illness. Adults and older children have diarrhea with severe abdominal cramps but no vomiting.
2. Bacterial Infection	*Salmonella, Shigella,* and *E. coli* are the best known bacterial causes of diarrhea, but *Campylobacter fetus* and *Yersinia enterocolitica* are being recognized with increasing frequency. Intermittent relapses with a chronic diarrheal picture are not uncommon.
3. Parasitic Infestation	Giardiasis, amebiasis, strongyloidiasis, hookworm infestation, and trichinosis may all cause chronic diarrhea with weight loss and abdominal distension.

4. Fungal Infection | *Candida* and *Histoplasma* are among the fungal pathogens.

B. Extraintestinal Infections | Many extraintestinal infections may be associated with diarrhea, especially in younger children. Otitis media, urinary tract infections, sepsis, and pneumonias are the most frequently recognized.

C. Carbohydrate Malabsorption | Watery, frothy stools that smell like vinegar and contain sugar should suggest this possibility. Lactose absorption is most frequently affected; congenital, acquired, and developmental lactose intolerances are well recognized. Sucrose, isomaltose, and glucose or galactose malabsorptions may be found.

D. Inflammatory Bowel Disease | Ulcerative colitis is characterized by abdominal cramps, tenesmus, and the passage of stools containing mucus and blood. In regional enteritis, the presentation may be more subtle with abdominal pain, fever of unknown origin, and weight loss or failure of development.

E. Cystic Fibrosis | Failure to thrive, recurrent pneumonias, and steatorrhea are the most frequent manifestations.

F. Celiac Disease | This disorder is now being recognized more frequently in the United States, but careful documentation is necessary. Diarrhea generally begins after the introduction of wheat-containing foods but is not a symptom in one third of affected children.

G. Maternal Deprivation Syndrome | Children with growth and developmental retardation secondary to psychosocial factors may present with chronic diarrheal stools.

H. Anatomic Abnormalities of the Bowel

1. Hirschsprung Disease (Congenital Megacolon) | The development of an enterocolitis in this disorder is particularly dangerous.

2. Short Bowel Syndrome

3. Blind or Stagnant Loop | Diarrhea, steatorrhea, abdominal distension, weight loss, and intermittent episodes suggestive of intestinal obstruction may be seen.

4. Malrotation and Partial Small Bowel Obstructions	The initial symptom may be diarrhea.
5. Enteric Fistulas	
6. Intestinal Lymphangiectasia	This disorder should be suspected in a child with edema, hypoproteinemia, steatorrhea, and loose stools.
I. Immune Deficiency	Diarrhea with failure to thrive, recurrent infections, and chronic cough should suggest any of several immune deficiency diseases.
1. IgA Deficiency	
2. Hypogamma-globulinemias or Agamma-globulinemias	
3. Combined Immunodeficiency	
4. Wiskott–Aldrich Syndrome	
5. Ataxia–Telangiectasia	
6. Defective Cellular Immunity	
7. Acquired Immune Deficiency Syndrome	
J. Endocrine Causes	
1. Hyperthyroidism	
2. Hypoparathyroidism	Diarrhea is unusual but may result from hypocalcemia. Seizures, tetany, and muscular cramps dominate the clinical picture.
3. Adrenal Insufficiency	Weakness, lethargy, vomiting, anorexia, and diarrhea are characteristic. Serum sodium levels are low; serum potassium levels are high.
K. Tumors	
1. Neuroblastoma; Ganglioneuroma; Ganglioneuroblastoma	

2. Carcinoid Tumors — These tumors are rare in children; findings may include episodes of cutaneous flushing, wheezing, and diarrhea.

3. Vasoactive Intestinal Peptide-Secreting Tumors — Findings include failure to thrive, abdominal distension, hypertension, sweating episodes, metabolic acidosis, and low serum potassium levels. Diarrhea may be intermittent at first but then becomes unremitting.

4. Intestinal Lymphosarcoma — Abdominal pain, malaise, anemia, and diarrhea are the primary features.

L. Pancreatic Disorders

   1. Exocrine Pancreatic Insufficiency — Malabsorption, failure to thrive, cyclic neutropenia, anemia, and metaphyseal dysostosis are found in the Schwachmann–Diamond syndrome.

   2. Chronic Pancreatitis

M. Hepatic Disturbances

   1. Hepatitis — Children with acute hepatitis may have diarrhea or constipation.

   2. Chronic Hepatitis

   3. Cirrhosis

   4. Bile Acid Deficiency — Steatorrhea develops along with anorexia and vomiting.

   5. Biliary Atresia — Progressively deepening jaundice, failure to thrive, malnutrition, and abdominal distension are prominent findings.

N. Protein–Calorie Malnutrition

O. Metabolic Disorders—Inherited

   1. Galactosemia — Jaundice, failure to thrive, cataracts, hepatomegaly, vomiting, and diarrhea are important findings. The urine should be checked for the presence of reducing substances.

   2. Tyrosinemia — Failure to thrive, vomiting, diarrhea, abdominal enlargement, edema, ascites, and hepatosplenomegaly are the leading symptoms.

   3. Methionine Malabsorption — This defect is characterized by diarrhea, convulsions, retardation, and a sweet odor to the urine.

4. Familial Protein Intolerance	Vomiting and diarrhea begin between 3 and 13 months of age.
5. Wolman Disease	Chronic diarrhea develops in the first few weeks of life. Hepatosplenomegaly and marked failure to thrive are found. Areas of calcification in the adrenal glands are seen on abdominal roentgenograms.
6. Abetalipoproteinemia	Ataxia, retinitis pigmentosa, and steatorrhea with acanthocytes on peripheral smear are clues.
7. Selective Malabsorption of Vitamin B_{12}	
8. Gaucher Disease	
9. Niemann–Pick Disease	
P. Vascular Disorders	
1. Mesenteric Artery Insufficiency	
2. Early Portal Hypertension	
3. Intestinal Ischemia	
Q. Miscellaneous Disorders	
1. Acrodermatitis Enteropathica	Perioral and perianal excoriations and vesicobullous lesions of the extremities with diarrhea, irritability, and alopecia should suggest this disorder. Dramatic improvement follows zinc therapy.
2. Zollinger–Ellison Syndrome	This disorder is associated with multiple gastric and peptic ulcers.
3. Scleroderma	Skin changes usually precede the intestinal manifestations.
4. Folic Acid Deficiency	
5. Neurofibromatosis	Café-au-lait macules and, after puberty, neurofibromas are present.
6. Familial Dysautonomia	Recurrent vomiting, aspiration, absent lacrimation, absent filiform papillae on the tongue,

emotional lability, and postural hypotension are associated findings.

7. Whipple Disease — This disorder, usually seen in adults, causes foul-smelling diarrhea with fever. An infectious pathogenesis is presumed.

8. Toxic Diarrhea — Diarrhea may be secondary to chemotherapy or irradiation.

9. Clostridium Difficile Toxin — A chronic watery diarrhea with poor weight gain may be caused by this toxin. Prior antibiotic therapy may or may not have preceded its onset. Oral vancomycin usually provides a cure.

SUGGESTED READINGS

Gall DG, Hamilton JR: Chronic diarrhea in childhood: A new look at an old problem. Pediatr Clin North Am 21:1001–1018, 1974

Gryboski JD: Chronic diarrhea. Current Probl Pediatr IX, No. 5, Mar 1979

Roy CC, Silverman A: Pediatric Clinical Gastroenterology, 3rd ed. St. Louis, CV Mosby, 1983

71

CONSTIPATION AND FECAL RETENTION

Although the old adage "one man's constipation may be another man's diarrhea" is a bit of an exaggeration, it serves to remind us that there are wide variations in normal elimination habits. In infancy, changes in stool type or frequency are common. In some families, excessive attention to elimination details may cause acceptable patterns to be perceived as abnormal.

Generally, constipation refers to a state in which the stools are hard, infrequent, and difficult to pass. The causes of constipation range from chronic stool-holding, in which huge fecal impactions may be found, to "spastic colon," in which scybalous (rabbit pellet-like) stools are characteristic; from dietary causes to metabolic disorders; and from neurogenic problems to psychogenic ones.

In 95% of neonates, meconium is passed within the first 24 hours of life; failure to do so requires careful evaluation and is considered separately in the following classification of causes of constipation. A careful history including diet and a description of the stools should not be neglected in any age group, nor should a family history of elimination patterns. A rectal examination is mandatory.

I. Delayed Passage of Meconium

A. Intestinal Obstruction	Infants with atresias, webs, volvulus, or other causes of obstruction may present with failure to pass stools as well as abdominal distension and vomiting. The passage of meconium does not rule out a high or low obstruction.
B. Meconium Ileus	Symptoms usually begin on the second day of life with abdominal distension and vomiting. Most affected infants have cystic fibrosis.
C. Hirschsprung Disease (Congenital Megacolon)	This disorder accounts for 20% to 25% of the cases of neonatal intestinal obstruction. Abdominal distension is followed by decreased appetite; the finding of bile-stained vomitus is common. Digital examination or saline enema

	may induce stool passage and relief of symptoms and signs. Occasionally, the disorder may not be diagnosed until later in life. The stools passed are never normal.
D. Meconium Plug	Plugs may block the intestines, especially in premature infants. Hirschsprung disease must always be considered.
E. Functional Ileus	Sepsis, respiratory distress syndrome, pneumonia, and electrolyte imbalance may be responsible for the ileus.
F. Small Left Colon Syndrome	Clinical presentation is typical of bowel obstruction. Barium enema demonstrates the markedly decreased caliber of the left colon. Maternal diabetes is common.
G. Drugs Administered to Mother	Magnesium sulfate, opiates, and ganglionic blocking agents given to the mother prior to delivery may cause delayed passage of meconium in the neonate.
H. Hypothyroidism	Prolonged jaundice, lethargy, and low body temperature are additional suggestive signs.

II. Physiologic Causes
A. Dietary Problems

1. Breast-Feeding	Breast-fed infants initially have frequent stools, often with every feeding; however, many at around 6 weeks of age begin to have prolonged periods, often many days, without the passage of stool.
2. Cow's Milk Ingestion	The casein curd, often difficult to digest, is one of the reasons why unaltered cow's milk often leads to constipation. Although this effect is most commonly seen in young infants, a high intake of milk or other dairy products at any age may result in constipation.
3. Low Dietary Roughage	A diet low in vegetable fiber or other bulk results in hard, difficult-to-pass stools. This is a common condition in children whose diet consists largely of milk, sugared cereal, and snack foods.
B. Deficient Fluid Intake	Any condition or illness that results in a reduced fluid intake or excessive fluid losses (*e.g.*, fever) may result in a decreased fecal bulk with less frequent elimination.
1. Febrile States	

2. Hot Weather
3. Insufficient
   Intravenous
   Fluids
C. Immobility   Constipation may be a problem in children
                             confined to bed, especially after surgery or
                             following the application of casts, especially
                             body casts.
D. Anorexia Nervosa

III. Voluntary Withholding

A. Megacolon With   A great deal has been written about the com-
   or Without Enco-   mon problem of the "stool hoarder." The
   presis   problem generally begins after $2\frac{1}{2}$ to 3 years of
                          age. Parental concern may not begin until the
                          child begins soiling the underwear because of
                          spillage around a huge fecal impaction dis-
                          tending the rectum. A rectal examination and
                          a careful history for possible precipitating
                          events are essential. Any of a number of
                          causes may result in painful defecation and
                          subsequent withholding, creating an ever-
                          increasing problem.

B. Painful Defecation
   1. Anal Fissure
   2. Perianal Der-
      matitis or Irri-
      tation
   3. Hemorrhoids
C. Intentional With-   This may occur during travel or at school,
   holding   with a change in environment, or during peri-
                         ods of family stress or upheaval.
D. Improper Toilet   Either failure to set standards or excessive
   Training   compulsion regarding training may cause con-
                         tipation.
E. Emotional Distur-
   bance
F. Severe Mental
   Retardation
G. Depression

IV. Neurogenic Disorders

A. Hirschsprung   Uncommonly the onset of symptoms is de-
   Disease (Congeni-   layed until after the newborn period. The con-
   tal Megacolon)   dition may have been obscured by repeated

digital examinations or enemas with relief of obstructive symptoms. Stools are infrequent and ribbonlike rather than the huge masses seen with the acquired form. Generally, the rectal ampulla is empty on digital examination.

B. Intestinal Pseudo-obstruction — This uncommon disorder of unknown cause with progressively severe motility problems leads to abdominal distension and failure to pass stools.

C. Cerebral Palsy — Children with the athetoid variety and those who are severely spastic are most likely to have constipation.

D. Myelomeningocele

E. Spinal Cord Injury

F. Sacral Agenesis

G. Diastematomyelia — The spinal cord may become tethered by bony spicules. There may be cutaneous abnormalities over the spine, as well as gait and urinary disturbances.

H. Spinal Dysraphism — Fibrous bands, lipomas, septa or dermal sinuses may cause traction or pressure lesions. Look for cutaneous clues over the spine.

I. Neurofibromatosis — Constipation or obstipation is an unexplained common association. Colonic neurofibromas may produce obstruction or an acquired megacolon.

J. Muscular Weakness — Various causes include the myotonias, prune belly syndrome, and muscular dystrophies. Lack of muscle power to create intra-abdominal pressure makes evacuation difficult.

K. Acquired Postganglionic Cholinergic Dysautonomia — Associated findings include bilateral internal ophthalmoplegia, impaired secretion of tears and saliva, and absence of sweating as well as gastrointestinal atony.

V. Endocrine and Metabolic Disorders

A. Hypothyroidism — Other features of hypothyroidism are generally more prominent than constipation.

B. Diabetes Mellitus — Constipation may be related to lack of adequate bowel water.

C. Pheochromocytoma — Affected children occasionally have severe constipation. More typical features include hypertension, headache, tachycardia, palpitations, nausea, and vomiting.

D. Hypokalemia — Reduced peristalsis or ileus may occur.

E. Hypercalcemia or Hypocalcemia — Children immobilized with casts, traction, and so forth, may develop hypercalcemia with its attendant problems, including constipation.

F. Conditions Associated with Polyuria — Polyuria results in deficient stool water. Diabetes insipidus and renal tubular acidosis may be causes.

G. Acute Intermittent Porphyria — Abdominal pain, vomiting, and constipation may be the initial manifestations.

H. Amyloidosis

I. Lipid Storage Disorders — Constipation may be a minor feature of some of these disorders.

VI. Miscellaneous Disorders

A. Anal or Rectal Stenosis — Stenosis is most commonly acquired rather than congenital, especially after imperforate anus repair or with neoplasms or pelvic abscesses.

B. Anteriorally Placed Anus — This may represent an aborted imperforated anus.

C. Dolichocolon — An abnormally long colon is often a familial trait. Increased extraction of water creates hard, compacted stools. Affected children require a high-bulk diet.

D. Appendicitis — Constipation is a minor feature, overshadowed by the abdominal pain.

E. Celiac Disease — A small number of children may have fecal impactions and vomiting, mimicking obstruction.

F. Scleroderma — Intestinal involvement may result in decreased intestinal motility.

G. Lead Poisoning

H. Viral Hepatitis — Diarrhea and constipation occur with equal frequency.

I. Salmonellosis — In the systemic form, fever for 1 to 3 weeks, rose spots, anorexia, splenomegaly, constipation, and leukopenia may be presenting signs.

J. Infant Botulism — Facial and ocular palsies, a poor suck, and hypotonia should suggest this possibility.

K. Tetanus

L. Chagas Disease

M. Drugs — Antihistamines, opiates, and phenothiazines may be constipating.

N. Meconium Ileus Equivalent | A significant number of children with cystic fibrosis may develop constipation to the degree of obstruction. This phenomenon may be due to the accumulation of intestinal luminal mucus that adheres to the intestinal wall and to which food adheres.

SUGGESTED READINGS

Bentley JFR: Constipation in infants and children. Gut 12:85–90, 1971

Fleisher DR: Diagnosis and treatment of disorders of defecation in children. Pediatr Ann 5:700–722, 1976

FECAL INCONTINENCE AND ENCOPRESIS

Most children achieve full bowel control and acquire regular bowel habits during the fourth year of life. Occasionally, episodes of fecal incontinence occur, and most parents are aware that these represent "accidents." When episodes of incontinence become frequent or regular, medical evaluation is required.

Encopresis refers to the voluntary or involuntary evacuation of feces into the underwear or in places that are not socially acceptable depositories. The most common cause of encopresis is a large fecal impaction, which in most cases develops after a series of painful defecations. A careful history will usually differentiate chronic constipation with characteristic overflow incontinence from those with a voluntary, anatomic, or neurologic cause.

I. Involuntary Causes

A. Chronic Constipation with Encopresis

This is by far the most common cause of fecal soiling. As the fecal impaction enlarges the anal sphincter becomes chronically stretched and unable to prevent spillage of stool. Two types of incontinence, which may coexist, have been reported: One is the rubbing of the hard fecal impaction as it extends through the anal sphincter onto the underwear, giving a linear caking of stool. The more common form is the frequent passage of small amounts of liquid stool around the bolus of impacted stool, causing soiling of the underwear. Abdominal and rectal examination will disclose the cause of the soiling. The causes of chronic constipation producing the encopresis are numerous (see Chap. 71, Constipation and Fecal Retention).

B. Diarrheal Conditions

During acute or chronic diarrheal diseases the child may not be able to voluntarily control the peristaltic rushes of liquid stool with the external anal sphincter. Although this is more likely to occur in young children, older children and adults with these diseases may occasionally lose control because of fatigue, inaccessibility of toilets, or general illness.

II. Voluntary Causes

A. Failure to Achieve Control

The child may never have been toilet trained for various reasons, such as family disinterest or resistance by the child to the training approach. The mentally retarded child may never achieve control.

B. Regressive Behavior

Previously toilet-trained young children may resume soiling at the time of stressful situations, such as birth of a sibling, illnesses, separations, death in the family, or moves.

C. Emotional Disturbances

The soiling may occasionally be a manifestation of severe psychologic problems.

III. Anatomic Causes

A. Anorectal Anomalies

Anatomic abnormalities such as perineal fistulas may result in soiling. Regional enteritis must be considered in the older child.

B. Scarring of the Anus

Control of defecation may be lost following anorectal surgery, particularly for imperforate anus.

IV. Neurogenic Causes

A. Diastematomyelia

Low back pain, progressive weakness of the lower extremities, and bladder and bowel incontinence may be present. Cutaneous changes over the spinal column may be a clue.

B. Myelomeningocele

C. Sacral Agenesis

D. Spinal Cord Injuries

E. Syringomyelia

F. Spinal Cord Tumors

Lipomas, teratomas, neurofibromas, gliomas, arteriovenous malformations, and other tumors may be associated with encopresis along with back pain, weakness of the lower extremities, and reflex or sensory changes. Cutaneous clues may be present over the spinal column.

G. Transverse Myelitis

A sudden onset of paralysis of the lower extremities occurs.

H. Epidural Abscess   Severe back pain over the infected area and lower extremity weakness are the more prominent symptoms.

I. Poliomyelitis

J. Infectious Poly-   Constipation is common; incontinence is rare.
neuritis

K. Osteomyelitis of   Swelling of surrounding structures may cause
Vertebral Body   impingement on the spinal cord.

L. Seizures   Fecal incontinence may occur during a convulsive episode.

73

GASTROINTESTINAL BLEEDING: HEMATEMESIS

Hematemesis, or the vomiting of bright red blood or coffee-ground material, quickens the pulse of all who see it. If significant blood loss occurs, tachycardia may occur as well. Hematemesis is so often a sign of a serious underlying disorder that it must be considered a medical emergency.

In the following classification of possible causes, neonatal hematemesis has been separated from that occurring in older infants and children. Swallowed blood, from epistaxis, for instance, must always be included in the differential diagnosis. The other causes are grouped by anatomic site or by hematologic origin.

In the past as many as one third to one half of cases of hematemesis in children were unexplained; however, newer techniques such as fiberoptic endoscopy may significantly lower this percentage. Unfortunately, hematemesis often occurs suddenly without warning in previously asymptomatic children. A careful history and physical examination may uncover subtle clues that may help in sorting out possible causes.

I. Neonatal Causes

A. Swallowed Maternal Blood
: The newborn may swallow maternal blood during the birth process. Almost always hematemesis of this variety occurs within the first 12 to 24 hours after birth. The Apt test, using the fact that fetal hemoglobin resists alkali denaturization, is helpful in documenting the presence of maternal blood.

B. Hemorrhagic Disease of the Newborn
: Otherwise healthy-appearing infants may vomit significant amounts of blood in the first few days of life. A bleeding site is not usually found; instead, there may be significant oozing from multiple foci. There may be evidence of bleeding from other areas of the body (umbilicus, penis if circumcision has been done, or puncture sites) or petechiae and purpura. Vitamin K deficiency is less common now, but

401

<table>
<tr><td></td><td>maternal aspirin ingestion during the few days prior to delivery or use of anticonvulsants or anticoagulants should be considered.</td></tr>
<tr><td>C. Hemorrhagic Gastritis</td><td>This disorder may occur in the sick neonate following a stressful delivery or a neonatal complication such as sepsis or meningitis.</td></tr>
<tr><td>D. Peptic Ulcer</td><td>Neonatal events may be stressful enough to result in ulcer formation or perforation.</td></tr>
<tr><td>E. Spontaneous Rupture of Esophagus</td><td>Occurrence is uncommon in infants, but this disorder should be suspected in the infant who appears well initially and then develops respiratory distress (secondary to the development of a tension pneumothorax), increased with feeding, and sometimes associated hematemesis.</td></tr>
</table>

II. Swallowed Blood

The site of bleeding may be in the upper respiratory tract, particularly with epistaxis or following dental extractions, tonsillectomy, and oral or pharyngeal lacerations.

III. Esophageal Disorders

<table>
<tr><td>A. Chalasia: Gastroesophageal Reflux</td><td>This condition is generally associated with small amounts of blood mixed in with the vomitus. Reflux of stomach acids into the esophagus results in erosions. Early symptoms may be vomiting after meals, irritability, poor appetite, recurrent coughing episodes, or pneumonitis.</td></tr>
<tr><td>B. Hiatus Hernia</td><td>Vomiting or excessive regurgitation after feedings may begin shortly after birth. Some infants have dysphagia, poor weight gain, and recurrent aspiration pneumonitis. The amount of blood in the vomitus is quite small.</td></tr>
<tr><td>C. Esophageal Varices</td><td>Massive hematemesis is the most frequent presentation. The two most common underlying conditions are portal vein thrombosis and hepatic cirrhosis. It is essential to obtain a careful neonatal history to uncover possible causes of long-standing portal vein thrombosis such as omphalitis, neonatal sepsis, diarrhea with shock, exchange transfusions, and umbilical vein catheterization. Hepatic cirrhosis may result from a host of disorders (see Chap. 63,</td></tr>
</table>

Ascites) including obstructive biliary disease, infections and inflammatory disorders, cardiovascular problems, genetic and metabolic disorders, and drugs. Some inherited causes of cirrhosis that may produce hematemesis and are worthy of consideration are cystic fibrosis, Wilson disease, alpha₁-antitrypsin deficiency, galactosemia, Gaucher disease, porphyria, and Rendu–Osler–Weber syndrome (hereditary hemorrhagic telangiectasia). Other less frequent presenting signs of portal hypertension include splenomegaly, prominent veins of collateral circulation over the abdominal wall, hepatomegaly, clubbing, and ascites.

D. Foreign Bodies

Ingested foreign bodies may cause lacerations along the alimentary tract with resultant bleeding.

E. Mallory–Weiss Syndrome

Excessive retching may cause a laceration at the gastroesophageal junction.

F. Corrosive Agents

Acid and alkali substances may produce significant bleeding as they erode through the mucosa.

G. Congenital Microgastria

In this rare disorder the stomach is small, resulting in reflux and esophagitis.

H. Esophageal Tumors

IV. Gastroduodenal Lesions

A. Peptic Ulcer

Symptoms may vary with the age of the child. Children under 3 years of age may have a poor appetite, vomiting, crying after meals, and abdominal distension; those 3 to 6 years of age often have vomiting related to eating, periumbilical pain, and pain that may awaken them at night. Children older than 6 years of age may complain of a burning or gnawing epigastric pain, most frequent after fasting or at night, that may occasionally be relieved by food or milk. In the Zollinger–Ellison syndrome, characterized by gastric hypersecretion, multiple duodenal or jejunal ulcers occur.

B. Stress Ulcers

These ulcers occur during times of other serious illnesses, such as central nervous system disease or burns.

C. Gastritis

Irritation of the stomach may follow ingestion of corrosives, aspirin, iron, acetaminophen, aminophylline, boric acid, fluoride, heavy metals, phenol, or bacterial food poisoning.

D. Gastric Outlet Obstruction

Small amounts of blood may appear in the vomitus in pyloric stenosis, antral ulcers, or pyloric webs.

E. Duplications

Esophageal or gastric duplications may become ulcerated and bleed. Abdominal pain or, occasionally, a palpable mass may be present.

F. Tumors

Leiomyomas, leiomyosarcomas, and lymphomas may erode vessels and cause hematemesis.

G. Infections
  1. Hemorrhagic Fevers

In various parts of the world the bites of ticks and mites may produce disorders characterized by fever, chills, muscle aches, headache, bleeding diatheses, hematemesis, and shock.

  2. Mycotic Infections

Debilitated patients are predisposed. Progressive sinusitis, cellulitis, and pneumonitis are common findings.

  3. Malaria
H. Drugs
  1. Theophylline
  2. Caffeine Intoxication
I. Pseudoxanthoma Elasticum

This rare disorder has skin changes resembling a plucked chicken in areas such as the neck and axillae. Alterations in elastic tissue of the gastrointestinal vessels may lead to bleeding.

V. Hematologic Disorders
A. Aplastic Anemia
B. Thrombocytopenia
C. Leukemia
D. Hemophilia
E. Disseminated Intravascular Coagulation

VI. Miscellaneous Disorders
A. Scurvy

The clinical presentation may mimic that of a peptic ulcer. There may be other signs of hemorrhage into the skin and periosteitis that may manifest as tender extremities.

B. Henoch–Schönlein Purpura — This disorder rarely causes hematemesis.

C. Pulmonary Bleeding — Hematemesis may occur in disorders that produce hemoptysis if the blood is swallowed.

D. Blunt Trauma to the Abdomen — Particularly, duodenal injuries may cause hematemesis.

E. Rendu–Osler–Weber Syndrome — Hereditary hemorrhagic telangiectasia is an autosomal dominant disorder associated with mucocutaneous telangiectasia.

SUGGESTED READINGS

Cox K, Ament ME: Upper gastrointestinal bleeding in children and adolescents. Pediatrics 63:408–413, 1979

Lamiell JM, Weyanot TB: Mallory–Weiss syndrome in two children. J Pediatr 92:583–584, 1978

Roy CC, Silverman A: Pediatric Clinical Gastroenterology, 3rd ed. St. Louis, CV Mosby, 1983

74

GASTROINTESTINAL BLEEDING: MELENA AND HEMATOCHEZIA

Hematemesis is generally associated with lesions located above the ligament of Treitz. Melena—the passage of black, tarry stools owing to the presence of blood altered by intestinal juices—and hematochezia—the passage of gross blood in the stool—may indicate bleeding in both upper and lower tracts. In fact, melena rather than hematemesis may be a presenting sign of upper tract bleeding. Hematochezia may also indicate brisk bleeding from the upper tract, when the transit time of gastrointestinal contents is short and may not allow the blood to change color.

The amount of blood passed, age of the patient, associated symptoms and condition of the patient, and location of the blood in the stool are important diagnostic considerations. In the past, gastrointestinal bleeding went unexplained in as many as half the cases; at present, with more sophisticated tools such as fiberoptic endoscopy, a definitive diagnosis should be possible more often.

The predominant causes of gastrointestinal bleeding vary with age. Some disorders listed in Chapter 73, Gastrointestinal Bleeding: Hematemesis, are repeated here in order to include the most common causes of bleeding in three age groups. Any disorder causing hematemesis however may also produce melena and hematochezia.

I. **Neonatal Period**
   A. Swallowed Maternal Blood
   B. Hematologic Problems
      1. Thrombocytopenia
      2. Hypoprothrombinemia
      3. Afibrinogenemia
   C. Trauma to Rectum   An anal fissure or more severe internal injuries may result from improper use of a rectal thermometer.

D. Gastroenteritis — Irritation or invasion of the gastrointestinal tract may occur during viral and bacterial infections, with milk allergy, or in isosensitization. Generally small amounts of blood are passed.

E. Necrotizing Enterocolitis — Occurrence is most common on the third to fifth day of life. Vomiting, abdominal distension, temperature instability, lethargy, and apnea are other symptoms. Diarrhea and later red to "currant jelly" stools may follow.

F. Peptic Ulcer

G. Severe Congenital Heart Disease — Ischemia of the bowel may occur with oozing of blood.

H. Midgut Volvulus — Intermittent episodes of bile-stained vomiting generally precede the onset of shock which occurs when the bowel twists on itself.

I. Acute Ulcerative Colitis — This disorder is rare in neonates. Signs include irritability and blood and mucus in the stool.

J. Intestinal Obstruction

K. Sepsis

L. Peritonitis

M. Hypoglycemia

II. Infancy

A. Anal Fissure — Fissure is the leading cause in this age group. Blood generally is present on the outside of the stool and is bright red. Constipation often leads to fissure formation.

B. Enterocolitis and Infectious Diarrheas — The amounts of blood passed are generally small. Fever and diarrhea are often present. Viruses and bacteria (especially *Salmonella*, *Shigella*, and *E. coli*) are the most common causes.

C. Esophagitis — See Chapter 73, Gastrointestinal Bleeding: Hematemesis.

D. Peptic Ulcer

E. Milk Allergy — The passage of small amounts of occult blood is common. Heiner syndrome is characterized by more active bleeding and a shock-like picture.

F. Intussusception — Intussusception must be suspected in the young child with episodic, crampy abdominal pain lasting 5 to 10 minutes during each attack. Vomiting, pallor, and lethargy are usually present. The passage of "currant jelly" stools is a later finding.

G. Meckel Diverticulum

This lesion is characterized by the painless passage of large amounts of bright to dark red blood in a previously well child. Symptoms begin in the first 2 years of life in half of the cases and occasionally may mimic those of appendicitis.

H. Gangrenous Bowel

Interference with the blood supply of the bowel, particularly with venous congestion, will eventually lead to the passage of blood.

I. Duplication of Bowel

This anomaly is particularly likely to be associated with bleeding if ectopic gastric mucosa is present in the duplication. A mass may be palpated on careful abdominal examination.

J. Volvulus

K. Esophageal Varices

L. Hemangiomata of Bowel

Occasionally cutaneous hemangiomas may be clues.

M. Acute Intestinal Ischemia

Clinical features include hematochezia, abdominal distension, and pneumatosis intestinalis. Stenosis of the superior mesenteric artery is a rare cause. Hypotension and necrotizing enterocolitis are other causes.

III. Childhood

A. Juvenile Polyps

The passage of blood, mixed in with the stool or on the outside, is painless; 75% of polyps are within 25 cm of the rectum.

B. Anal Fissures

C. Peptic Ulcers

D. Inflammatory Bowel Disease

   1. Ulcerative Colitis

Most frequent symptoms include loose stools, weight loss, rectal bleeding, abdominal pain, growth failure, tenesmus, arthritis, and uveitis. Onset may be insidious or acute.

   2. Regional Ileitis

Diarrhea, abdominal pain, weight loss, anemia, fever, rectal bleeding, growth failure, and arthritis are the primary symptoms.

E. Esophageal Varices

F. Meckel Diverticulum

G. Blood Dyscrasias
   1. Thrombocytopenia
   2. Leukemia
   3. Hemophilia

H. Intestinal Duplication

I. Hemorrhoids

J. Intestinal Foreign Bodies

K. Lymphosarcoma

L. Henoch–Schönlein Purpura   Rash, abdominal pain, arthritis, and nephritis should suggest this disorder.

IV. Miscellaneous Causes

A. Polyposis   Other types of intestinal polyposis may rarely produce gastrointestinal bleeding.

    1. Familial Polyposis   Inheritance pattern is autosomal dominant, with a high incidence of intestinal carcinoma. Diarrhea is a common early symptom. Polyps may number in the hundreds.

    2. Peutz–Jeghers Syndrome   Polyps are in the upper intestine; melanotic patches occur on the oral mucosa.

B. Hemolytic–Uremic Syndrome   The clinical picture develops after an episode of diarrhea. Affected children present with pallor, edema, and symptoms resembling those of an acute glomerulonephritis. Thrombocytopenia is present along with the hemolytic anemia.

C. Intestinal Parasitism   Blood loss is either occult or small in amount. Diarrhea, abdominal cramps, and weight loss may be present. In the United States, amebiasis, hookworm, and whipworm infestations are the most frequent parasitic causes of blood in the stool.

D. Hemangiomas and Telangiectasias   These disorders are associated usually with painless bleeding. Gastrointestinal hemangiomas may be associated with cutaneous lesions. The Rendu–Osler–Weber syndrome (hereditary hemorrhagic telangiectasia) is an autosomal–dominant disorder associated with mucocutaneous telangiectasia. Cavernous hemangiomas may extend throughout the intestinal submucosa and are commonly associated with cutaneous lesions as well.

E. Nodular Lymphoid Hyperplasia

This disorder is often preceded by an infectious diarrheal disease. Small, sessile, polypoid lesions are found in the colon and rectum. The bleeding is painless and in small amounts.

F. Cryptitis

Inflammation may be caused by constipation or diarrhea. Symptoms include pain on defecation, rectal burning, and tenesmus.

G. Diverticulitis

This disorder, rare in children, may produce a clinical picture of a "left-sided appendicitis."

H. Uremia

I. Scurvy

J. Blunt Injury to the Bowel

Injury to the bowel wall may result in hematomas with associated bleeding into the intestinal lumen.

K. Scorpion Bite

L. Necrotizing Enterocolitis

Older infants and children may also develop this condition. Sudden abdominal distension and pneumatosis intestinalis are other features.

M. Pseudoxanthoma Elasticum

The alteration of elastic tissue in gastrointestinal vessels may lead to bleeding. Skin changes, which are usually not recognizable until the second decade, present as yellowish papules resembling a plucked chicken on the neck, below the clavicles, in the axillae, perineum, and thighs.

N. Chronic Granulomatous Disease (CGD)

Gastric outlet obstruction, resulting from granulomatous inflammation of the antral wall, may be the first clinical manifestation of CGD. Vomiting, anorexia, and poor weight gain are other features.

V. Mimics

It is important to ascertain that the black tarry or bright red stool color is due to blood.

A. Black Stools
  1. Licorice
  2. Bismuth

Peptobismol is a commonly used over-the-counter preparation.

  3. Iron
  4. Charcoal

B. Red Stools
  1. Food Coloring   Kool-aid, Frankenberry cereal, and a host of
     Additives   others may be responsible.
  2. Red Beets
  3. Tomatoes

SUGGESTED READINGS

Berman WF, Holtzapple PG: Gastrointestinal hemorrhage. Pediatr Clin North Am 23:885–895, 1971

Liebman W: Diagnosis and management of upper gastrointestinal hemorrhage in children. Pediatr Ann 5:690–699, 1976

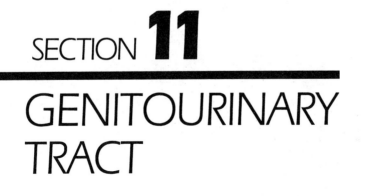

SECTION **11**

GENITOURINARY TRACT

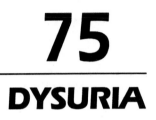

DYSURIA

Painful urination is most frequently attributed to infectious causes. Urethral or perineal irritation, however, may be an even more common cause. The perineum should be closely inspected, the urinary stream observed if possible, and urine obtained for microscopic examination and culture.

I. Infectious Causes

A. Urinary Tract Infection	Bladder infections, usually bacterial in origin, are a common cause of dysuria. Urinary frequency, lower abdominal pain, and enuresis may also be present.
B. Hemorrhagic Cystitis	Onset is usually sudden, with frequency and dysuria. Suprapubic pain, enuresis, and fever are less common. Most cases are thought to be of viral origin.
C. Urethritis	Pain on urination and a urethral discharge suggest gonococcal or chlamydial urethritis.
D. Herpes Simplex	Herpetic lesions in the periurethral area will cause pain on urination.
E. Varicella	Young girls with varicella may have periurethral lesions that are painful on urination. In some cases urinary retention may occur.
F. Renal Tuberculosis	This is a rare cause of dysuria. Most cases are asymptomatic and are discovered during the evaluation of sterile pyuria.
G. Prostatitis	This uncommon disorder may affect adolescent boys. Fever and chills may be associated with low back pain and testicular aching. On rectal examination the prostate is enlarged, boggy, and tender. Gonorrheal organisms are the most common pathogen, but others have been described.
H. Vaginitis	In adolescent girls dysuria in most cases is secondary to a gynecologic infection.

II. Irritation

A. Trauma	Trauma to the perineum may cause urethral irritation and dysuria. The injury may occur

415

after a fall against a bicycle frame or a direct kick to the perineum, or it may follow sexual abuse. Masturbation may cause urethral irritation and transient dysuria. Occasionally, the urethra may be irritated by insertion of a foreign body.

B. Primary Irritant Dermatitis

This condition occurs primarily in infants and young children in diapers. Prolonged contact of the skin with urine or leaching out of detergents from diapers may cause local irritation and pain on urination. Other irritants include perfumes, deodorants, and chemicals found in some soaps, feminine hygiene deodorants, and spermicides.

C. Meatal Ulceration

Infant boys may develop meatal ulcers from contact with diapers.

D. Bubble Bath

Any strong detergent used in bath water may cause a chemical urethritis.

E. Shampoo

Urethritis may be caused by shampoo used to wash the child's hair while the child is sitting in the tub.

F. Diarrhea

Any severe diarrhea may produce local irritation of the perivaginal and periurethral area.

G. Urinary Calculi

Pain on urination may occur during passage of a stone. Hematuria is almost always present.

H. Pinworms

Pinworm infestation is more likely to be a cause in young girls. The pinworms may migrate out of the anus at night and enter the urethra, occasionally causing irritation. Night crying in young girls should suggest the possibility of pinworms, which may be seen upon inspection of the hymenal ring.

I. Meatal Stenosis

True stenosis is a debated cause of dysuria in boys. Splaying of the urinary stream may cause a burning sensation. The meatal opening is a pinhole rather than a slit.

J. Urethral Stricture

Stricture formation may follow trauma or irritation. The quality of the urinary stream should be checked.

III. Miscellaneous Causes

A. Bladder Outlet Obstruction

Symptoms include dysuria, urinary hesitancy, and sometimes dribbling.

B. Bladder Diverticulum

Dysuria, lower abdominal pain, urinary frequency, and difficulty in initiating urination are possible symptoms.

C. Appendicitis	If the inflamed appendix or a periappendiceal abscess lies low in the iliac fossa, urination may be frequent and painful. Any pelvic abscess may produce similar symptoms.
D. Drugs	Various drugs may cause cystitis with resulting dysuria. Amitriptyline hydrochloride, an antidepressant, may cause dysuria and urinary retention.
E. Reiter Disease	Occurrence is uncommon in children. The classic triad of symptoms is arthritis, urethritis, and conjunctivitis.
F. Urethral Prolapse	This disorder has primarily been described in young, black females. A purplish, mulberry-like mass, usually bloody, is found on perineal inspection.
G. Acute Nephritis	Acute glomerulonephritis is rarely associated with dysuria.

76

PYURIA

Pyuria, or the presence of white blood cells in the urine, is frequently equated with a urinary tract infection, either bacterial or nonbacterial. However, a variety of disorders may lead to pyuria. Fever is probably the most common cause of pyuria. True bacterial infection must be documented by a urine culture and colony count.

Pyuria is defined as the presence of 5 or more white blood cells per high-powered field (HPF) of urine; the specimen for examination must be 5 ml carefully collected by the clean-catch method and then centrifuged at 3000 rpm for 3 minutes. Leukocytes from sources other than the urinary tract, such as found in vaginal leukorrhea or balanitis, must not be mistaken for those from the urinary tract.

I. Infection
  A. Urinary Tract Infection
    1. Pyelonephritis — Pyuria cannot be equated with infection; from 20% to 30% of urinary tract infections are *not* associated with pyuria. Pyelonephritis is likely to produce systemic signs such as fever and chills; gastrointestinal symptoms and back pain are common.
    2. Cystitis — Bladder infections may be bacterial or viral. Dysuria and frequency are common complaints.
    3. Renal Abscess
    4. Urethritis — Urethral discharge is typical. Nonspecific urethritis is probably most commonly caused by *Chlamydia* infection.
    5. Tuberculosis — Renal tuberculosis must be considered in cases of sterile pyuria.
    6. Blastomycosis — Disseminated blastomycosis, though rare, may involve the urinary tract.
  B. Systemic Infection
    1. Gastroenteritis — Pyuria may occur in viral infections of the gastrointestinal tract.

2. Other Systemic Infections — Pyuria may be found in other systemic infections, particularly those associated with high fever.

II. Nephropathies

A. Glomerulone-phritis — (See Chap. 77, Hematuria.)

  1. Acute Glomerulonephritis — Hematuria and proteinuria are more prominent, but the number of white blood cells may be increased significantly.

  2. Chronic Glomerulonephritis

  3. Lupus Nephritis

B. Hereditary Disorders

  1. Alport Syndrome — Affected children most commonly present with gross hematuria, especially with intercurrent upper respiratory infections. Striking pyuria may be found. Deafness may occur in late childhood or adolescence.

  2. Nail–Patella Syndrome (Arthro-onychodysplasia) — In this disorder, inherited as an autosomal dominant trait, small or atrophic patellae, nail dysplasia, elbow deformities, and the presence of iliac horns are features. The nephropathy may be benign or progressive, leading to chronic renal insufficiency.

  3. Renal Tubular Acidosis — Permanent distal RTA may have a low level proteinuria and pyuria. The urinary pH is 6.0 to 6.5 with a low blood pH and hyperchloremia. Growth retardation may be the only abnormality. Nephrocalcinosis is almost constant.

  4. Polycystic Kidney Disease — In the infantile form, inherited as an autosomal-recessive trait, early onset with abdominal masses is characteristic.

III. Irritation

A. Chemical Irritation — Urethritis and cystitis may be caused by irritation from strong detergents such as bubble bath.

B. Masturbation — Irritation of the urethra may produce pyuria.

C. Instrumentation

D. Calculi — Stones may be formed in or cause irritation to

various parts of the urinary tract. Hematuria is commonly associated with the pyuria.

IV. Other Causes

A. Fever	Pyuria commonly occurs in febrile states.
B. Dehydration	
C. Urethral Stricture	Only boys are affected. The severity of the stricture usually dictates symptoms such as poor urinary stream, dribbling of urine, and occasionally dysuria.
D. Urinary Tract Tumor	Bladder tumors are rare but may cause pyuria.
E. Lymphoma	Renal involvement may occur, resulting in pyuria and proteinuria, sometimes with palpable kidneys, hypertension, and azotemia.
F. Bladder Diverticuli	
G. Renal Papillary Necrosis	
H. Intramuscular Iron Injection	
I. Oral Polio Vaccine	
J. Sarcoidosis	The kidneys are rarely affected. The extent of renal involvement may be correlated with the degree of hypercalcemia. Cough, weight loss, and chest pain are the most common symptoms.

SUGGESTED READING

Pryles CV, Lustik B: Laboratory diagnosis of urinary tract infection. Pediatr Clin North Am 18:233–244, 1971

77

HEMATURIA

Hematuria, or the presence of blood in the urine, may be gross or microscopic; it may also be symptomatic or asymptomatic. However, the nature of the hematuria may vary during the course of the related disease.

A number of studies of hematuria in children have found prevalence rates of less than 0.5% for both sexes combined. Ingelfinger and colleagues[1] reported gross hematuria in 1.3 per 1000 pediatric emergency room patients. Vehaskari and colleagues[2] screened an unselected population of over 8000 school children and found that in 1.1%, 2 or more urine specimens revealed microscopic hematuria, defined as 6 or more red blood cells (RBC) per 0.9 mm^3 of fresh uncentrifuged midstream urine. Other studies of hematuria in children have used different criteria, such as more than 3 RBC per high-powered field (HPF) of urine centrifuged at 2500 rpm for 5 minutes, with the supernatant poured off leaving 0.2 ml. The use of urine dipsticks may disclose as few as 3 RBC per HPF.

There are a few rules of thumb that can aid in the differentiation of renal from extrarenal causes of hematuria (Table 77-1).

Hematuria without proteinuria does not rule out a renal cause, but a combination of persistent proteinuria and hematuria must be considered presumptive evidence of renal parenchymal disease.

I. Immunologic Injury

A. Acute Glomerulonephritis (Poststreptococcal)	This disorder may follow pharyngeal or skin infection. Streptococcal serum antibody titers are usually elevated. Various signs and symptoms include fever, headache, malaise, ab-

Table 77-1. Differentiating Renal from Extrarenal Causes of Hematuria

	RENAL CAUSES	EXTRARENAL CAUSES
Three-tube Test	Number of RBCs similar in each tube	Increased RBCs in tube I or III
Color	Brown and smoky	Pink or red
RBC Casts	May be present	Absent
Clots	Generally absent	May be present
Pain	Not usually present	May be present
Edema	May be present	Not usually present
Hypertension	May be present	Not usually present

B. Primary Persistent Glomerulonephritis
1. Focal Proliferative
2. Membranous
3. Membranous Proliferative
4. Diffuse Proliferative
5. IgA–IgG Mesangial Nephropathy (Berger)

dominal pain, periorbital edema, and convulsions. (See IIB)
Several types have been described; the clinical picture in one may resemble that in another, so that differentiation is difficult.

C. Henoch–Schönlein Disease

The presence of petechial or purpuric lesions, primarily involving the lower extremities, should suggest this diagnosis. Abdominal pain and arthritis are common features.

D. Collagen–Vascular Diseases
1. Systemic Lupus Erythematosus

Renal involvement occurs eventually in most patients with lupus.

2. Polyarteritis Nodosa

The most common clinical features include fever, signs of cardiac failure, abdominal complaints, and a diffuse maculopapular rash.

E. Subacute Bacterial Endocarditis

The nephritis may be the result of septic emboli or immune complexes. There may be subtle changes in heart sounds or evidence of microembolic phenomena in the skin.

F. Goodpasture Syndrome

The combination of hemoptysis, anemia, and renal disease suggests this disorder.

G. Nephrotic Syndrome

Hematuria is uncommon in NIL disease but is more common in a secondary nephrotic syndrome.

H. "Shunt" Nephritis (Ventriculojugular Shunt Infection)

Immune complexes against bacteria infecting the shunt, usually staphylococcal, may develop. Anemia, splenomegaly, and arthritis may also be present.

I. Wegener Granulomatosis

Renal vasculitis is responsible for the glomerulopathy. Necrotizing granulomas occur in the upper and lower respiratory tract.

II. Infectious Diseases

A. Pyelonephritis (Acute or Chronic) Hematuria is frequently present during active infections.

B. Nephritis Associated with Infection

   1. Bacterial Infections Staphylococcal, pneumococcal, brucellar, and meningococcal infections may be associated with hematuria.

   2. Viral Infections Hepatitis B, mumps, echovirus and Coxsackie virus infections, rubeola, and varicella–zoster are examples.

   3. Other Infections Syphilis, malaria, toxoplasmosis, leptospirosis, and rickettsial infection have been implicated.

C. Renal Tuberculosis This is an uncommon cause but should be considered when sterile pyuria is a finding.

D. Hemorrhagic Cystitis The origin is probably viral. Signs of lower urinary tract infection are common.

E. Urethroprostatitis A tender prostate is found on rectal examination.

F. Chlamydia A urethritis produced by this common, sexually transmitted pathogen, may present with dysuria and hematuria. Small clots in the urine are common.

G. *N. Gonorrhoeae* Macroscopic hematuria, with a purulent urethral discharge and dysuria, may result from the toxic action of this bacterium on the urethral epithelium.

H. Shistosomiasis

III. Familial and Congenital Urinary Tract Disorders

A. Chronic Hereditary Nephritis Various types have been described, some benign and some progressive and fatal. Alport syndrome, inherited as a sex-linked dominant trait, is associated with deafness in 30% to 40% of cases; cataracts are a finding in 10%. Affected men die younger than women of renal failure, but usually do not until the fourth or fifth decade. In cases of unexplained hematuria, urine of family members should be examined.

B. Benign Familial Hematuria Microscopic hematuria, almost always a finding, may become gross with intercurrent systemic infection; proteinuria is unusual. The inheritance pattern is autosomal dominant.

C. Polycystic Disease of the Kidney

   1. Infantile Form — Early death is common. The kidneys are usually easily palpable; liver cysts are common. Inheritance pattern is autosomal recessive.

   2. Adult Form — Onset of symptoms including hypertension may be delayed until after the fourth decade; 10% die in the first decade of cerebral aneurysms. Inheritance pattern is autosomal dominant.

D. Congenital Urinary Tract Abnormalities — Structural aberrations may lead to hematuria. Posterior urethral valves may go unnoticed. Hematuria may occur after trauma in disorders such as hydronephrosis.

E. Nail–Patella Syndrome — Dystrophic nails and absent or hypoplastic patellae are the prominent external signs of this disorder inherited as an autosomal dominant trait. The onset of nephritis is late.

IV. Bleeding or Vascular Disorders

A. Coagulation Disorders

   1. Coagulation Factor Deficiencies

   2. Platelet Deficiencies

B. Hemoglobinopathies

   1. Sickle Cell Trait — Hematuria is uncommon in sickle-cell disease.

   2. Sickle Cell–Hemoglobin C Disease (S–C Disease)

   3. Sickle Cell–Thalassemia Disease

   4. Hemoglobin C Disease

C. Vascular Abnor-
   malities

1. Hemangi- omas	Occasionally cutaneous hemangiomas may also be present.

2. Hereditary
   Hemorrhagic
   Telangiectasia
   (Rendu–
   Osler–Weber
   Syndrome)
	Telltale purplish telangiectasia are found on the skin, particularly the mucous membranes. Inheritance pattern is autosomal dominant.

3. Renal Vein Thrombosis	This is more likely to occur in dehydrated infants or infants of diabetic mothers. Diminished urine output with an enlarging flank mass strongly suggests this diagnosis.

4. Varices of the
   Renal Pelvis
   or Ureter	

V. Neoplastic Disease

A. Renal Neo- plasms	Children with Wilms tumors rarely have hematuria, whereas children with renal cell carcinoma commonly do. The hematuria is usually painless.
B. Leukemia	
C. Bladder Tumors	

VI. Urinary Tract Trauma

A. Direct Trauma	Football, lacrosse, or any contact sport (including many noncontact varieties), as well as accidents, battering, and the like, may cause urinary tract injury and hematuria.
B. Indirect Trauma	Hematuria may follow episodes of shock or anoxia.
C. Renal Stones	Colicky flank pain is characteristic if a stone becomes lodged in a ureter. Bladder stones may otherwise be asymptomatic. The presence of stones may indicate pyelonephritis, structural abnormalities, or cystinuria.
D. Foreign Bodies	Urethral foreign bodies are more common in girls than boys.

E. Meatal or Peri-
   neal Excoria-
   tions
	These lesions are most prevalent in infant boys in diapers.

F. Masturbation	Masturbation may cause microscopic hematuria; sperm are usually present on microscopic examination.
G. Prolapsed Urethra	Inspection reveals a purplish periurethral mass in a young girl.

VII. Drug-Induced Injury

Several drugs must be monitored for their nephrotoxic effects. Hematuria may be related to large doses or long-term therapy with methicillin, sulfonamides, and mercurial diuretics.

VIII. Miscellaneous Causes

A. Exercise	The heavier the exercise, the more likely is the tendency for hematuria. Almost 20% of marathon runners will have microscopic hematuria that clears within 48 hours of the race.
B. Hydronephrosis	Acquired structural anomalies of the urinary tract may also be associated with hematuria.
C. Menstruation	In any postmenarchal girl in whom urinalysis shows hematuria, menstruation is the most likely cause of the spurious presence of heme in the urine.
D. Hemolytic–Uremic Syndrome	This occurs most commonly in young infants, usually following an acute gastroenteritis. Pallor and oliguria are presenting features. Thrombocytopenia and a hemolytic anemia with bizarre-shaped red blood cells on peripheral smear are characteristic.
E. Allergy	Rarely, allergic reactions result in the passage of blood in the urine.
F. Polyps	
G. Congestive Heart Failure	
H. Scurvy	
I. Emotional Factors: Autoerythrocyte Sensitization	This is a bizarre disorder characterized by spontaneous bleeding, especially in the skin, seen primarily in young women with psychological problems.
J. Hypercalcuria	The site and mechanism of injury are not clear. Children with unexplained hematuria should be evaluated for hypercalcuria. Children with juvenile rheumatoid arthritis seem more prone to this problem.
K. Sarcoidosis	

IX. Recurrent Monosymptomatic (Essential, Benign, Idiopathic) Hematuria

Hematuria may be recurrent, especially associated with upper respiratory infections. The etiology is unknown.

X. Mimics of Hematuria

A. Urate Crystals	Urate crystals may precipitate in an acid urine, giving the appearance of a pink sediment.
B. Hemoglobinuria	This may occur with blood dyscrasias, severe infections, burns, or transfusion reactions.
C. Myoglobinuria	Occurrence is most likely in the postinfluenzal syndrome and during malignant hyperthermia.
D. Porphyrinuria	Children with congenital erythrocytic porphyria pass a bright red urine.
E. "Beeturia"	Certain people after ingesting red beets will excrete the coloring in the urine. In children, this usually indicates iron deficiency.
F. Biliuria	
G. Povidone–Iodine (Betadine)	Results of a dipstick test may be positive for blood if this agent is present in the urine.
H. Drugs	Phenytoin, phenothiazines, and pyridium are examples.
I. Food Dye	
J. Red Diaper Syndrome	*Serratia marcescens* in the stool may impart a reddish color to diapers after hours of incubation in the diaper pail.

REFERENCES

1. Ingelfinger JR, Davis AE, Grupe WE: Frequency and etiology of gross hematuria in a general practice setting. Pediatrics 59:557–561, 1977
2. Vehaskari VM, Rapola J, Koskimies O et al: Microscopic hematuria in school children: Epidemiology and clinicopathologic evaluation. J Pediatr 95:676–684, 1979

SUGGESTED READINGS

James JA: Proteinuria and hematuria in children: Diagnosis and assessment. Pediatr Clin North Am 23:807–816, 1976

Kallen RJ: What's causing the hematuria. Contemp Pediatr 3:55–71, 1986

Stapleton FB, Roy S, Noe HN, Jerkins G: Hypercalcuria in children with hematuria. N Engl J Med 310:1345–1348, 1984

West CD: Asymptomatic hematuria and proteinuria in children: Causes and appropriate diagnostic studies. J Pediatr 89:173–182, 1976

78

CHANGES IN URINE COLOR

The color of the urine may range from pale yellow or almost colorless to amber, depending on the amount of liquid ingested and the types of foods eaten. Various dyes in foods and drink and certain drugs and diseases may also cause discoloration of the urine.

This chapter highlights only a few of the causes of discolored urine. A more complete listing can be found in the text by Shirkey.[1]

I. Red Urine
   A. Heme
      1. Hematuria
      2. Hemoglobin-uria   Intravascular hemolysis occurring in various disorders may result in the passage of a pink to red wine urine. The plasma also takes on a pinkish color.
   B. Myoglobinuria   This occurs during muscular necrosis, such as after trauma, ischemia, intense exercise, and ingestion of drugs such as alcohol or barbiturates, and in inflammatory and degenerative diseases of muscle. Characteristic symptoms include muscle weakness, tenderness, and edema.
   C. Urate Crystals   This cause is most prevalent in newborns, but a pinkish sediment of urate crystals may also appear in urine specimens refrigerated for later urinalysis.
   D. Food Pigments
      1. Beets   About 10% of the population will have "beeturia" normally following the ingestion of red beets, but the incidence is greatly increased in children with iron deficiency.
      2. Blackberries
      3. Anthocya-nine   This is a pigment found in berries.
   E. Dyes
      1. Aniline   Aniline dyes are used in candies.
      2. Rhodamine B   This dye is used to color foods and drinks.
      3. Pyridium

4. Phenol-
   phthalein
5. Congo Red

F. Drugs
   1. Pyrvinium
      Pamoate
   2. Phenothia-
      zines
   3. Deferox-   Urine discoloration may occur when serum
      amine (Des-   iron levels are elevated.
      feral)
   4. Methyldopa
      (Aldomet)
   5. Senna

G. Porphyrins   The passage of a pink to red urine may be the
                     first sign of congenital erythropoietic porphy-
                     ria in the neonatal period. Photosensitivity
                     and hirsutism occur later. In all probability the
                     "werewolves" of old probably were afflicted
                     with this malady. Children with other forms
                     of porphyria are less likely to pass red or pink
                     urine.

H. Other Causes
   1. *Serratia mar-* This is a nonpathogenic chromobacterium that
      cescens   produces a red pigment when grown aerobi-
                       cally, particularly on wet diapers (red diaper
                       syndrome).
   2. Biliuria   A reddish yellow color may be present.

II. Green Urine

A. Food Color   Excessive ingestion of Clorets, containing chlo-
                     rophyll, has been reported to produce a green
                     urine.

B. Biliverdin   Biliverdin may be passed in the urine in disor-
                     ders producing chronic obstructive jaundice.

C. Drugs
   1. Amitrypty-
      line Hydro-
      chloride
      (Elavil)
   2. Methocarba-
      mol (Ro-
      baxin)

D. *Pseudomonas*
   Infection

E. Other Causes
   1. Phenol
   2. Resorcinol
   3. Tetrahydro-
      naphthalene
   4. Methylene
      Blue

III. Blue Urine
A. Methylene Blue
B. Triamterene
   (Dyrenium)
C. Doan's Kidney
   Pills
D. Blue Diaper   A bluish discoloration of the diaper may be
   Syndrome   caused by the dye indigotin, an oxidative
                    product of indican, produced in a defect in
                    tryptophan absorption.

IV. Dark Brown or Black Urine
A. Hematuria   Decomposition of hemoglobin to acid hematin
                    results in a Coca–Cola-colored urine.
B. Drugs
   1. Metronida-
      zole (Flagyl)
   2. Nitrofurans
      (Nitrofuran-
      toin [Fura-
      dantin] and
      others)
   3. Methocarba-
      mol (Ro-
      baxin)
   4. Quinine
   5. Phenacetin
C. Dyes   Aniline dyes, used to color candies, may pro-
                    duce a dark urine.
D. Other Causes
   1. Nitrates
   2. Naphthol
   3. Phenols
   4. Rhubarb
   5. Alkaptonuria   Homogentisic acid produces a dark color of
                     the urine only after the specimen stands for
                     hours.

6. Cascara
7. Chlorinated Hydrocarbons
8. Carotene Ingestion of foods containing large amounts produces discoloration.
9. Vitamin B Complex
E. Melanoma Widely disseminated melanoma may result in excretion of a dark urine.

V. Yellow Urine
A. Riboflavin
B. Picric Acid (Trinitrophenol)
C. Jaundice

VI. Orange Urine
A. Sulfisoxazole-Phenazopyridine (Azogantrisin)
B. Pyridium
C. Rifampin

VII. Milky White Urine
A. Pus
B. Phosphate Crystals
C. Chyle

VIII. Purple Urine
Phenolphthalein

REFERENCE

1. Shirkey HC: Drugs that discolor the urine and feces. In Shirkey HC (ed): Pediatric Therapy, pp 163–166. St. Louis, CV Mosby, 1980

SUGGESTED READING

Cone TE Jr: Some syndromes, diseases and conditions associated with abnormal coloration of the urine or diaper. Pediatrics 41:654–658, 1968

79

ENURESIS

Unfortunately the cause of enuresis in most cases is not clear. To the urologist, obstructive disorders of the urinary tract seem the most likely explanation; the psychiatrist may favor an emotional origin. The pediatrician may well subscribe to the theory of developmental delay of bladder control, although the pathophysiologic mechanisms involved are somewhat nebulous.

Each case of enuresis must be evaluated with consideration of the many possible causes, about which a great deal has been written (see the Suggested Reading list for a few examples). A careful history must be obtained, and a thorough physical examination including observation of the urinary stream must be performed.

By $3\frac{1}{2}$ years of age, approximately 75% of children are dry by day and night. At 5 years of age, 10% to 15% of children still wet the bed at night; in 5%, nocturnal enuresis remains a problem at age 10; and at 15 years of age, 1% of children may still be enuretic. Affected boys outnumber girls. There is a strong hereditary background: 32% of fathers and 20% of mothers have a history of enuresis. About two thirds of monozygotic twins are concordant for enuresis; dizygotic twins are likely to be discordant.

Some researchers prefer to separate enuretic children into primary and secondary groups. Primary enuretics are those who never have achieved a period of consistent dryness; secondary enuretics are those who relapse after a period of dryness generally of 6 months or longer. Children with congenital abnormalities resulting in enuresis or those with maturational delay in bladder control are more likely to be primary rather than secondary enuretics.

Despite the long list of possible causes, developmental or maturational delay is responsible for most cases of enuresis. Many organic abnormalities have been suggested as possible causes, but most reports of valves, strictures, contractures, and the like are anecdotal or come from studies that lacked appropriate controls. A history of poor urinary stream, dribbling, daytime incontinence, or urinary tract infection suggests the need for further evaluation.

I. Developmental Delay

Most pediatricians subscribe to this theory, which is supported by hereditary data, the demonstration of small functional bladder capacity, urinary frequency and urgency, and the fact that most children eventually attain control with maturation. Despite the urinary frequency, the 24-hour output of urine is not increased, and the urinary stream and neurologic examination are normal. Although most children in this group have primary enuresis, one fourth to one third have a dry period of several months or more before relapsing; from 10% to 25% also have encopresis.

II. Psychogenic Enuresis

A. Toilet Training — Some cases are felt to be related to pressures experienced by the child around the time of toilet training—either premature training, excessive parental rigidity, associated punishment, or excessive leniency.

B. Emotional Stress — Bladder control may never be attained or may be lost because of various stressful conditions: illness, separation from parents, birth of a sibling, death of a family member, or fear of abandonment.

C. Psychological Disturbances — These are an uncommon cause, but may be a factor in severe cases.

III. Organic Abnormalities

A. Obstructive Lesions

  1. Chronic Constipation — Children with known or unsuspected constipation may have enuresis as well as encopresis. Resolution of the constipation may control the enuresis.

  2. Urethral Valves — A poor urinary stream and dribbling may be findings.

  3. Ectopic Ureters — In girls, dribbling or constant wetting may occur because of vaginal placement of the ureter.

  4. Diverticulum of Anterior Urethra

  5. Urethral Stricture

  6. Meatal Stenosis — There may be no relationship to enuresis, since meatotomy usually does not solve the problem.

  7. Contraction of Bladder Neck

  8. Bladder Diverticuli

9. Prostatic Tumor or Abscess

10. Hydrocolpos or Hematocolpos

Examination may reveal absence of hymenal patency or the presence of a perineal bulge.

11. Labial Atresia

12. Marked Phimosis

B. Neurogenic Disorders

1. Myelomeningocele

2. Sacral Agenesis

3. Occult Neuropathic Bladder

Clinical manifestations include diurnal wetting, encopresis, urinary tract infections, trabeculated bladder, vesicourethral reflux, upper tract deterioration, and "emotional imbalance."[1] The etiology is uncertain, but perhaps this disorder represents one end of the spectrum of developmental delay.

4. Seizures

Incontinence may be a sign of nocturnal seizures, but this is unusual.

5. Spinal Cord Injuries

6. Spinal Cord Tumors

Various types of tumors include gliomas, neurofibromas, teratomas, lipomas, and arteriovenous malformations. Back pain, encopresis, lower extremity weakness, reflex or sensory changes, bony abnormalities of spinal column, or cutaneous abnormalities may be findings

7. Diastematomyelia

There may be cutaneous abnormalities over the spinal column. Low back pain or progressive weakness of legs may be present.

8. Spinal Dysraphism

Fibrous bands, lipomas, septa, or dermal sinuses may cause traction or pressure lesions. Look for discolorations, hair, or lumps over the vertebral column.

C. Infections

1. Urinary Tract Infections

Cystitis, urethritis, or trigonitis may be associated with enuresis, but infection may not be the primary cause.

2. Osteomyelitis of Vertebral Body	Compression of the spinal cord by the infection is the cause.
3. Spinal Epidural Abscess	Exquisite pain over the infected area is the predominant symptom.
D. Disorders Associated with Polyuria and Polydipsia	The possibilities are numerous (see Chap. 18, Polydipsia). Diabetes mellitus or insipidus, sickle-cell anemia, and renal disorders are included in this group.

IV. Miscellaneous Causes

A. Allergies	Some authors believe various allergies, particularly hidden food allergies, are responsible for some cases. Elimination diets, particularly of milk, chocolate, or eggs, may be tried.
B. Obesity	In extremely obese girls, urine may be trapped in the vagina during micturition. Subsequently they may have wetting upon standing.
C. Global Retardation	
D. Obstructive Sleep Apnea	Children who develop hypoxemia as a result of intermittent upper-airway obstruction while sleeping may have enuresis. Snoring with obstructive-type breathing patterns may be the clue.
E. Giggle Micturition	Giggle micturition is an unusual form of incontinence with complete emptying of the bladder brought on by giggling or hearty laughter. The loss of urine is sudden, involuntary, and uncontrollable.

REFERENCE

1. Hinman F: Urinary tract damage in children who wet. Pediatrics 54:142–150, 1974

SUGGESTED READINGS

Cohen MW: Enuresis. Pediatr Clin North Am 22:545–560, 1975

Foxman B, Valdez RB, Brook RH: Childhood enuresis: Prevalence, perceived impact, and prescribed treatments. Pediatrics 77:482–487, 1986

O'Regan S, Yazbeck S, Hamberger B et al: Constipation: A commonly unrecognized cause of enuresis. Am J Dis Child 140:260–261, 1986

80

PRECOCIOUS PUBERTY

Precocious puberty refers to the appearance of signs and symptoms of puberty earlier than expected. In the United States, breast development in girls before 8 years of age and the appearance of pubic hair in boys before 10 years of age are generally considered to be abnormal, and investigation for the underlying cause is recommended.

In this chapter, true isosexual precocity is considered separately from incomplete forms. Sexual precocity is more common in girls than boys, and in most cases it is idiopathic. True sexual precocity in boys is less likely to be idiopathic and demands careful investigation. The Suggested Reading list at the end of this chapter gives a few sources for review of the laboratory methods required for precise definition of the causes of precocity.

Particular attention should be paid to premature thelarche and premature pubarche, which are briefly discussed here. Differentiation of incomplete forms of precocity from true isosexual precocious puberty is mandatory.

I. True Isosexual Precocious Puberty

A. Idiopathic Precocity (Constitutional)

Cryptogenic or idiopathic precocious puberty is a diagnosis of exclusion. In girls it is by far the most common cause, accounting for as many as 80% of the cases. In boys, however, the reverse is true: Only 20% of the cases are idiopathic, and the rest are secondary to underlying central nervous system, adrenal, or other causes. The first sign of pubertal development may be breast development or labial enlargement in the girl, pubic hair in either sex, testicular or phallic enlargement in the boy, and a growth spurt in both sexes. The true incidence of idiopathic precocious puberty is unknown, however, since occult lesions may be found at routine autopsy in these children years later. Occult hypothalamic hamartomas may be responsible for many of these cases. Hung and colleagues[1] have recommended computed tomography in the evaluation of cases in which a cause cannot be found.

B. Disorders of the Central Nervous System

   1. Familial Trait   Premature activation of the hypothalamic-pituitary axis with subsequent stimulation of the gonads occurs in boys but is apparently uncommon in girls.

   2. Tumors   A number of tumors may stimulate the hypothalamic-pituitary-gonadal axis. Neurologic and ophthalmologic signs and symptoms are important clues, but some tumors may be completely asymptomatic. The following tumors may trigger precocious puberty: gliomas, astrocytomas, ependymomas, pinealomas, suprasellar cysts, and craniopharyngiomas. Hamartomas usually produce an early onset of sexual maturation, before 2 years of age; the other tumors usually cause this symptom later. Pineal tumors producing sexual precocity have been described only in boys.

   3. Infections   Precocious puberty may follow central nervous system insults such as encephalitis, tuberculous meningitis, and brain abscesses.

   4. Head Trauma

   5. Hydrocephalus   Various causes of hydrocephalus have been associated with precocious puberty, including congenital syphilis and toxoplasmosis.

   6. Diffuse Cerebral Atrophy

   7. Tuberous Sclerosis   Hypopigmented macules, ash-leaf patches, facial papules (adenoma sebaceum), and seizures are prominent signs of this disorder inherited as an autosomal dominant trait.

   8. Sarcoid Granulomas

C. Adrenal Causes

   1. Tumors   The feminizing effects of adrenal tumors are difficult to differentiate from hypothalamic (idiopathic) precocious puberty. Urinary 17-ketosteroids are increased in both but not suppressed by dexamethasone in adrenal tumors. Adrenal tumors can cause either virilization or feminization of either sex.

   2. Congenital Adrenal Hy-   The virilization of genitalia in boys may not be noticeable at birth but appears later. Affected

perplasia (Adrenogenital Syndrome)

  3. Corticosteroid-Treated Congenital Virilizing Adrenal Hyperplasia

D. Ovarian and Testicular Causes

  1. Ovarian Tumors

  2. Testicular Tumors

  3. Peutz–Jegher Syndrome

E. Miscellaneous Causes

  1. Hypothyroidism

  2. Polyostotic Fibrous Dysplasia (McCune–Albright Syndrome)

girls undergo virilization *in utero* and thus have ambiguous genitalia at birth.

In a number of infant girls who were somewhat virilized and advanced in general development but not treated with glucocorticoids until after infancy, onset of thelarche and menarche was reported to occur early.

These are a rare cause of true isosexual precocity. The tumors generally are responsible for incomplete precocity as a result of estrogen production, with breast enlargement, some nipple development, and vaginal mucosa changes. Ovarian cysts are most common, followed by granulosa or theca cell tumors. Most of these tumors are palpable on bimanual examination. Urinary estrogen levels are greatly increased.

In idiopathic sexual precocity both testes are enlarged. Unilateral enlargement suggests a Leydig cell tumor. Virilizing adrenal hyperplasia is usually associated with small testes, but adrenal rests of aberrant tissue may cause bilateral enlargement in some of these cases.

The presence of ovarian tumors has been described in several patients. Some males have had Sertoli cell tumors. Oral melanosis and intestinal polyposis are the clues.

Severe congenital hypothyroidism may be associated with sexual precocity and galactorrhea in girls. The clinical signs of hypothyroidism are usually obvious.

This syndrome, often associated with precocious puberty, features bony lesions, often causing bending or bowing of limbs, abnormal gait, or pathologic fractures, and large patches of skin pigmentation with an irregular border. In girls the first sign of precocious puberty may be menarche. In boys, the development

	of precocious puberty rarely begins before 8 years of age.
3. Russell–Silver Syndrome	Low birth weight, short stature, a triangular face, and a large-appearing head are characteristic. Asymmetry and the early onset of puberty have been reported.
4. Exogenous Hormones	Estrogens in contraceptive pills, foods, medications, and even hand creams contaminated by estrogens, have been implicated. Increased pigmentation of the areolae and external genitalia is a common finding.
5. Gonadotropin-Producing Tumors	
a. Hepatoblastoma	This tumor is seen only in boys with precocious puberty. Physical findings include an enlarged liver that is sometimes nodular, phallic and muscular enlargement, and advanced skeletal growth, with little or no testicular enlargement.
b. Chorioepitheliomas	These rare but highly malignant tumors produce large amounts of gonadotropic substances.
c. Teratoma	Reported tumors have been presacral in location, and some have produced increased chorionic gonadotropins.
6. Neurofibromatosis (Von Recklinghausen Disease)	Hypothalamic gliomas associated with neurofibromatosis may cause precocious puberty. The presence of 6 or more smooth-edged café-au-lait spots is an important skin clue.

II. Premature Thelarche

This benign disorder usually occurs before 4 years of age and may be unilateral or bilateral. It is not accompanied by other signs of puberty. The bone age is not advanced, urinary 17-ketosteroid excretion is not increased, gonadotropins are low or absent, and the vaginal smear shows no estrogen effect. The breast enlargement is nonprogressive and may regress. The onset of puberty is not advanced. Premature thelarche must be differentiated from true precocious puberty, ovarian cysts, and ovarian tumors, which are associated with other estrogen effects.

III. Premature Pubarche (Adrenarche)

This disorder predominantly occurs in girls and is occasionally associated with mental deficiency or preceding cerebral damage. It is defined as the appearance of pubic or axillary hair without other signs of virilization or feminization before the age of 8 years. The bone age and height age are slightly advanced, and urinary 17-ketosteroid levels are slightly high. Pregnanetriol and gonadotropic hormones are not found in the urine. This disorder must be differentiated from true precocious puberty or if clitoral enlargement is present, from congenital adrenal hyperplasia, adrenal carcinoma, or a virilizing ovarian tumor.

IV. Incomplete Sexual Precocity

A. Feminizing Disorders
    1. Ovarian Cysts — Ovarian cysts may enlarge and produce enough estrogen to induce signs of feminization, usually breast enlargement, nipple development, and vaginal mucosal effects.
    2. Granulosa or Theca Cell Tumors — These rare tumors produce estrogen. The majority are palpable on bimanual examination.
    3. Rare Sources of Estrogen — Gonadoblastomas, lipoid tumors, cystadenomas, and ovarian carcinomas are examples.
    4. Exogenous Estrogens

B. Disorders with Virilization — Both ovarian and adrenal disorders may promote incomplete sexual precocity with virilization.
    1. Ovarian Tumors — Arrhenoblastoma, lipoid tumors, cystadenomas, ovarian carcinomas, and gonadoblastomas are examples.
    2. Adrenal Carcinoma — Signs of glucocorticoid excess may also be present with growth failure, obesity, moon facies, and other cushingoid features. Urinary excretion of 17-ketosteroids and pregnanetriol is not suppressed by dexamethasone.
    3. Congenital Adrenal Hyperplasia (Adrenogenital Syndrome)

REFERENCE

1. Hung W, August GP, Brallier DR et al: Computerized tomography in the evaluation of isosexual precocity. Am J Dis Child 134:25–27, 1980

SUGGESTED READINGS

Moore DC, Sizonenko PC, Ferrier PE: Disorders of sexual maturation. In Kelley VC (ed): Practice of Pediatrics, Vol 7, Chap 54, pp 1–44. Hagerstown, Harper & Row, 1987

Styne DM, Kaplan SL: Normal and abnormal puberty in the female. Pediatr Clin North Am 26:123–148, 1979

81

PUBERTAL DELAY

Puberty is considered to be delayed when there are no signs of sexual development at 12 to 13 years of age in girls or at 13 to 14 years of age in boys. An abnormality in pubertal development should also be considered if more than 5 years has elapsed between the onset of breast development and the occurrence of menarche in girls or between the start of enlargement of testes in boys and the completion of genital growth.

Delayed puberty is more common in boys than in girls and is usually a result of constitutional delay; a family history of a similar delay is especially helpful in making this diagnosis. In girls with pubertal delay a demonstrable cause, such as X chromosomal abnormalities, is likely to be found. Chronic systemic diseases also frequently result in a delay of sexual development.

I. Constitutional Delay

Constitutional or physiologic delay of sexual development is the most common cause of pubertal delay in boys. The diagnosis is one of exclusion; a history of similar delay in other family members is helpful. The hypothalamus and pituitary fail to stimulate gonadal development.

II. Gonadal Defects

A. Chromosomal Abnormalities

1. Turner Syndrome and X Chromosomal Abnormalities	These are the most common causes of hypogonadism and delayed adolescence in girls; probably mosaics are more common than the 45X karyotype. There is a great variation in the phenotypic picture such as webbed neck, shield chest, high-arched palate, cubitus valgus, and multiple nevi. Girls with an XO karyotype are rarely taller than 63 inches.
2. Klinefelter Syndrome (XXY Karyotype)	Diagnosis is rarely possible before puberty because there is no characteristic phenotype. This disorder should be suspected in boys with pubertal delay who are tall with euchnoid proportions and have gynecomastia and

small, atrophic testes (less than 2 cm in
length).

3. Mixed Go-
nadal Dys-
genesis (45X/
46XY Karyo-
type)

Affected children usually present at puberty
with an unmasculinized Turner syndrome
phenotype or some sexual ambiguity.

B. Prepubertal Cas-
tration

1. Congenital
Anorchia

The testes are absent.

2. Testicular
Atrophy

This may occur *in utero* or following testicular
torsion or hemorrhage before puberty.

3. Ovarian At-
rophy

This condition may be associated with other
endocrinopathies such as Hashimoto thyroiditis, Addison disease, and hypoparathyroidism
or may be the result of ovarian trauma.

C. Swyer Syn-
drome

The phenotype is female with a 46XY karyotype. Streak gonads are present. The disorder
is inherited as an X-linked recessive trait.

D. Reifenstein Syn-
drome

Testicular hypoplasia and sclerosis with gynecomastia at adolescence and a variable degree
of hypospadias are features.

E. Cytotoxic Drugs

The gonads may be damaged by cytotoxic
agents used in the treatment of neoplasia,
blood disorders, or collagen–vascular diseases.

III. Pituitary Defects

A. Pituitary Dys-
genesis

Other features of panhypopituitarism are
present long before pubertal delay becomes a
concern.

B. Pituitary Tu-
mors

C. Functional De-
fects

There may be complete failure of production
of gonadotropic hormones.

IV. Hypothalamic Defects

A. Congenital
Anomalies

1. Kallmann
Syndrome

This disorder represents a familial metabolic
defect of gonadotropin-releasing factor. Key
features include a decreased or absent sense of
smell and, in some cases, a complaint of inability to taste. There is a family history of
infertility.

2. Septo-Optic Dysplasia	Midline malformations may be associated with hypothalamic-pituitary deficiencies. The septum pellucidum may be absent, and optic dysplasia may be present. Vision is often impaired.
3. Encephalocele	Hypothalamic structures may be involved.
4. Congenital Hydrocephalus	
B. Hypothalamic Tumors	
1. Craniopharyngioma	Usual features include growth failure, symptoms of increased intracranial pressure, and visual disturbances.
2. Gliomas of the Optic Chiasm	
3. Histiocytosis X	Diabetes insipidus and growth failure are more notable than eventual sexual infantilism.
4. Other Tumors	
C. Hypothalamic Trauma	Injuries to the hypothalamus may occur as a result of blunt trauma to the head, hemorrhage, or infection.

V. Other Endocrinopathies

A. Hypothyroidism	This is an uncommon cause of delayed puberty. Growth failure and delayed bone age are common.
B. Congenital Adrenal Hyperplasia (Adrenogenital Syndrome)	Deficiency of 17-α-hydroxylase is associated with gonadal failure and hypertension.
C. Addison Disease	
D. Cushing Syndrome	

VI. Chronic Disease

Any chronic disease may potentially be associated with a delay in pubertal development.
  A. Chronic Malnutrition

    B. Anorexia Nervosa
    C. Celiac Disease
    D. Inflammatory Bowel Diseases
    E. Chronic Pulmonary Disorders
    F. Chronic Renal Failure
    G. Neoplasia
    H. Collagen–Vascular Disorders
    I. Hemoglobinopathies
    J. Sickle-Cell Disease

VII. Failure to Reach Menarche

    A. Testicular Feminization — The karyotype is 46XY, but the testes fail to respond. The phenotype is female with good breast development but little or no axillary or pubic hair. The vagina is short. Inguinal hernias may contain testes. The usual presenting complaint is failure to reach menarche.

    B. Polycystic Ovary Disease

    C. Anatomic Defects
        1. Imperforate Hymen
        2. Transverse Vaginal Septum
        3. Congenital Absence of Uterus — Renal, skeletal, and cardiac anomalies may also be present.

VIII. Miscellaneous Disorders

    A. Prader–Willi Syndrome — Short stature, hypotonia, hypogonadism, and obesity are the characteristic features.

    B. Laurence–Moon–Biedl Syndrome — This disorder inherited as an autosomal-recessive trait is characterized by short stature, polydactyly, obesity, mental retardation, and retinitis pigmentosa.

C. Pseudopseudo-
hypoparathy-
roidism
    Obesity, mental retardation, delayed puberty, short hands, and round facies are present.

D. Fabry Disease
(Angiokeratoma
Corporis Diffu-
sum)
    This is a rare disorder with progressive symptoms and signs including hypertension, renal disease, seizures, and crises of excruciating extremity pains. Angiokeratomas (tiny angiomas) become diffuse on the skin.

SUGGESTED READINGS

Frasier SD: Pediatric Endocrinology. New York, Grune & Stratton, 1980

Reindollar RH, McDonough PG: Etiology and evaluation of delayed sexual development. Pediatr Clin North Am 28:267–286, 1981

Styne DM, Kaplan SL: Normal and abnormal puberty in the female. Pediatr Clin North Am 26:123–148, 1979

82

AMENORRHEA

As a symptom, amenorrhea reflects an underlying pathologic process. It is also a normal state for the first 10 to 16 years of life. Some adolescents who visit pediatricians with concern over the failure to reach menarche simply have a physiologic delay in beginning menstruation, which may be familial. Attention to details of secondary sexual development is important in determining whether this delay is physiologic. Other adolescents may have experienced menarche but have not had another period for 4 to 6 months; here again the cause may be physiologic, anovulatory menstrual cycles.

Amenorrhea may be primary or secondary. In the evaluation of primary amenorrhea, it is important to distinguish patients with full development of secondary sexual characteristics from those with a prepubertal appearance: Girls who fail to show any development of secondary sexual characteristics by 14 years of age require investigation for endocrine, chromosomal or hypothalamic-pituitary problems, whereas, adolescents who have attained full secondary sexual development without the onset of menstruation within a year or so should have a careful examination for anatomic causes of menstrual failure.

Secondary amenorrhea is a far more common complaint than primary amenorrhea. Irregular menstrual periods are common for the first few years after menarche because of anovulatory cycles. Psychogenic interference with hypothalamic function is also a common cause of missed periods. Various stresses, depression, and dietary misadventures may result in secondary amenorrhea. Naturally of great concern to the parents is the fear of pregnancy as the cause.

In this chapter, pathologic conditions that should be considered in the differential diagnosis have been divided into those causing primary and secondary amenorrhea.

I. Primary Amenorrhea
    A. Physiologic Causes

1. Delayed Menarche	Menarche may occur normally between 10 and 16 years of age. Failure to show any signs of pubertal development by 14 years of age requires investigation, however. Anatomic causes should be suspected in the adolescent

who has attained full breast and pubic hair development without menarche within the next year. Examination for other signs of normal pubertal development is often helpful in determining whether the delay in menarche is physiologic. A family history of similar delays in the mother, aunts, or siblings is obviously important.

2. Pregnancy

Although uncommon, pregnancy as a cause of primary amenorrhea must also be considered in the sexually active adolescent.

B. Anatomic Causes

If the secondary sexual development is complete, anatomic causes of failure to menstruate must be considered first.

1. Imperforate Hymen

The typical complaint is lower abdominal pain, sometimes at monthly intervals, in a 14- or 15-year-old. There also may be urinary difficulties. A bluish bulge may be seen when the labia are separated.

2. Vaginal Atresia

In the Mayer–Rokitansky–Kuster–Hauser syndrome the uterus varies from normal to streak, to complete absence. Ovarian function is normal. Associations with renal, skeletal, and other anomalies are frequent.

3. Congenital Atresia of Cervix

4. Absent Uterus

C. Chromosomal Abnormalities

1. Turner Syndrome

The classic phenotype, with short stature, webbed neck, shield chest, increased carrying angle of the arms, short fourth and fifth metacarpals, increased nevi, and a history of lymphedema at birth, is difficult to miss. Most cases are not so well defined. Short stature in an adolescent with deficient sexual development indicates the need for chromosomal studies.

2. Turner Syndrome Variants

The clinical picture may range from that of Turner syndrome, to some degree of masculinization, to a normal female appearance.

a. Mosaics

b. X Chromosomal Abnormalities

      c. Balanced X Autosomal Translocations

D. Gonadal Problems

1. Pure Gonadal Dysgenesis	Secondary sexual maturation is delayed or absent. Affected girls may be tall. On laparoscopy only gonadal streaks are found.
2. Resistant Ovaries Syndrome	Although lutenizing hormone (LH) and follicle-stimulating hormone (FSH) levels are increased, the ovarian follicles fail to respond. Ovarian biopsy is required to distinguish this disorder from pure gonadal dysgenesis.
3. Testicular Feminization	Affected children are phenotypic "females" with an XY karyotype. They have excellent breast development but infantile nipples, absent pubic and axillary hair, a short, blind vagina, and an absent or rudimentary uterus. There is often a positive family history on the maternal side.
4. Incomplete Testicular Feminization	Here there is also an XY karyotype, but hirsutism, clitoral enlargement, and absence of breast development are features.
5. True Hermaphroditism	Most affected children have some virilization, usually incomplete, and are raised as boys. Breasts develop at puberty.
6. Ovarian Tumors	Granulosa cell tumors secrete estrogens at a high level that is constant. Androgen-producing tumors are associated with virilization.
7. Stein–Leventhal Syndrome	The amenorrhea is usually secondary.
8. Ovarian Failure	This disorder may follow radiation treatment for an abdominal malignancy in infancy or childhood or the use of chemotherapy.

E. Hypothalamic-Pituitary Causes

    1. Congenital Disorders

a. Panhypopituitarism	Sexual infantilism, as well as growth deficiency and evidence of other endocrine deficiencies, usually suggests this disorder before delayed menarche becomes a concern.
b. Laurence–Moon–Biedl Syndrome	Features include obesity, mental deficiency, polydactyly or syndactyly, retinal pigmentation, and hypogonadism with genital hypoplasia.

c. Prader–Willi Syndrome	Hypotonia, obesity, short stature, retardation, and small hands and feet are characteristic features.
d. Hypogonadotropic Hypogonadism	This disorder produces sexual infantilism with normal or increased height; plasma levels of luteinizing hormone are low. It may occur alone or be associated with a, b, or c above.
e. Olfactogenital Syndrome	In this form of hypogonadotropic hypogonadism, the sense of smell is decreased or absent.

2. Acquired Disorders

Suprasellar of Infrasellar Tumors	Craniopharyngiomas, gliomas, and other tumors are rare causes of primary amenorrhea. Visual field defects, symptoms of diabetes insipidus, lethargy, and rarely obesity may be additional features.

3. Psychogenic Amenorrhea

a. Stress	Reactions to stress of various types may involve primary but more commonly secondary amenorrhea. Depression over family conflicts, moves, school, and so forth may delay the onset of menses.
b. Anorexia Nervosa	
c. Obesity	For unexplained reasons, marked obesity may be associated with amenorrhea.

F. Endocrine Disorders

1. Congenital Adrenal Hyperplasia (Adrenogenital Syndrome)	Affected children may have a partial defect in adrenal steroid synthesis and may develop clitoromegaly and subsequent virilization at puberty.
2. Hypothyroidism	This condition is more likely to produce menstrual irregularities rather than amenorrhea.
3. Hyperthyroidism	Hyperthyroidism resulting from toxic goiter is more often associated with amenorrhea than with menstrual irregularities.
4. Diabetes Mellitus	Long-standing, untreated diabetes mellitus with growth failure is now rare.
5. Cushing Syndrome	Truncal obesity, hypertension, and a falling-off of growth velocity are among the preceding symptoms and signs.

6. Addison Disease	Symptoms may suggest anorexia nervosa, but the presence of lethargy and fatigue accompanied by hyperpigmentation of the skin should alert the physician to this possibility.

G. Other Causes

1. Chronic Debilitating Disease	Various chronic diseases may affect menarche. Among the more common disorders are Crohn disease, chronic liver disease, and celiac disease.
2. Autoimmune Disorders	Rarely, the ovary may be affected by the production of antibodies directed against it, resulting in amenorrhea. There may also be associated adrenal or parathyroid antibodies.

II. Secondary Amenorrhea

A. Physiologic Causes

1. Anovulatory Cycles	Menstrual irregularity is common during the first few years after menarche. Delays between periods may range up to 6 months.
2. Pregnancy	Pregnancy must always be considered, especially in the sexually active adolescent. A urine test for pregnancy is a quick screening method.

B. Hypothalamic-Pituitary Causes

1. Psychogenic Factors	Emotional factors are common causes of secondary amenorrhea. Depression from moves, family disruption, separation from home, and so forth may be associated with menstrual failure.
2. Anorexia Nervosa	
3. "Crash" Diets	
4. Pseudocyesis	There may be all the signs of pregnancy without positive results of a pregnancy test or enlargement of the uterus as seen on ultrasonogram.
5. Tumors	Tumors are a rare cause of secondary amenorrhea. The presence of galactorrhea, however, should suggest a pituitary tumor.
6. Pituitary Failure	Hypopituitarism may result from infarction of the pituitary gland.

C. Gonadal Disorders

1. Ovarian Neoplasms	Granulosa cell tumors may keep estrogen levels constantly high, preventing sloughing of

the endometrium. Androgen-producing tumors produce increasing signs of virilization.

2. Stein–Leventhal Syndrome (Polycystic Ovary Disease)

Half of the women with this syndrome present with amenorrhea. Infertility is a more common initial complaint. Obesity, virilization, and hirsutism are common. the LH/FSH ratio is greater than 2.5/1.

3. Premature Ovarian Failure

This is an unusual cause of secondary amenorrhea. Premenopausal symptoms may be present.

4. Autoimmune Disease

Antibodies directed against the ovary may be responsible for the development of amenorrhea. Other endocrine glands may also be affected.

D. Endocrine Disorders

1. Thyroid Disorders

Hyperthyroidism is much more likely than hypothyroidism to be associated with amenorrhea.

2. Adrenal Disorders

Hypoadrenocorticism (Addison disease) and excessive production of corticosteroids (as in Cushing syndrome) are uncommon causes of amenorrhea.

E. Miscellaneous Causes

1. Systemic Illness

Chronic, severe, and debilitating illnesses often may be associated with cessation of menstrual periods.

2. Uterine Infections

Severe infections of the endometrial cavity may result in scarring or the formation of synechiae.

3. Oral Contraceptives

Amenorrhea may follow cessation of oral contraceptives, particularly in young women who began taking these hormones before normal hypothalamic rhythm had been established.

4. Obesity

The cause of amenorrhea in obese adolescents has not been well defined. In some cases depression over a poor body image may affect hypothalamic centers.

5. Chiari–Frommel Syndrome

This unusual and poorly explained disorder occurs in the postpartum period and is characterized by amenorrhea and persistent galactorrhea. Affected women are usually moderately obese and slightly hirsute.

SUGGESTED READINGS

DeKoos EB: Primary amenorrhea. Pediatr Ann 4:12–25, 1975

Dewhurst CJ: Amenorrhoea and the paediatrician. Pediatr Clin North Am 19:605–618, 1972

Emans SJH, Goldstein DP: Pediatric and Adolescent Gynecology, 2nd ed. Boston, Little, Brown & Co, 1982

Grodin JM: Secondary amenorrhea in the adolescent. Pediatr Clin North Am 19:619–630, 1972

83

ABNORMAL VAGINAL BLEEDING

Vaginal bleeding may be the result of physiologic alterations or indicative of significant pathology. In the newborn period, withdrawal of maternal hormones is the most common cause, whereas in adolescence dysfunctional uterine bleeding accounts for most cases. Premenarchal children with vaginal bleeding almost never have functional causes.

I. Neonatal—Maternal Hormones

Vaginal bleeding, usually spotty, is a relatively common phenomenon in newborns following withdrawal of maternal hormones. Estrogen effects such as hypertrophy of the labia minora and leukorrhea are almost universally present in newborn females.

II. Preadolescent Vaginal Bleeding

A. Foreign Bodies	A foul-smelling, bloody discharge should raise the possibility of a foreign body. Occasionally, material may be milked from the vagina by a rectal examination.
B. Trauma	Vaginal lacerations may occur as a result of injuries, such as falls or by masturbation; but sexual abuse must always be considered.
C. Urethral Prolapse	Careful perineal examination should disclose a mulberry-like hemorrhagic mass surrounding the urethral opening.
D. Excoriations	Pruritus may lead to scratching severe enough to cause bleeding of the vulvar mucosa.
E. Infections	See the section on vulvovaginitis (Chap. 84).
F. Pinworms	Rarely, significant infestation of the vagina may cause vaginal irritation and bleeding.
G. Precocious Puberty	Functional vaginal bleeding may be the result of true sexual precocity. Other signs of sexual development should be noted.
H. Sarcoma Botryoides	A rare malignant rhabdomyosarcoma that can involve the vagina, cervix, uterus, or bladder. A polypoid, grapelike mass is found on exami-

nation. This tumor is rarely found in the vagina beyond childhood.

III. Adolescent Vaginal Bleeding

A. Dysfunctional Uterine Bleeding (DUB)

The vast majority of abnormal vaginal bleeding in adolescents is due to DUB, but other causes must always be considered. DUB is defined as bleeding that occurs in cycles <20 days or >40 days; lasts longer than 8 days; has blood loss >80 ml; or is associated with anemia.

The cause is thought to be a failure of feedback resulting in estrogen stimulation of the endometrium unopposed by progesterone. Anovulatory cycles are common in the perimenarchal age group.

B. Pregnancy

A pregnancy test should be performed in any teenager who has reached Tanner stage III despite denial of sexual activity. Twenty percent of pregnancies are associated with some bleeding, but incomplete or threatened abortions, ectopic pregnancy, molar pregnancy, or complications of legal or illegal abortions must always be considered.

C. Trauma

Vaginal lacerations may be secondary to sexual abuse, rape, or masturbation.

D. Foreign Bodies

Tampons, diaphragms, contraceptive sponges, and other materials retained in the vagina may lead to chronic irritation and bleeding, usually accompanied by a foul discharge.

E. Infections
  1. Trichomonas
  2. Chlamydia
  3. Gonorrhea

Cervical friability or endometritis may lead to spotting in pelvic inflammatory disease.

F. Medications
  1. Contraceptives

Mid-cycle bleeding is relatively common with oral contraceptives. Break-through bleeding occurs with missed doses. Intrauterine contraceptives should not be used in adolescents.

  2. Other

Anticoagulants, gonadal and adrenal steroids, reserpine, phenothiazines, monoamine, oxidase inhibitors, morphine, and anti-cholinergic medications have been associated with bleeding.

3. Salicylates — Decreased platelet adhesiveness secondary to salicylates may result in prolonged or heavy menstrual periods.

G. Bleeding Disorders — Consider this group strongly if anemia is present.
  1. Thrombocytopenia — Thrombocytopenia may be hereditary or acquired.
  2. Von Willebrand Disease
  3. Factor IX Deficiency
H. Cervical Problems
  1. Cervical Polyp
  2. Hemangioma
  3. Cervical Friability — This may occur in an area of squamous metaplasia.
I. Uterine Myomas — Uterine myomas are unusual in adolescents.
J. Ovarian Disorders
  1. Functional Ovarian Cysts — Most functional ovarian cysts are follicular and represent failures of ovulation.
  2. Corpus Luteum Cyst — This cyst may mimic an ectopic pregnancy by presenting with amenorrhea and an adrenal mass followed by vaginal bleeding and abdominal pain on rupture of the cyst.
  3. Ovarian Tumors — Careful palpation for abdominal masses should be performed.
  4. Polycystic Ovary Disease — Amenorrhea is a much more common problem, but a significant amount of functional uterine bleeding occurs. Obesity, hirsutism, and virilization are other findings.

K. Hypothalamic-Pituitary-Gonadal Dysfunction
  1. Chronic Illness — Chronic illness often causes amenorrhea but may be associated with abnormal frequency or amounts of bleeding.
  2. Other — Emotional stress, eating disorders, crash diets, obesity, and exercise generally result in amenorrhea, but abnormal bleeding may also occur.
  3. Prolactinoma — Prolactinoma is the most common pituitary tumor associated with menstrual irregularities. The first sign is irregular bleeding followed by oligomenorrhea and then amenorrhea.

L. Adrenal Disorders
    1. Addison Disease — Abnormal vaginal bleeding occurs in about one quarter of the cases.
    2. Congenital Adrenal Hyperplasia — Abnormal bleeding may occur in late onset disease or in previously diagnosed patients who are noncompliant with replacement steroid medications.

M. Thyroid Disorders
    1. Hyperthyroidism
    2. Hypothyroidism — Excessive bleeding may be the first sign.

N. Miscellaneous
    1. Endometriosis — Although cyclic or acyclic pain, bladder dysfunction, gastrointestinal distress, and dyspareunia are more common symptoms, irregular bleeding may be a presentation.
    2. Diethylstilbestrol — Estrogens used in mothers to suppress abortion may have caused changes in the fetus that later can present as bleeding. Cervical adenosis occurs in as many as 35% of exposed female fetuses. Adenocarcinoma is much rarer.

SUGGESTED READINGS

Anderson MM, Irwin CE Jr, Snyder DL: Abnormal vaginal bleeding in adolescents. Pediatr Ann 15:697–707, 1986
Litt IF: Menstrual problems during adolescence. Pediatr Rev 4:203–212, 1983

84

VAGINAL DISCHARGE AND VULVOVAGINITIS

The most common gynecologic complaint in childhood is a vaginal discharge or irritation and pruritus of the vulvar area. Normal physiologic leukorrhea of the premenarchal adolescent must be differentiated from pathologic conditions such as irritative and infectious causes of vulvovaginitis.

The most common cause of vulvovaginitis is a nonspecific bacterial infection. Nonspecific means that a mixture of organisms, particularly coliform bacteria, are cultured from the vaginal smear. This type of infection often follows a primary irritative problem with the secondary introduction of bacteria from the anal area. Specific bacterial infections such as streptococcal or gonococcal, among others, may also be found. The presence of a bloody vaginal discharge, particularly if malodorous, strongly indicates the presence of a foreign body. A careful history may suggest causes of irritation.

I. Physiologic Leukorrhea

The discharge is clear to whitish and mucoid; it is nonirritating and reflects the response of the cervix to rising estrogen levels. On Gram stain many epithelial cells but no bacteria are found.

A. Neonatal Leukorrhea	Most newborn female infants have a thick discharge as a result of maternal estrogen effect.
B. Pubertal Leukorrhea	Onset of the discharge is usually a few months before menarche.
C. Precocious Puberty	

II. Irritation

A. Foreign Body	If the foreign material remains in the vagina long enough, the discharge will become malodorous and bloody. Wads of toilet paper are the most frequent foreign bodies found in prepubertal children and forgotten tampons in postpubertal adolescents.
B. Chemicals	Bubble bath, various soaps, colored toilet paper, and feminine deodorant sprays may be irritating to the perineal area.

C. Tight Undergarments — Particularly synthetic fabrics such as nylon that do not absorb secretions may cause irritation or promote bacterial or fungal overgrowth.

D. Masturbation — Excoriations or irritation from masturbatory activity may lead to secondary infection.

E. Poison Ivy

F. Neurodermatitis; Atopic Dermatitis; Seborrheic Dermatitis — Pruritus producing scratching may lead to lichenification, continuing the itch–scratch–itch cycle, and may predispose to secondary infection.

G. Drug Reactions — Local and rarely systemic reactions to drugs may produce a discharge. Drugs such as Mycolog, used for "diaper dermatitis," may produce local sensitization to its many ingredients.

H. Psoriasis — Local irritation may be the result of "napkin psoriasis."

I. "Sandbox" Vaginitis — Little girls sitting and playing in sand or dirt may develop irritation from particulate matter trapped in the vagina.

J. Sexual Abuse — Chronic irritation may be the result of unsuspected sexual molestation.

K. Scabies

L. Obesity — Trapping of urine, resulting in reflux into the vagina, may cause a chronic irritation.

M. Lichen Sclerosis et Atrophicus — An ivory white, atrophic, hour-glass appearance in the perineum should suggest this diagnosis. Pruritus is frequently present.

III. Infection

A. Nonspecific Vaginitis — This disorder most likely represents a mixed infection with coliforms, streptococci, *Hemophilus vaginalis,* and other bacteria; it is the most common cause of pathologic vaginal discharge in prepubertal children. The discharge is usually gray and malodorous but is generally nonirritating and nonpruritic.

B. Gonococcal Infection — The vaginal discharge is thick and purulent; dysuria is often present. Although it is most common in the postpubertal age group, young children may be infected as well.

C. β-Hemolytic Streptococcal Infection — The infection may or may not be associated with a pharyngeal streptococcal infection.

D. Shigella   Diarrhea is uncommon. Most affected children do not have pain, pruritus, or dysuria; almost one half have a bloody discharge.

E. Diphtheria   The infection may be primary but is usually secondary to nasopharyngeal infection. A thick, whitish gray adherent membrane may be seen.

F. Mycoplasma   Consider this diagnosis if routine cultures are negative.

G. Other Bacteria   *S. pneumoniae, N. menigitidis, S. aureus, H. influenzae,* and *Yersinia* have also been implicated. *Gardnerella vaginalis* is more likely to be found in an adolescent who presents with a profuse, pruritic, and often foul-smelling vaginal discharge.

H. Syphilitic   Chancres or luetic condylomata are possible causes.

I. Herpes Simplex   Grouped vesicles and ulcers should suggest this diagnosis.

J. Moniliasis   Predisposing factors include removal of normal flora by systemic antibiotics, increased heat and moisture in the perineum due to tight-fitting undergarments, diabetes mellitus, and oral contraceptives. The vulvae are erythematous, pruritic, and irritated, and a white, cheesy discharge is present.

K. Trichomoniasis   Postmenarchal girls are those usually affected. The discharge is frothy and profuse with local erythema.

L. Chlamydia   This organism must be considered in any nonspecific discharge.

M. Pinworms   The tiny ubiquitous thread-like worms do not in themselves cause a vulvovaginitis, but the associated pruritus causes scratching and the transferral of bacteria from the perineum to the vulva.

IV. Discharge Associated with Systemic Illness
Several systemic illnesses may be associated with a vaginal discharge.
  A. Measles
  B. Scarlet Fever
  C. Varicella
  D. Typhoid
  E. Smallpox

V. Anatomic Abnormalities

Abnormalities may introduce bacteria or allow bacterial overgrowth.

A. Rectovaginal Fistula

B. Labial Agglutination   Fusion of the labia may trap urine or secretions in the vagina, resulting in secondary infection.

C. Aberrant Urethral Orifices   Constant dribbling of urine should be a clue to this diagnosis.

D. Urethral Prolapse   This problem is acute; a bloody discharge is present. A periurethral mulberry-like purplish mass is found on inspection.

VI. Miscellaneous Causes

A. Tumors   Sarcoma botryoides is the most common, albeit rare, malignant neoplasm of the lower genitourinary tract in infants and children. The discharge is frequently bloody, and a polypoid mass is found in the vagina.

B. Condyloma Acuminata   Venereal warts may extend into the vagina and may be associated with a discharge.

C. Vaginal Polyps

SUGGESTED READINGS

Altchek A: Pediatric vulvovaginitis. Pediatr Clin North Am 19:559–580, 1972

Emans SJ: Vulvovaginitis in children and adolescents. Pediatr Rev 2:319–326, 1981

Emans SJ, Goldstein DP: The gynecologic examination of the prepubertal child with vulvovaginitis: Use of the knee-chest position. Pediatrics 65:758–760, 1980

Murphy TV, Nelson JD: *Shigella* vaginitis in 38 prepubertal patients. Pediatrics 63:511–516, 1979

85

SCROTAL SWELLING

Scrotal swelling may or may not be accompanied by pain. The acute onset of painful swelling necessitates the rapid differentiation of testicular torsion from epididymo-orchitis. Clinical distinction of these disorders is often difficult. A radionuclide testicular scan and ultrasonography may be helpful adjunctive diagnostic procedures, but the consequences of delaying surgical exploration in testicular torsion are too severe should these tests not give a clear answer.

Testicular tumors usually present as nonpainful masses. An old adage states that testicular masses are generally malignant, whereas extratesticular ones are usually benign.

I. Anatomic Abnormalities

A. Hydrocele	The mass, which does not change in shape or size with crying or straining, is painless, soft, and fluid-filled; it is not reducible, and it transilluminates easily. Hydroceles may occur following trauma or may be associated with and obscure testicular tumors.
B. Hernia	The bulge may or may not extend into the scrotum. The testis should be palpable below the mass. Coughing or straining may increase the size of the swelling.
C. Testicular Torsion	The onset of pain associated with torsion is usually acute. The scrotal skin quickly becomes edematous and discolored. Nausea, vomiting, and fever are frequent. Elevation of the testis increases the pain.
D. Torsion of Testicular Appendix	The onset of testicular pain is more gradual and less intense than in testicular torsion. A pea-sized mass may be palpable on the testis. The scrotum may be edematous in a small area overlying the mass.
E. Varicocele	This disorder has been estimated to occur in 10% of boys during puberty. The scrotal mass feels like a bag of worms and is usually on the left side. The swelling is without symptoms.

II. Infectious Causes

A. Epididymitis — The pain is slower in onset than in testicular torsion, from which this condition must be separated. An enlarged, tender epididymis may be palpated distinct from the testis. The scrotum may be red and parchment-like but is not edematous. Fever, chills, dysuria, a urethral discharge, and inguinal pain are common. This infection is uncommon before puberty unless a urinary tract infection is present or urethral instrumentation has been performed. *E. coli* and *N. gonorrhoeae* are the most common pathogens.

B. Orchitis — Testicular pain, scrotal swelling, chills, and often rectal pain are present. The pain is often relieved with testicular elevation. Orchitis is rarely found in prepubertal boys. The most common cause is mumps virus; Coxsackie virus, Echovirus, and gonorrheal infections are rarer causes.

C. Scrotal Cellulitis — Swelling, pain, and edema may be associated with spreading infection of the skin of the scrotum and perineum.

III. Neoplasia

A. Testicular Tumors — The most common sign is painless, indurated, unilateral testicular enlargement. The masses are generally firm and nontender to palpation. Some tumors are associated with sexual precocity or gynecomastia. Although testicular tumors are rare in children, painless testicular enlargement should not be ignored. A hydrocele occurs frequently with the tumor.

B. Testicular Leukemia — The usual presenting sign is a painless swelling later in the course of leukemia. Testicular relapse is the second most common type of extramedullary relapse.

IV. Miscellaneous Causes

A. Edema — Any disorder causing generalized edema may be associated with marked scrotal swelling.

B. Idiopathic Scrotal Edema — This unexplained, uncommon disorder may be confused with more serious causes of scrotal swelling. Affected children are otherwise well when they develop bilateral or unilateral, nontender but erythematous swelling of the scrotum. The problem resolves in 48 hours.

C. Henoch–Schönlein Purpura — Intense swelling of the scrotum may suggest testicular torsion, but the enlargement is bilateral. The purpuric rash may appear later in its typical distribution.

D. Trauma — The history of the trauma is important. The scrotum may be ecchymotic and swollen.

E. Traumatic Hematocele and Hydrocele — Blood or fluid in the scrotal sac may be the result of trauma.

F. Healed Meconium Peritonitis — Scrotal masses are usually noted at birth. The problem may be secondary to an intrauterine volvulus, intussusception, intestinal atresia or stenosis, or cystic fibrosis. Intraperitoneal calcifications are present on roentgenographs.

G. Cysts or Angiomas

H. Sarcoidosis — A rare presenting sign of sarcoidosis in adolescence may be a paratesticular mass. Perihilar adenopathy is usually present.

I. Elephantiasis — Scrotal swelling may follow disruption of lymphatic drainage by the parasite responsible for filariasis.

J. Fat Necrosis

K. Hypertriglyceridemia — Other features may include episodic abdominal pain, eruptive xanthomas, and hepatosplenomegaly.

SUGGESTED READING

Stillwell TJ, Kramer SA: Intermittent testicular torsion. Pediatr 77:908–911, 1986

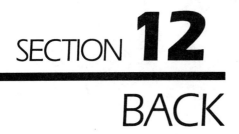

SECTION 12
BACK

86

BACK PAIN

Back pain in a child requires careful evaluation, because this symptom is usually the result of a serious underlying disorder, although the disorder may be psychogenic. Examination may reveal other signs and symptoms, such as abnormalities in gait or in the configuration of the back (subtle changes in contour may offer localizing clues) or tenderness on palpation. The skin overlying the spine should be carefully inspected for dimples, tufts of hair, hemangiomas, and other cutaneous changes, any of which may denote developmental defects. The lesions causing back pain may also produce neurologic changes in the extremities or bladder or bowel dysfunction.

I. Trauma

A. Ligamentous or Muscle Strain
History of a fall, unusual exercise, or other forms of trauma should be sought. There may be a localized tenderness and a paravertebral muscle spasm. Strain is probably the most common cause of back pain.

B. Prolapse of Intervertebral Disc
This is an uncommon lesion in children. There is almost always a history of injury. The lower lumbar area is usually involved; pain may be local or radiate to the legs.

II. Infections

A. Myalgias
Muscle pain may be associated with a multitude of viral and bacterial infections. Aches are not limited to the paravertebral muscles.

B. Urinary Tract Infection
Back pain may be the primary complaint; a urine culture should be done.

C. Diskitis
Aching pain in the lower back radiates to the flanks, abdomen, and lower extremities. The young child may refuse to walk. Illness may be associated with low-grade fever, irritability, and lethargy. Back motion is limited.

D. Osteomyelitis of Vertebra
Localized tenderness is present at a specific level. The spine is held rigid because of muscle spasm. Systemic signs are often absent.

E. Tuberculosis
This is a less common cause of back pain today. Dull local pain is present over the in-

	volved vertebrae; there may be a localized swelling. Destruction of vertebrae may cause pressure on the spinal nerves. The gait is stiff; the back is held rigid.
F. Spinal Epidural Abscess	There are generally exquisite pain and tenderness on palpation over the site of the abscess, as well as rapidly developing signs of spinal cord dysfunction such as paraparesis, loss of bladder and bowel control, and sensory changes.
G. Brucellosis	Small abscesses may develop in the vertebrae. This disorder is generally associated with widespread lymphadenopathy and hepatosplenomegaly; it is transmitted from animals including cows, goats, and pigs.
H. Acute Transverse Myelopathy	This rare disorder is preceded by an upper respiratory infection. Back pain may be an early sign, but progressive weakness develops in 1 or 2 days.
I. Iliac Osteomyelitis, Sacroiliac Joint Infection	These are frequently confused with appendicitis or septic arthritis of the hip.

III. Neoplastic Disorders
A. Benign Tumors

1. Osteoid Osteoma	The onset of pain is gradual; it is worse at night and is often relieved by aspirin. Palpation discloses localized tenderness. Roentgenograms reveal a small translucent area with surrounding dense bone.
2. Benign Osteoblastoma	Symptoms are similar to those of osteoid osteoma, but the lesion is larger with less adjacent bone density seen on x-ray films.
3. Eosinophilic Granuloma	Usually only one vertebra is involved with collapse, but intervertebral disk spaces are maintained. The condition may be asymptomatic, or there may be backache and postural change.
4. Aneurysmal Bone Cyst	A cystic expansile lesion in a vertebra may cause neurologic symptoms.
5. Neurenteric Cysts	Signs of cord dysfunction are present.

B. Malignant Tumors
1. Ewing Sarcoma

2. Osteogenic
Sarcoma
C. Metastatic Tu-
mors
1. Neuroblastoma
2. Wilms Tumor

D. Spinal Cord Tumors	Symptoms may be subacute or chronic. Gliomas are most common, followed by neurofibromas, teratomas, and lipomas. Developmental defects may be associated with cutaneous changes. There are signs of cord compression with changes in gait, bladder and bowel dysfunction, localized tenderness, and scoliosis. A deformity of the foot such as cavus or cavovarus is a frequent presenting complaint.
E. Leukemia and Lymphoma	Pain may be fleeting and is not localized. Rarely spinal cord compression may occur producing typical signs of spinal cord tumors.

IV. Bony Abnormalities

A. Scheuermann Disease (Vertebral Osteochondrosis)	This disease produces a round-back deformity. Several vertebrae may be wedged anteriorly. The pathophysiologic mechanism is thought to be prolapse of the nucleus pulposis into the vertebral body, possibly owing to osteoporosis.
B. Spondylolisthesis	Pain is caused by anterior displacement of vertebrae; usually the fifth lumbar slides forward on the first sacral. Sciatica, increased lumbar lordosis, and tight hamstrings are often present.
C. Spondylolysis	The defect in the pars interarticularis without vertebral slipping is probably the result of a stress fracture. Low back pain, sometimes with radiation down the leg, is common. The pain is increased by activity.
D. Osteoporosis	Fractures are more likely to occur in osteoporotic bones present in disorders such as Cushing syndrome, osteogenesis imperfecta, homocystinuria, Turner syndrome, malabsorption, and immobilization. Idiopathic juvenile osteoporosis has its onset between 8 and 14 years of age and is self-limited.
E. Scoliosis	Back pain is present only in severe cases.

V. Psychogenic Pain

Back pain may be associated with reaction to stressful situations. This cause should always be considered if the patient's affect is inconsistent with symptoms or if findings are unexplainable. A careful history must be obtained.

VI. Miscellaneous Causes

A. Anklyosing Spondylitis	Affected children are usually boys; arthritis in hips or knees and loss of mobility of the back may be findings.
B. Chronic Hemolytic Anemias	Signs of cord compression may result from extramedullary hematopoiesis in the extradural space.
C. Calcification of Intervertebral Disks	Back pain is localized, with loss of mobility due to muscle spasm. The cause is unknown. Fluffy calcification in the disk space on x-ray films may not appear for 1 to 2 weeks following onset of pain.
D. Diastematomyelia	A developmental defect causes a cleft in the cord by bone, cartilage, or fibrous septum. Cutaneous abnormalities over the affected area may be apparent. Low back pain is aggravated by cough or sneeze. Bladder dysfunction or slowly progressive weakness of the legs may be noted.
E. Arteriovenous Malformation of Cord	Symptoms are usually slow to develop. Low back pain is common, with progressive gait and bladder or bowel dysfunction. There may be a cutaneous angioma over the cord lesion.
F. Limb–Girdle Muscular Dystrophy	This is not a single disease entity but a group of dystrophies and myopathies, usually with an autosomal recessive inheritance pattern. First symptoms usually appear during the second decade; an early sign is difficulty in climbing stairs or rising from the floor. Low back pain may be the source of either complaint. Pseudohypertrophy is sometimes present. Deep tendon reflexes are difficult to elicit.
G. Multiple Epiphyseal Dysplasia	The most prominent symptoms are painful joints (usually the hips, knees, and ankles) with some decreased mobility. Back pain is frequent. The gait may be waddling.

87

SCOLIOSIS

Scoliosis is defined as any lateral curvature of the spine from its normal straight position. The incidence of scoliosis in school children has been estimated to be nearly 10%. The leading cause of this problem, comprising 60% to 80% of cases, is idiopathic scoliosis. Although most children who have idiopathic scoliosis require no therapy, close follow-up is recommended in order to detect undue progression of the curvature. Scoliosis in an adolescent is not necessarily idiopathic, however; in fact, it may be a sign of an occult neuromuscular disorder.[1]

Screening for scoliosis has become part of routine school testing in many states. The ease, rapidity, and effectiveness of these screening programs has fostered their popularity. The clinical examination for scoliosis should include a general inspection of the erect child for an obvious deformity of the spine, for shoulder height discrepancy, for prominence of one scapula, and for asymmetry of the hips; comparison of the distances between the arm and trunk on each side; and, most important, an inspection for hemithorax prominence on forward bending of the trunk at the waist.

The following classification divides the causes of scoliosis into nonstructural and structural. Nonstructural curves produce no rotary deformity on forward flexion or upon lying down. Structural curves imply a fixed deformity.

I. Nonstructural Causes

A.	Primary Postural Scoliosis	This condition is seen most commonly in children between 10 and 15 years of age. The shoulders may be rounded, or one hip may seem more prominent than the other. The apparent curvature disappears on forward flexion or on lying down.
B.	Secondary Postural Scoliosis	The curvature is a result of other conditions, such as leg length discrepancy. The curve disappears on forward flexion.
C.	Hysterical Scoliosis	In this unusual type, the scoliosis is not present on forward flexion.

II. Structural Causes

A. Idiopathic Scoliosis

The cause is probably genetic in 90% of cases.

1. Infantile Scoliosis

This type is noted in the first 3 years of life; it is rare in the United States and more common in boys than girls. In most cases, the curvature lessens with age.

2. Juvenile Scoliosis

This type is defined as that appearing in the 4- to 10-year-old age group. Boys and girls are equally affected.

3. Adolescent Scoliosis

This is the most common type occurring in children older than 10 years of age. Girls outnumber boys 5 to 7 to 1. The condition generally goes unnoticed until the adolescent growth spurt.

B. Congenital Scoliosis

Scoliosis may be associated with vertebral anomalies such as hemivertebrae, wedge vertebrae, congenital bars, or failure of vertebrae segmentation. Other significant congenital defects, such as of the heart or genitourinary system, or other bony abnormalities may be present. These disorders may be complicated by diastematomyelia, spinal lipomas, and other defects.

C. Neuromuscular Origin

1. Neuropathies

a. Cerebral Palsy

Structural scoliosis occurs in 15% to 25% of children with cerebral palsy, more commonly in the more severely affected, especially those with spastic quadriplegia.

b. Poliomyelitis

This disease is now an uncommon cause. Deformity occurs a year or two after the acute illness.

c. Myelomeningocele

This lesion may be obvious or occult. Overlying skin defects, lower extremity weakness, neurologic changes, and bladder and bowel difficulties may be present.

d. Friedreich Ataxia

Ataxia develops in the first or second decade; deep tendon reflexes are hypoactive. Pes cavus and kyphoscoliosis develop in almost all patients.

e. Charcot–Marie–Tooth Disease

Atrophy of the peroneal muscles gives a stork-leg appearance. Progressive weakness affects the lower and later the upper extremities.

f. Juvenile Spinal Muscle Atrophy — Onset of weakness ranges from early childhood to late adolescence. Signs of this disorder are often mistaken for muscular dystrophy.

g. Spinal Cord Injury — Scoliosis will develop in almost half of the patients with cord injuries.

h. Syringomyelia — Scoliosis may be a presenting sign before sensory changes are noted.

i. Diastematomyelia — There may be cutaneous defects or changes over the site of the bony abnormality.

2. Myopathies

a. Duchenne Type Muscular Dystrophy — Scoliosis occurs later, particularly when the patient is confined to a wheel chair.

b. Limb–Girdle Muscular Dystrophy — Onset of symptoms is later than in the Duchenne type. Proximal muscle weakness is greater than distal.

c. Arthrogryposis — Multiple contractures are present at birth. Anterior horn cell loss may create muscle imbalance, leading to scoliosis.

D. Neurofibromatosis — This disorder accounts for approximately 2% of cases of scoliosis; in half of these, a slowly progressive curve similar to the idiopathic variety develops. More significant, however, is the type with a short, sharply angular curve in the thoracic spine. Café-au-lait spots and axillary freckling are important cutaneous clues.

E. Mesenchymal Origin

1. Marfan Syndrome — Almost 50% of affected children develop scoliosis in infancy or early childhood. Dislocated lens, spiderlike fingers and extremities, and a high-arched palate are features.

2. Ehlers–Danlos Syndrome — Hyperlaxity of joints and skin is characteristic.

3. Congenital Laxity of Joints — Skin hyperelasticity is not part of this disorder.

F. Trauma

1. Direct Vertebral Trauma — Fractures or wedging of vertebral bodies or nerve root irritation may cause scoliosis.

2. Irradiation — Destruction of the vertebral growth plates, especially in treatment of Wilms tumor, produces curvature later.

3. Extravertebral Trauma	Severe trunk burns or thoracic surgery may result in scoliosis.
G. Tumors	
1. Intraspinal Tumors	Various types of tumors may result in scoliosis. Sensory and motor changes in the lower extremities and bladder and bowel incontinence may also occur.
2. Osteoid Osteoma	Vertebral body tumors may cause paraspinal muscle spasm and resultant scoliosis. Pain is often worse at night and is relieved by aspirin.
H. Miscellaneous Causes	
1. Rickets	Scoliosis may develop late if the condition is untreated. Epiphyseal enlargement, bowing of long bones, growth retardation, apathy, and muscle weakness are among the features.
2. Osteogenesis Imperfecta	Collapse of vertebrae following fractures may result in scoliosis.
3. Scheuermann Disease	This disease causes the adolescent round-back deformity; it rarely causes scoliosis.
4. Achondroplasia	Of affected children, 25% will develop scoliosis in late childhood.
5. Klippel–Feil Syndrome	Short neck with decreased movement is typical; cervicothoracic scoliosis may also be present.
6. Sprengel Deformity	Congenital high scapula is almost always associated with cervical or thoracic spine abnormalities.
7. Cleidocranial Dyostosis	This disorder features hypoplastic or absent clavicles, large head with delayed closure of the fontanel, and a narrow chest.
8. Hyperphosphatasia	This condition is characterized by fever, pain, and bone fragility with frequent fractures. Stature is short, limb bones are thickened, and sclerae are bluish.
9. Hypervitaminosis A	Features include dry skin, thickened bones, and often increased intracranial pressure.
10. Hypothyroidism	
11. Congenital Indifference to Pain	
12. Juvenile Rheumatoid Arthritis	

| 13. Mucopolysac- charidoses | In type VII, progressive scoliosis may be the initial presenting sign. Hepatosplenomegaly, short neck, and cloudy corneae develop gradually. Type VI (Maroteaux–Lamy) also has scoliosis as a clinical feature. |
| I. Syndromes Associated with Scoliosis | Scoliosis has been described in a number of malformation syndromes[2]; other features of these syndromes are more striking than the scoliosis. |

Conradi–Hunermann Syndrome
Diastrophic Dwarfism
Basal Cell Nevus Syndrome
Coffin–Lowry Syndrome
Cohen Syndrome
Pseudoachondroplastic Spondyloepiphyseal Dysplasia
Craniocarpaltarsal Dystrophy (Freeman–Sheldon Syndrome)
Aarskog Syndrome
Camptomelic Dwarfism
Cri du Chat Syndrome

Hallermann–Streiff Syndrome
Fetal Trimethadione Syndrome
Larsen Syndrome
Metaphyseal Dysplasia (Pyle Disease)
Prader–Willi Syndrome
Rubinstein–Taybi Syndrome
Seckel Syndrome (Bird-headed Dwarfism)
Stickler Syndrome
Turner Syndrome
XXXXY Karyotype
XXY Karoytype

III. Transient Structural Scoliosis

A. Inflammation	A lateral curvature can be produced by irritation from empyema or a perinephric abscess.
B. Torticollis	
C. Sciatic Scoliosis	Pressure of an intervertebral disk on nerve roots may produce a scoliosis.

REFERENCES

1. Rothner AD, Keim H, Chutorian AM: Occult neuromuscular disease in 100 consecutive patients with scoliosis. J Pediatr 86:748–750, 1975
2. Smith DW: Recognizable Patterns of Human Malformation, 3rd ed. Philadelphia, WB Saunders, 1982

SUGGESTED READINGS

Sharrard WJW: Paediatric Orthopaedics and Fractures, 2nd ed. Oxford, Blackwell Scientific Publications, 1979
Winter RB: Spine deformity in children: Current concepts of diagnosis and treatment. Pediatr Ann 5:96–111, 1976

88

KYPHOSIS AND LORDOSIS

Curvature of the spine may occur in anterior and posterior directions as well as laterally as in scoliosis. Most children with kyphosis, a posterior curvature of the spine, or lordosis, an anterior curvature of the spine, have postural deformities. Pathologic or fixed deformities, however, may result from various disorders, many of which are listed below.

I. Kyphosis

A. Poor Posture

Poor posture accounts for most cases of kyphosis, especially in adolescence when concern about appearance is most prevalent. Obviously, postural kyphosis is not fixed and can easily be corrected. The problem is finding the appropriate method of encouragement or exercises to maintain an appropriate appearance.

B. Scheuermann Disease (Juvenile Kyphosis)

This poorly understood disorder usually develops about the time of puberty. The posture is poor, and a round-back deformity is apparent. Fatigue and discomfort in the area of kyphosis are common and increased on standing. Full correction cannot voluntarily be obtained. One or more of the thoracic vertebrae have a wedged-shaped appearance on roentgenograms due to diminished anterior height. The cause is unknown. Lumbar lordosis is often accentuated.

C. Congenital Kyphosis

The kyphosis is noted in infancy and usually progresses with age, especially after the child begins to walk and stand. The cause, a structural abnormality of the spine, is apparent on roentgenographic examination. This deformity is painless in childhood but may become painful during adolescence and adulthood. Compression of the spinal cord may occur.

D. Neuromuscular Problems

Spinal deformities may be caused by almost any neuromuscular disorder in a growing child. Important causes include cerebral palsy,

E. Myelomeningocele

F. Infection

G. Skeletal Dysplasias

    1. Spondyloepi-
       physeal Dys-
       plasia

    2. Mucopolysac-
       charidoses

    3. Diastrophic
       Dwarfism

    4. Diaphyseal
       Dysplasia
       (Engelmann
       Disease)

    5. Kniest Dwarf-
       ism

    6. Achrondro-
       plasia

    7. Cleidocranial
       Dystosis

    8. Cockayne Syn-
       drome

    9. Neurofibroma-
       tosis

    10. Noonan Syn-
        drome

H. Metabolic and
   Endocrinologic
   Disorders

post-traumatic paralysis, spinal muscular atrophy, myotonic dystrophy, and poliomyelitis.
Kyphotic defects may be present at birth secondary to vertebral disruption or may develop later associated with muscle weakness.
Destruction of vertebrae from infectious causes may lead to kyphosis, or spasm of paravertebral musculature may be responsible for the abnormality. Tuberculosis is the archetypical cause but is much less common today than previously. Tuberculous spondylitis or Pott's disease may affect any level of the spine and is often insidious in onset.
A host of skeletal disorders may involve the vertebral column and produce kyphosis. A radiographic skeletal survey will help to differentiate the various types.

Kyphosis is especially likely to be a finding in Hurler syndrome (Type I), Morquio syndrome (Type IV), Maroteaux–Lamy syndrome (Type VI), and Type VII.

1. Hypothyroid-
   ism
2. Gaucher Dis-
   ease
3. Ehlers–Danlos
   Syndrome
4. Marfan Syn-
   drome
5. Homocystinuria
6. Osteogenesis
   Imperfecta
7. Juvenile Osteo-
   porosis

I. Tumors — Benign or malignant tumors, either primary or metastatic, may cause a kyphotic deformity. Intraspinal tumors must always be considered.

J. Iatrogenic Kypho-
   sis
   1. Radiation Ther- — Damage to vertebral growth plates may follow
      apy   radiation therapy, resulting in kyphosis.
   2. Surgery — Surgical removal of parts of the vertebral column may lead to kyphosis.

II. Lordosis

A. Physiologic Lordo- — An exaggerated lumbar lordosis is common in
   sis   toddlers.

B. Compensatory — A compensatory lumbar lordosis frequently
   Posture   accompanies kyphotic disorders such as Scheuermann disease.

C. Neuromuscular — Lumbar lordosis is prominent and progressive
   Disorders   in muscular dystrophy and often accompanies cerebral palsy, spinal injuries with paralysis, and poliomyelitis.

D. Spondylolisthesis — A slipping forward of the vertebral column at the lumbosacral junction can be secondary to congenital sacral defects or the result of trauma or of developmental or acquired bone defects. Poor posture and an increased lumbar lordosis may be the only complaints. Back-ache, often with radiation down the legs, oc-curs in the second and third decades.

E. Bilateral Flexion — An increased pelvic inclination, the result of
   Contractures of   hip flexion contractures, will produce a com-
   the Hips   pensatory lumbar lordosis. Flexion contrac-

	tures may occur in juvenile rheumatoid arthritis, other hip dysplasias, and cerebral palsy.
F. Myelomeningocele	Lordosis is the most common spinal deformity in this disorder and is compensatory in nature.
G. Inflammatory Processes	Spasm of paravertebral muscles from inflammatory processes in the spine may cause an accentuated lordosis. In diskitis, an inflammation of the intervertebral disk space, symptoms of backache, pain radiating to the legs, and, occasionally, lower extremity muscle weakness are common.
H. Skeletal Dysplasias	
1. Achondroplasia	Lumbar lordosis is exaggerated in this disorder because of fixed flexion of the hips and some thoracolumbar kyphosis.
2. Cleidocranial Dysostosis	Major features include a large head with a delayed closure of the anterior fontanel and hypoplastic clavicles.
3. Spondyloepiphyseal Dysplasias	

SUGGESTED READING

Lovell, WW, Winter RB: Pediatric Orthopedics. Philadelphia, JB Lippincott, 1978

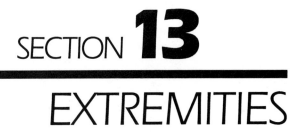

SECTION **13**

EXTREMITIES

89

LEG PAIN

Leg aches are common in children. Fortunately, in most cases the episodes are short-lived and the cause is benign, probably related to trauma or exercise. Should the limb pain continue or become increasingly severe or recurrent, an investigation for an underlying disorder is mandatory.

Many of the disorders listed in Chapter 90, Limp, and Chapter 91, Arthritis, produce leg pain, and they are not repeated here. The primary purpose of this chapter is to suggest possible causes for the kind of leg pain that is often referred to as "growing pains."

The physician is often faced with a dilemma of how far to proceed with the diagnostic evaluation. The leg pain associated with most disorders in this chapter can be differentiated from growing pains by careful evaluation including history and physical examination, with special attention to pain location and systemic symptoms, and a few laboratory studies such as roentgenograms, blood count, and sedimentation rate.

I. Idiopathic Leg Pain ("Growing Pains")

Leg pain is often attributed to this rather nebulous entity. As many as 10% to 20% of children may complain of vague leg pain on a recurrent basis, sometimes in association with headaches and abdominal pain. Various criteria have been suggested for differentiation of this symptom complex from serious underlying disorders. The pains are usually intermittent and bilateral and located deep in the legs, most commonly in the thigh or calf. Joint pain is rare and points to other diagnoses. Although the pains may occur at any time of the day or night they typically occur only at night, either when the child is falling asleep or actually wakening the child from sleep; usually they last $\frac{1}{2}$ to 1 hour and may respond to rubbing, heat, or analgesics. Systemic signs and symptoms are absent, and roentgenographic findings and the sedimentation rate are normal. The etiology has still not been determined, but most researchers agree that the pain is not due to "growth"; excessive exercise or trauma, hidden food allergy, or emotional factors have been suggested.

II. Trauma

Trauma is probably the most common cause of leg pain. Often, superficial clues such as bruises are present, or there may be a history of an episode of physical trauma.

A. Muscle or Bone
   Bruises

B. Fractures   The prototype in this category may be the
                             stress fracture produced by running on a hard
                             surface for a prolonged period. The pain is
                             localized rather than diffuse and bilateral. Ini-
                             tial roentgenograms may be normal.

C. Pathologic Frac-   Bone cysts or areas of fibrous dysplasia may
   tures   make the bone susceptible to fracture from
                             minimal trauma.

D. Osteoporosis   Fractures are more likely to occur in osteopo-
                             rotic bone. Causes include Cushing syndrome,
                             osteogenesis imperfecta, homocystinuria,
                             Turner syndrome, malabsorption and immobi-
                             lization. Idiopathic juvenile osteoporosis has
                             its onset between 8 and 14 years of age and is
                             self-limited.

E. Muscle Injections

III. Leukemia and Lymphoma
Leg pain—the result of leukemic infiltrate in the bone—may be an
early symptom of leukemia or lymphoma. Systemic signs such as fever, weight loss, and adenopathy may not be present. Occasionally,
radiolucent lines in the metaphyseal areas may be seen.

IV. Bone Tumors
A. Malignant Tu-   Characteristically, the pain is persistent and of
   mors   increasing severity. Osteogenic sarcoma and
                             Ewing tumor are the most common. Roent-
                             genograms should be obtained in any child
                             complaining of localized bone pain.

B. Benign Tumors   Benign neoplasms are more likely to be pain-
                             less unless they are associated with a patho-
                             logic fracture or the result of some mechanical
                             difficulty. These are two notable exceptions:

   1. Osteoid Os-   The pain associated with this tumor is char-
      teoma   acteristically worse at night than during the
                             day and is usually relieved by aspirin. On ro-
                             entgenographic examination a small radiolu-
                             cent nidus is surrounded by a rim of sclerotic
                             bone.

   2. Benign Osteo-   This lesion is larger than the osteoid osteoma,
      blastoma   the nature of the pain is not so well defined,
                             and the surrounding bone is less sclerotic.

| C. Metastatic Tumors | Neuroblastoma is one of the more common metastatic bone tumors that may produce leg pain. |

V. Infection and Inflammation

A. Osteomyelitis	Infection in the bone is usually localized and is associated with tenderness and swelling over the lesion, but not always with systemic signs. A bone scan rather than roentgenograms is much more likely to reveal early changes.
B. Myositis	Pyogenic infection of muscle or myositis as a result of a systemic infection, such as the severe calf tenderness associated with influenza, may produce leg pain with significant tenderness.
C. Tuberculosis	Limb pain without systemic symptoms may be a presenting complaint.
D. Syphilis	The great mimic may produce a periostitis with severe pain and pseudoparalysis, particularly in congenital infections.
E. Trichinosis	Severe muscle pain is one of the characteristic findings, as well as fever, periorbital edema, and eosinophilia.

VI. Miscellaneous Causes

A. Hypermobility Syndrome	Children with evidence of hypermobility may present with leg and joint aches without other obvious causes.
B. Shin Splints (Anterior and Posterior Compartment Syndromes)	Hypertrophy or swelling of muscles of the lower leg will lead to muscle cramping and pain on sudden resumption of excessive exercise.
C. Scurvy	This disorder is rarely seen in North America. Subperiosteal hemorrhages produce exquisite tenderness in the limbs.
D. Hypervitaminosis A	The excessive intake of vitamin A may result in bone pain as well as symptoms of increased intracranial pressure.
E. Caffey Disease (Infantile Cortical Hyperostosis)	Although onset of symptoms in this uncommon disorder is usually before 6 months of age, failure to recognize early signs may suggest osteomyelitis in older infants with involvement of the lower extremities.

F. Sickle-Cell Disease

This disorder should be considered in black children with painful extremities and anemia.

G. Gaucher Disease

Bone lesions may suggest osteomyelitis in the early stages because of the severe pain, tenderness, swelling, erythema, and heat. The spleen is usually enlarged, and the skin develops a yellowish color.

H. Melorheostosis

This rare disorder is characterized by longitudinal thickening of the shaft of long bones, usually of one limb. The pain may be severe, and underlying skin is often tense, shiny, and indurated.

I. Engelmann Disease (Diaphyseal Dysplasia)

This is another rare disorder characterized by symmetric enlargement and sclerosis of the shafts of the major long bones and changes in the skull as well. Affected children usually present with difficulty in walking because of limb pain.

J. Multiple Epiphyseal Dysplasia

Painful joints, sometimes enlarged in size, are a leading symptom. The hips, knees, or ankles are most commonly affected, and there may be some restriction in mobility. Back pain is common; the gait may be waddling. Roentgenograms show irregular, small, flat, or fragmented epiphyseal ossification centers.

K. Stickler Syndrome (Hereditary Artho-ophthalmopathy)

Features may include a marfanoid habitus with large joints and hyperextensible knees, elbows, and finger joints. The joints are sometimes painful; morning stiffness is common. The midface is flat, the chin is small, and clefting is common. Congenital myopia is common; conductive hearing loss may be present. Inheritance pattern is autosomal dominant.

L. Foods

Several observers have reported unexplained leg pains that seem to be related to the ingestion of potatoes, tomatoes, egg plants, and peppers.

M. Spinal Cord Tumor

Radicular or back pain are common presentations.

N. Renal Tubular Acidosis (RTA)

In adolescents and adults osteomalacia with bone pain and pathologic fractures is a cardinal sign of distal RTA. Growth retardation may be the only early finding.

O. Chemical Preservatives

Inhalation of smoke from the burning of outdoor grade lumber may cause muscle aches, pains, and cramps as well as rashes, hair loss, seizures, red eyes, and other symptoms.

P. Ehlers–Danlos Syndrome — Leg cramps, particularly of the calves, are frequent. Types with increasing hypermobility have increasing symptoms.

Q. Pseudoxanthoma Elasticum — A rare, AR disorder, in which alterations in elastic tissues of vessels may lead to gastrointestinal bleeding and episodes similar to intermittent claudication. Skin changes occur after the second decade and give a plucked chicken-like appearance in localized areas.

SUGGESTED READINGS

Calabro JJ, Wachtel AE, Holgerson WB et al: Growing pains: Fact or fiction? Postgrad Med 59 (2):66–72, 1976

Orlowski JP, Mercer RD: Osteoid osteoma in children and young adults. Pediatrics 59:526–532, 1977

Passo MH: Aches and limb pain. Pediatr Clin North Am 29:209–219, 1982

Peterson HA: Leg aches. Pediatr Clin North Am 24:731–736, 1977

Teotia, M, Teotia SPS, Singh RK: Idiopathic juvenile osteoporosis. Am J Dis Child 133:894–900, 1979

90

LIMP

Fortunately, the cause of limp in most children is fairly straightforward. A thorough history and physical examination usually reveal the origin of the problem. The type of gait responsible for the limp should be observed by having the child walk unencumbered by clothing in a hallway; the gait may suggest a foot, knee, or hip problem. The presence of systemic symptoms usually indicates a more complex problem than simple trauma. The extremities should be carefully palpated; changes in temperature, coloration, and evidence of swelling should be noted. All joints should be put through range of motion to elicit possible subtle manifestations in other areas.

The following classification of disorders associated with limp in childhood has been modified from an approach by Salter.[1] Painful and nonpainful causes of limp are the two main categories.

It is important to remember that pain may be referred. A painful knee may result from hip disease. A child with hip complaints may have an intraabdominal or a spinal disorder. Signs of trauma responsible for a painful limp may be subtle. An unusual or new activity—for instance, hitting a bucket of golf balls or raking pine needles—may result in toxic synovitis. A sudden twisting motion may produce the notorious incomplete, undisplaced "toddler's fracture" of the tibia, which is inapparent on initial roentgenograms.

I. Painful Causes of Limp
A. Trauma

1. Local Superficial Lesions	Sometimes the cause is so obvious that it may be overlooked. Skin irritation from a tight shoe or a shoe defect, lacerations or foreign bodies in the foot, or plantar warts may be the cause.
2. Ligamentous Strains and Sprains	Ankle and knee injuries are common and may mimic fractures. Joints are often swollen and sometimes bruised.
3. Tendon Disorders	Achilles tendonitis is characterized by sudden acute pain in the tendon; there is pain on palpation, but plantar flexion is usually strong. Rupture of the Achilles tendon, in which there is a lack of forceful plantar flexion, is uncommon.

4. Muscle Bruising	There is usually a history of trauma; purpura of the skin may be present. Tenderness of affected muscle is usual.
5. Fractures	Fractures must be considered in any painful limp. Careful palpation of the extremity may localize the fracture site. Stress fractures may occur in joggers or children involved in athletics; the pain may not be severe. "Toddler's fracture" is an undisplaced, often spiral fracture; radiologic confirmation may be lacking early on; it occurs typically in the tibia.
6. Child Abuse	There may be muscle bruising, sprains, or fractures. The history may not fit the injury; there may be other evidence of abuse present.
7. Injections	Limp is typically seen in toddlers after booster DPT injections. Gluteal injections may irritate the sciatic nerve; the large muscle mass of the thighs is the preferred injection site to avoid this problem.
8. Subluxation of Patella	Adolescent girls are most commonly affected; the knee suddenly gives way, followed by swelling of the joint. The patella is usually not displaced at the time of examination for the acute problem, but can be subluxed easily.

B. Inflammatory Conditions

1. Toxic Synovitis	The hip is the most common site by far. This condition follows trauma or viral infection; fever and systemic signs are usually absent. There is pain on abduction and internal rotation of the hip. It may predispose to Legg–Calvé–Perthes disease.
2. Acute Rheumatic Fever	Migratory joint pain or swelling is typical. Diagnosis must be based on the Jones criteria. Pain is usually out of proportion to findings.
3. Juvenile Rheumatoid Arthritis	There are many different presentations; one or many joints may be involved. This is a diagnosis of exclusion; pain is usually not exquisite.
4. Systemic Lupus Erythematosus	Arthritis or arthralgias and muscle weakness are common. There may be other clues.
5. Polyarteritis Nodosa	There may be diffuse symptoms, secondary to vasculitis of medium-sized and small arteries.

6. Dermatomyositis	Weakness is more pronounced in proximal muscles than distal; there is often pain on palpation of muscles, as well as erythematous scaling papules over elbows, knees, and knuckles.
7. Henoch–Schönlein Purpura	A petechial or purpuric rash is characteristic; abdominal pain; arthritis, nephritis, and tissue swelling may be other features.
8. Serum Sickness	Findings may include urticaria, arthralgias or arthritis, fever, and lymphadenopathy. The disorder is most commonly associated with drug use.
9. Ulcerative Colitis; Regional Enteritis	Arthritis or arthralgias may be associated.
10. Lupoid Hepatitis	Arthritis or arthralgia with jaundice and hepatosplenomegaly are common.

C. Infections

1. Osteomyelitis	Usually, localized pain, fever, and an elevated sedimentation rate are present. At times osteomyelitis may mimic septic arthritis. The infection may be in the pelvis or vertebral column rather than the bones of the lower extremity.
2. Septic Arthritis	Onset is usually acute; the infection is generally monarticular and very painful. Gonococcal arthritis may be migratory.
3. Acute Myositis	This disorder follows a viral illness, usually influenza. There is severe pain in the calves; creatine phosphokinase levels are elevated.
4. Pyomyositis	This is an uncommon localized muscle infection.
5. Diskitis and Intervertebral Disc Infection	Back pain is usual; pain may be referred to the hips. The child may refuse to walk.
6. Epidural Abscess	Exquisite back pain, with sensory changes in the lower extremities, is typical.
7. Acute Appendicitis	Psoas irritation may alter gait.
8. Retroperitoneal Masses	Pain from infection or inflammation may be referred to the hip. The abdomen should be palpated carefully for masses.
9. Acute Iliac Adenitis	Suppuration of lymph nodes may irritate the hip capsule, with resultant limp. Careful palpation along the ileum may detect the swelling associated with the adenitis.

D. Aseptic Necrosis and Osteochondritis

1. Legg–Calvé-Perthes Disease	The femoral epiphysis is involved; the condition may be totally asymptomatic; it is most common in boys 4 to 8 years of age.
2. Osgood–Schlätter Disease	The tibial tuberosity is painful. Limping may occur after heavy exercise; usually boys 11 to 15 years of age are affected.
3. Freiberg Disease	The head of the second metatarsal is involved; there is pain on palpation. It is more common in girls 12 to 15 years of age.
4. Köhler Disease	Osteochondrosis of the tarsal navicular bone causes a mild limp; it is seen usually in boys 3 to 6 years of age.
5. Sever Disease	Calcaneal apophysitis, with pain on heel palpation, is seen primarily in boys 8 to 12 years of age.
6. Osteochondritis Dissecans	The knee is most commonly involved; there is a history of locking of the joint, as well as intermittent swelling.
7. Chondromalacia Patellae	Scoring of the cartilaginous surface of the patella produces a grating sensation when the patella is moved back and forth over the knee joint. Pain is worse after exercise.
8. Larsen–Johansson Disease	There is pain, and tenderness over the lower pole of the patella, with swelling of the adjacent soft tissues. Boys between 10 and 14 years of age are most commonly affected. Limp with inability to kneel and run is typical.
9. Sinding–Larsen Disease	Avulsion of patellar ligament may occur, especially in cerebral palsy.

E. Neoplasms

1. Leukemia	Leg pain and limp may be presenting signs, both of which may suggest arthritis.
2. Malignant Bone Tumors	Osteogenic sarcoma, Ewing sarcoma, and metastatic neuroblastoma are examples.
3. Benign Bone Tumors	Osteoid osteoma, eosinophilic granuloma, and fibrous dysplasia may cause limp.

F. Hematologic Conditions

1. Hemophilia	Hemarthrosis is usually obvious.
2. Sickle-Cell Anemia	The hand–foot syndrome in toddlers may be secondary to bone infarction. The symmetric swelling is painful.

3. Phlebitis	There is tenderness of involved veins with local swelling.
4. Scurvy	Limp is secondary to periosteal hemorrhage.
5. Hypervitaminosis A	Bone pain may occur with intoxication. Signs of pseudotumor cerebri may be present.

II. Nonpainful Causes of Limp

A. Neurologic Disorders

1. Flaccid Paralysis	Limp is due to weak muscle groups. Poliomyelitis was the most common cause prior to routine vaccination programs.
2. Spastic Paralysis	Jerky gait is accentuated on running. Cerebral palsy is the most common cause. Increased muscle tone and hyperreflexia are other features.
3. Ataxia	Causes may be drugs, infection, or heredity. The gait is unsteady and broad-based.
4. Involvement of Spine	Intraspinal masses, diastematomyelia, lesions of the cauda equina, herniated disk, and spondylolisthesis may cause limp. A careful neurologic examination is mandatory.

B. Muscle Disorders

1. Muscular Dystrophy	Limp is secondary to muscle weakness; there may be pseudohypertrophy of calf muscles. Numerous other primary muscle disorders with weakness may produce an abnormal gait.
2. Arthrogryposis	The etiology is unclear; it may be neurogenic or muscular. There is a lack of full muscular extension due to contractures.

C. Joint Disorders

1. Stiffness or Contractures	These disorders may be seen in several inherited diseases, such as mucopolysaccharidoses.
2. Instability	Congenital dislocated hip may produce a waddling gait. Results of the Trendelenberg test are positive. Severe hyperextensibility of joints may also be a cause. The condition may occur with Ehlers–Danlos syndrome or severe pes planus.

D. Bony Deformities

1. Leg Length Discrepancies	
2. Slipped Femoral Capital Epiphyses	Onset in most cases is insidious; adolescents 11 to 15 years of age, often obese, are those most often affected. The limp may be painful.

3. Coxa Vara	In this congenital condition, the head of the femur is at a more acute angle; the gait is waddling.
4. Knock Knees	Severe knock knees may cause an unsteady gait.
5. Blount Disease	Unilateral or bilateral bowing of tibia and beaking of proximal tibial epiphysis on roentgenograms are findings.
6. Torsional Deformities of Lower Extremities	
7. Epiphyseal Dysplasias	Symptoms may mimic those of Legg–Calvé–Perthes disease. Hereditary multiple epiphyseal dysplasia, Gaucher disease, hypothyroidism, and sickle-cell disease should be considered.
8. Postmeningococcal Skeletal Dystrophy	Symmetrical epiphyseal–metaphyseal lesions and asymmetrical destruction of major epiphyses may follow sepsis and DIC, especially with meningococcal infections. Months to years later these children may present with a limp, bow-legs, asymmetric limbs, and short stature.
E. Functional States	
1. Hysteria	This cause is uncommon in young children.
2. Mimicry	The limp is likely to occur intermittently or to vary in form.

REFERENCE

1. Salter RB: Gait disturbances and limp in childhood. In Green M, Haggerty RJ (eds): Ambulatory Pediatrics, pp 232–236. Philadelphia, WB Saunders, 1968

91

ARTHRITIS

Joint complaints are common in children; fortunately, in most cases the problem is transient and is the result of trauma or exercise. Arthritis, defined as swelling of a joint or limitation of motion accompanied by heat, pain, and tenderness, is much less common than arthralgia (joint pain), but it requires a thorough investigation to arrive at its cause.

The causes of arthritis are numerous. Of causes of monarticular disease, traumatic arthritis is still the most common, but septic arthritis is a serious disorder that must be diagnosed and treated early. The incidence of acute rheumatic fever is lessening, but that of juvenile rheumatoid arthritis (JRA) appears to be increasing. Unfortunately, the diagnosis of JRA is one of exclusion and requires the presence of swelling involving one or more joints for 6 weeks. These criteria create unsettling feelings in the physician who is evaluating the recent onset of joint swelling in a child. How extensive must the laboratory investigation be?

Many disorders can be easily excluded from consideration. Others, such as the viral arthriditides, may be more common than realized; fortunately, these rarely are long-lasting. The reactive arthriditides, such as with *Salmonella*, *Shigella*, or *Yersinia* infections, present interesting material for future investigation. Certain segments, of the population, such as those with the histocompatibility locus B-27, seem to be prone to develop arthritis following certain environmental insults, such as infection and as yet undetermined other factors.

I. Rheumatic Diseases

A. Juvenile Rheumatoid Arthritis

Criteria for the diagnosis of JRA include a chronic arthritis lasting more than 6 weeks in at least one joint and the exclusion of other possibilities. There are no confirmatory diagnostic tests. JRA has three general forms (1) systemic, characterized by prominent constitutional symptoms and, eventually, involvement of multiple joints; (2) polyarticular, with involvement of more than four joints, often symmetric in distribution and frequently affecting the hands, and with minor systemic manifestations; and (3) pauciarticular, with involvement of four or fewer joints, and rarely with systemic signs and symptoms.

B. Acute Rheu-
matic Fever

Diagnosis is based on confirmation of a pre-ceding streptococcal infection and the Jones criteria. The arthritis is typically migratory and lasts 3 to 5 days at most in each joint; the du-ration of arthritis in all joints does not exceed 1 month. The joints are usually very painful, occasionally have areas of erythema, and most frequently are not greatly swollen. The arthri-tis is not destructive.

C. Systemic Lupus
Erythematosus
(SLE)

Joint disease is the most common presentation of SLE. Fever, rashes or alopecia, weakness or fatigue, weight loss, photosensitivity, and neurologic complaints may be present. The antinuclear antibody titer is almost invariably elevated, but this finding is not specific for SLE.

D. Polyarteritis

Prominent findings include fever, myalgias, abdominal pain, bizarre skin rashes including unusual erythema multiforme, petechiae or purpura, and painful nodular swellings along the course of blood vessels in some patients. Urinary sediment abnormalities are often present. Arthritis is less frequent than arthral-gias, and the arthritis may be migratory. Hy-pertension and seizures are common.

E. Dermatomyo-
sitis

Symmetric, progressive muscle weakness is characteristic. The muscles may be tender to palpation. The classic skin rashes, erythema over the knuckles, scaly erythematous papules over the elbows, and a discoloration of the eyelids are found in three fourths of the cases. A few patients will have objective evidence of arthritis, particularly of the knees.

F. Scleroderma
  1. Linear or
     Localized
     Scleroderma

Linear sclerotic areas of skin or multiple patches of sclerosis are found in this form, which is much more common than progres-sive systemic sclerosis. One third of patients will develop active synovitis at some time dur-ing the course of their disease, in either a polyarticular or pauciarticular distribution.

2. Progressive Systemic Sclerosis	In this form skin symptoms are prominent and are characterized by a progressive tightening, usually symmetric in distribution. Raynaud phenomenon may precede the sclerosis; gastrointestinal disturbances and pulmonary, cardiac, and renal involvement develop. Arthritis is not common, but arthralgias and contractures of joints are often present.
G. Ankylosing Spondylitis	Back pain is a frequent presenting complaint. The sacroiliac and spinal apophyseal joints eventually become involved, but in children, initial involvement is often peripheral, asymmetric, and limited to a few large joints such as the hips, knees, and rarely small joints. Affected boys outnumber girls by 10 to 1, and 90% of affected children have HL-A B-27. In some cases, the clinical presentation is recurrent attacks of acute iridocyclitis.
H. Mixed Connective Tissue Disease	Signs and symptoms of this curious disorder may be identical to those in a number of other disorders. The arthritis affects multiple joints and commonly the small joints. Skin changes may be consistent with scleroderma; serositis, hepatosplenomegaly, lymphadenopathy, Raynaud phenomenon, and abnormal esophageal motility may be found.
I. Henoch–Schönlein Purpura	This relatively common vasculitis of unknown etiology is often categorized with the rheumatic diseases. The rash—purpuric, petechial or occasionally eczematous—is characteristic and is most prominent on the lower extremities, although it sometimes occurs on the arms and face, and rarely on the trunk. Arthritis, involving a few joints, occurs in about 40% of the cases. Abdominal pain, nephritis, hypertension, and unusual areas of edema are frequently found.

II. Other Related Conditions

| A. Inflammatory Bowel Disease | A peripheral arthritis involving a few large joints, of short duration, may be seen in about 20% of children with Crohn disease or ulcerative colitis. The arthritis may precede the bowel symptoms but usually does not. |

B. Psoriatic Arthritis	Pauciarticular arthritis, especially involving the distal interphalangeal joints, is occasionally seen in children with psoriasis. The arthritis may precede the skin disorder. There are few systemic symptoms.
C. Sarcoidosis	The most consistent features of childhood sarcoidosis are fever, weight loss, anorexia, dyspnea, cough, and lymphadenopathy. The arthritis is often monarticular at onset and relatively painless. A papular skin rash or uveitis should suggest this possibility.
D. Stevens–Johnson Syndrome	This hypersensitivity reaction characterized by erythema multiforme-like lesions, often progressing to bullae and extensive mucocutaneous lesions, can be triggered by drugs, infections (especially herpes simplex), and sometimes other connective tissue disorders. Arthritis may be part of the clinical picture.
E. Mucocutaneous Lymph Node Syndrome (Kawasaki Disease)	Criteria for diagnosis of this relatively recently described disorder include fever lasting more than 5 days, a polymorphous rash, conjunctival injection, cracking of the lips, pharyngitis, and cervical adenopathy. Arthralgias or arthritis may be found. Up to 40% of cases develop an arthritis late in the febrile stage that usually lasts 2 to 4 weeks.
F. Chronic Active Hepatitis	Arthritis or arthralgia may be confined to a single joint, but often several joints are involved, usually the large ones. Anorexia, weight loss, and jaundice are other features.
G. Sjögren Syndrome	This syndrome may be seen in other rheumatic disorders, particularly rheumatoid arthritis. The triad of characteristic findings is keratoconjunctivitis sicca (dry eyes), xerostomia (dry mouth) and salivary gland enlargement.
H. Reiter Disease	An episode of diarrhea frequently precedes onset of arthritis with marked swelling of joints (particularly those of the lower extremity), conjunctivitis, and urethritis.
I. Behçet Syndrome	The primary symptoms of this rare disorder include recurrent aphthous stomatitis, genital ulceration, and iritis. Skin lesions (particularly pustular and ulcerative ones), erythema multi-

forme, and erythema nodosum are seen along with an arthritis, which is usually pauciarticular.

J. Giant Cell Arteritis

Early symptoms include fever, weakness, arthralgias or frank arthritis, myalgias, cough, and skin rashes.

K. Wegener Granulomatosis

Arthritis and arthralgias are usually overshadowed by evidence of upper and lower respiratory tract necrotizing granulomas and renal vasculitis.

III. Arthritis Associated with Infections

A. Bacterial Infections

An important cause of arthritis that needs immediate attention is septic arthritis caused by various bacteria. In over 90% of the cases, involvement is monarticular, and usually the joint is exquisitely painful. Among the more common pathogens are *Staphylococcus*, *Hemophilus influenzae*, *Streptococcus*, and *Neisseria gonorrhoeae*.

B. Viral Infections

Arthritis has been reported to occur in a large number of viral infections including rubella (after immunization as well), mumps, mononucleosis, and varicella. The joint symptoms usually last less than 6 weeks and are often pauciarticular. Infections by hepatitis A and B viruses may have as a prodrome a serum sickness-like syndrome with urticaria and the swelling of multiple joints.

C. Mycobacterial Infections

The arthritis is usually monarticular but may be polyarticular. Systemic signs may be minimal, and results of the skin test are negative in the first 6 weeks of illness.

D. Mycoplasmal Infections

A migratory polyarthritis, often with an urticarial rash, is usual. Pneumonia is common. One half of the cases have effusion. Recovery occurs when the respiratory infection clears.

E. Fungal Infections

Usually the infections involve bone before invading contiguous joints. Arthritis has been described with coccidioidomycosis, cryptococcosis, histoplasmosis, actinomycosis, and blastomycosis.

F. Reactive Arthritis

Children with invasive bacterial infections, such as meningococcal illnesses, *H. influenzae* type B meningitis, and *N. gonorrhoeae* may develop a nonsuppurative arthritis involving multiple joints later in the course of antibiotic therapy or up to a few weeks after completion of therapy. Immune complexes have been found in both blood and synovial fluid in some cases.

Acute infections such as pharyngitis, scarlet fever, and bacteremias may also be associated with synovitis involving single joints, multiple joints, or migratory in nature.

Various gastrointestinal infections, including *salmonella, shigella, brucella, yersinia,* and *campylobacter* have been implicated. Persons with the histocompatibility locus B-27 seem particularly predisposed.

G. Parasitic Infestations
A pauciarticular, self-limited arthritis has been described with *Giardia lamblia* infestation.

H. Syphilitic Infection

I. Osteomyelitis
Chronic osteomyelitis occurring near a joint may produce a reactive, sterile arthritis. In young children a septic arthritis may be produced by contiguous spread.

J. Miscellaneous Infections
Periarticular cellulitis may mimic a septic arthritis. A psoas abscess or retroperitoneal lymph node infection may stimulate a reactive arthritis of the hip joint.

K. Lyme Disease
The arthritis is sudden in onset, monarticular or oligoarticular and occasionally migratory. The knees are most commonly involved. The arthritis may last 1 day to 3 months and sometimes recurs for years.

L. Toxic Shock Syndrome
Hypotension, rash, and multiple other signs overshadow the arthritis.

IV. Neoplastic Disorders

A. Leukemia
A number of children, much to the consternation of the examining physician, may have arthritis as a presentation of leukemia. The arthritis is usually polyarticular but may be migratory; it is monarticular in 5% of the cases. Severe joint pain is frequent, and the rheumatoid factor may be present. Hematologic abnormalities may offer a clue, particularly anemia and thrombocytopenia.

B. Lymphoma

C. Neuroblastoma

V. Trauma

A. Joint Injury	Direct trauma to a joint is the most common cause of monarticular arthritis.
B. Transient Synovitis	This is a frequent cause of limp and hip pain in young children. The synovitis is probably secondary to any of a number of factors including trauma or viral infections.

VI. Allergic Reactions

A hypersensitivity arthritis or serum sickness may result in the swelling of multiple joints lasting from a few days to several weeks. The joint swelling may be associated with edema of the hands and feet or periorbital area. Urticarial or erythema multiforme rashes are common.

VII. Immunologic Causes

A. Subacute Bacterial Endocarditis	
B. Ventriculojugular Shunt Infections	Chronic infections, especially with coagulase-negative staphylococci, may induce the formation of immune complexes with arthritis and nephritis.
C. Immunodeficiency Syndromes	Up to 20% of children with hypogammaglobulinemia or agammaglobulinemia may develop a chronic polyarthritis mimicking juvenile rheumatoid arthritis.
D. Complement Deficiency	A polyarticular arthritis has been described with a hypomorphic variant of C3 associated with chronic glomerulonephritis.

VIII. Metabolic and Endocrine Disorders

A. Gout	This is an unusual cause of arthritis in children.
B. Hyperlipoproteinemia	Type II and Type IV disorders may be associated with an oligoarticular arthritis, but usually in adults.
C. Gaucher Disease	Arthritis is rare, but bone pain may result from infiltration of the bone marrow with storage cells.
D. Lipogranulomatosis	Lumpy masses over the joints develop in infancy along with a hoarse cry, restricted joint

movement, and recurrent infections; early death is common.

E. Thyroid Disorders — Joint swelling has been described both in hypothyroidism and hyperthyroidism but is an unusual manifestation.

F. Mucopolysaccharidoses — Restricted joint motion and swelling may occur in these disorders, which should be obvious from dysmorphic features.

G. Fabry Disease (Angiokeratoma Corporis Diffusum) — Nodular angiectases of the skin are noted at about 10 years of age. Attacks of burning pain of the hands and feet are often the presenting complaint.

H. Hyperparathyroidism

I. Primary Hyperoxaluria (Oxalosis) — This is a rare cause of acute arthritis. Renal findings with hematuria, nephrolithiasis, and renal failure are more common presentations.

IX. Hereditary Disorders

A number of inherited disorders may be associated with joint symptoms, although many feature arthralgias, bony prominence, or intermittent swelling rather than a florid arthritis.

A. Sickle-Cell Disease — The hand–foot syndrome, painful swelling of the hands and feet, is seen in young children with SS hemoglobin. Avascular necrosis due to sickling may produce painful attacks in older children as well, but usually in other areas.

B. Hemophilia — Clinical signs of hemarthrosis may mimic an acute arthritis.

C. Familial Mediterranean Fever — This uncommon but striking disorder is characterized by acute, recurrent attacks of fever, serositis, and arthritis. The fever lasts 24 to 48 hours and is accompanied by peritonitis, pleuritis, synovitis, and often an erysipelas-like erythema. The joint involvement tends to be monarticular.

D. Marfan Syndrome

E. Ehlers–Danlos Syndrome — The joint hyperextensibility may lead to dislocations and traumatic effusions.

F. Homocystinuria — Affected children have a marfanoid habitus, but the joints tend to have a restricted rather than hyperextensible mobility.

G. Stickler Syndrome (Hereditary Arthroophthalmopathy)	The large joints may be prominent, and joint pains may be present. Generally, affected children have flat facies, depressed nasal bridge, deafness, myopia, and hypotonia. The joints tend to be hyperextensible.

X. Mimics of Arthritis

A. Hypermobility Syndrome	Children with joint hypermobility commonly present with leg and joint aches, sometimes with joint effusions, mimicking arthritis.
B. Subluxation of Patella	
C. Chondromalacia Patellae	This relatively common cause of knee pain rarely may produce effusions; it may be a familial trait or occur after trauma.
D. Osteochrondritis Dissecans	
E. Idiopathic Chondrolysis	Pain and limp in adolescence, with progressive loss of articular cartilage and loss of hip mobility, are characteristic features.
F. Popliteal (Baker) Cysts	
G. Carpal–Tarsal Osteolysis	This rare disease results in gradual disintegration of the carpal and tarsal bones. Other joints may be involved as well; with a clinical picture simulating that of rheumatoid arthritis.
H. Hypertrophic Osteoarthropathy	Arthralgia and occasionally a polyarthritis may precede the appearance of clubbing of the fingers.
I. Tietze Syndrome	The cause of the pain and swelling of costochondral junctions is unknown.

XI. Miscellaneous Causes

A. Cystic Fibrosis	Recurrent painful joint swelling has been reported in children with cystic fibrosis. Usually one or a few joints are involved during each short-lived episode.
B. Thorn-Induced Arthritis	Unusual bacterial pathogens may be introduced into a joint by penetration with a thorn.
C. Whipple Disease	This rare disorder is characterized by diarrhea, malabsorption with steatorrhea, progressive weight loss, anemia, increased skin pigmentation, and joint symptoms, either arthralgias or arthritis. A gram-positive organism has been found on intestinal mucosal biopsies.

| D. Villonodular Synovitis | This uncommon lesion produces masses of nodular synovium, resulting in a swollen joint. Aspirated synovial fluid is often dark and serosanguineous. Usually only one joint is affected. |
| E. Neuropathic Arthropathy | Swollen, tender, warm joints may result following recurrent episodes of inapparent trauma secondary to lack of sensory innervation (Charcot joint). |

XII. Psychogenic Pain

Children may complain of joint pain as part of a conversion reaction. The joints are not swollen, hot, or erythematous, and the sedimentation rate is normal.

SUGGESTED READINGS

Proceedings of the Conference on the Rheumatic Diseases of Childhood. Schaller JG, Hanson V (Co Chrm). Arthritis Rheum 20 (Suppl 2), Mar 1977

Rush PJ, Shore A, Inman R et al: Arthritis associated with *Haemophilus influenzae* meningitis: Septic or reactive? J Pediatr 109:412–415, 1986

92

FRAGILE BONES/
RECURRENT FRACTURES

Physicians caring for children must be acutely aware of the possibility of child abuse in any child with a bone fracture. Occasionally other underlying problems with bone fragility are responsible. Most of these disorders can be separated by a careful history, and a physical and radiologic examination.

I. Trauma

A. Child Abuse

The suspicion of abuse must always be entertained in children with trauma or fractures, particularly if the alleged history does not seem to fit the findings. Other manifestations such as failure to thrive, cutaneous lesions, poor hygiene as well as other high risk notations should be made.

B. Accidents

The "accident-prone" child may be unlucky enough to have repeated fractures.

II. Disorders with Osteoporosis

A. Osteogenesis Imperfecta

Undoubtedly many variants of osteogenesis imperfecta exist, but four general syndromes are often proposed.

1. Type I (Congenita Tarda)

This is a dominantly inherited syndrome with osteoporosis leading to bone fragility. The sclerae are distinctly blue and hearing loss is common in the patient or the family. Other features include joint hypermobility, skeletal deformities, and easy bruisability. Fractures may be present at birth or begin at any time during infancy or childhood. Most patients are short in stature. The bones are usually slender, but otherwise relatively unremarkable. The family history is a key to diagnosis.

2. Type II (Congenita)

This autosomal recessive disorder is characterized by extreme bone fragility. Intrauterine or early infant death usually occurs. Wormian

	bones of the skull and marked deformities of the limbs are present. The skin is frequently fragile as well.
3. Type III (Congenita Tarda)	This is also an autosomal recessive variety characterized by severe bone fragility with multiple fractures and resultant severe, progressive deformities of the limbs and bones. The sclerae become progressively less blue with age. Growth failure is marked.
4. Type IV (Congenita Tarda)	A dominantly inherited osteopenic type with variable severity. The sclerae are not abnormally blue after early infancy. The incidence of hearing loss is low. Postnatal short stature is common as is bowing of the legs.
B. Immobilization Osteoporosis	Bone reabsorption continues in face of reduction of bone cell formation of matrix. When activity is resumed fractures may result. Children with paralytic disorders such as myelomeningocele, poliomyelitis, cerebral palsy, and arthrogryposis are particularly prone to fractures.
C. Exogenous Corticosteroids	Osteoporosis with bone fragility is a well recognized complication of steroid therapy.
D. Cushing Syndrome	Adrenocortical excess often leads to osteoporosis and fractures, particularly vertebral compressions.
E. Idiopathic Osteoporosis	The usual onset of this uncommon disorder is between 8 and 14 years of age. Fractures of the vertebrae and metaphyseal areas of long bones are most common. The disorder is self-limited and improves during adolescence. Low calcitriol has been found in some patients.
F. Rickets	
1. Type I (Vitamin D Deficiency)	Osteoporosis may lead to fragile bones although other features of D-deficiency rickets are usually more obvious. The deficiency may be the result of a lack of sunlight exposure, dietary lack, vitamin D malabsorption, liver disease, anticonvulsant drugs, renal disease, and vitamin D dependency.
2. Type II (Primary Phosphate Deficiency)	A host of disorders with different mechanisms resulting in phosphate deficiency may be seen. Disorders with renal tubule reabsorption problems include Fanconi syndrome (e.g., cystinosis, tyrosinosis, Lowe syndrome, and

so forth); renal tubular acidosis; genetic primary hypophosphatemia and hypophosphatemia associated with "nonendocrine" tumors. Phosphate deficiency or malabsorption may occur with parenteral hyperalimentation, low phosphate feeding in premature infants, and secondary to gastrointestinal binding with aluminum hydroxide.

G. Protein–Calorie Malnutrition

Osteopenia may result from severe malnourishment with resultant fragile bones. Diminished formation of collagen matrix as well as calcium deficiency may be operative.

H. Scurvy

Lack of vitamin C results in osteopenia with loss of trabecular structure and thinning of the cortices. Periosteal hemorrhages and submetaphyseal rarefraction are characteristic.

I. Copper Deficiency

Distorted bones, the result of osteopenia, are rarely due to a copper deficiency. Chronic intestinal malabsorption and Menke syndrome may be causes.

J. Homocystinuria

Osteoporosis leading to compression deformity of the vertebrae is a major manifestation of this inborn error. Dislocated lenses, thromboembolic phenomenon, and mental retardation are other features.

K. Primary Hyperphosphatasia

This rare disorder is characterized by proliferation of poorly mineralized subperiosteal osteoid. Bone thickening, pain, fractures, and deformity often result. The serum alkaline phosphatase is markedly high.

L. Osteoectasia

This autosomal recessive disorder is characterized by small stature, large skull, progressive bowing of the legs and arms with pain, tenderness, and muscle weakness. The calvarium is thickened and tubular bones are expanded but demineralized.

M. Hyperparathyroidism

Hypercalcemic symptoms, anorexia, weakness, constipation, and polyuria overshadow bony problems. Bone pain, particularly in the back and lower extremities, is probably the result of microfractures. Pathologic fractures of long bones and vertebral compression may also occur. Radiographs show diffuse demineralization as well as localized areas of subperiosteal resorption.

N. Congenital Cutis
   Laxa and Os-
   teoporosis

One case of apparent autosomal recessive inheritance has been described. The osteoporosis was incapacitating with multiple fractures.

III. Disorders with Osteosclerosis

A. Osteopetrosis

Dense, marble-like bone is the classic radiologic appearance of this autosomal recessive
disorder. Despite the density, the bone is brittle. The bone marrow is crowded out resulting
in progressive anemia, thrombocytopenia, and
propensity to infection. Sight and hearing are
lost due to narrowing of cranial nerve foramina.

B. Pyknodysostosis

This rare disorder features short stature and
craniofacial disproportion. The cranial sutures
are widened and the fontanel remains open.
The entire skeleton is dense.

C. Dysosteosclerosis

This rare autosomal recessive disorder includes short stature, a failure to erupt permanent teeth, optic atrophy from sclerosis of the
base of the skull, and other cranial nerve involvement. The bones are dense with vertebral platyspondyly and phalangeal tuft resorption.

IV. Miscellaneous Disorders

A. Primary Oxalosis

This rare inborn error results in widespread
deposition of calcium oxalate crystals throughout the body. Symptoms usually begin before
age 5, with nephrolithiasis and resulting urinary tract problems. Pathologic bone fractures
occur later through cystic areas.

B. Pyle Disease

Marked flaring occurs at the metaphyses of
tubular bones. Severe genu valgum develops
early in life. There is an increased tendency to
fractures of long bones.

C. Trichorhinopha-
   langeal Syndrome

Fractures are more frequent in this inherited
disorder which features a pear-shaped, bulbous nose, a long philtrum, a thin upper lip,
and thin scalp hair. Multiple exostoses are
common.

D. Polyostotic Fi-
   brous Dysplasia

Pathologic fractures are prone to occur in the
structurally unsound bone. McCune–Albright
syndrome should be considered if hyper-

pigmented patches of skin and signs of endocrinopathy are present.

E. Bone Cysts and Tumors — Bone fragility occurs with a number of bony lesions, benign and malignant.

F. Dyskeratosis Congenita — Skin findings predominate in this rare disorder that affects mostly males. Atrophy and pigmentation give the skin a reticulated pattern. Nail dystrophy occurs during childhood. The teeth are defective with early decay.

SUGGESTED READINGS

Harrison HE, Harrison HC: Disorders of calcium and phosphate metabolism in childhood and adolescence. Philadelphia, WB Saunders, 1979

Marder HK, Tsang RC, Hug G, Crawford AC: Calcitriol deficiency in idiopathic juvenile osteoporosis. Am J Dis Child 136:914–917, 1982

93

ASYMMETRY

Asymmetry of body parts exists in everyone to a minor degree. The left leg is usually longer than the right, and the right arm longer than the left; fortunately, this asymmetry is usually not noticeable. True, readily apparent asymmetry is unusual.

The following classification divides asymmetry into two types: hemihypertrophy and hemidystrophy. In some cases, it may be difficult to tell whether one side is hypertrophic or the other is atrophic. In many of the disorders associated with asymmetry, the presence of other signs and symptoms provides diagnostic clues. Particularly noteworthy, however, is the association of congenital hemihypertrophy with tumors, especially Wilms' tumor and adrenocortical neoplasms.

I. Hemihypertrophy

A. Idiopathic

Overgrowth of body parts may be localized to one area or involve an entire half of the body, or portions of the body on both sides may be affected. There is considerable variability in the severity of this deformity. Occurrence seems to be sporadic, although affected siblings have been described. Other associated abnormalities have been described in a significant number of cases, including mental retardation in as many as 25%, pigmented skin lesions, hemangiomas, and genitourinary anomalies. A distressing association of hemihypertrophy with neoplasms has also been described, most commonly Wilms' tumor, but also adrenocortical tumors and, less frequently, hepatoblastomas.

B. Disturbances of Bone Growth
   1. Long-Standing Hyperemia

Overgrowth of a part may result from increased blood flow to growing bone. Causes may include arteriovenous fistulas, chronic osteitis, tuberculosis, arthritis, healing fractures, and neoplasms.

2. Neurofibroma- tosis	This relatively common inherited disorder is characterized by multiple café-au-lait spots and later by the appearance of neurofibromas. A wide array of associated deformities and tumors may occur, including hemihypertrophy as well as bony reduction deformities.
C. Hemihypertrophy Associated with Soft Tissue Abnormalities	
1. Lymphedema	An extremity may appear hypertrophied because it is edematous (see Chap. 11, Edema).
2. Klippel–Trenaunay–Weber Syndrome	Hemihypertrophy may be associated with cutaneous hemangiomas, varicose veins, other cutaneous defects, visceromegaly, and a host of other anomalies.
3. Epidermal Nevus Syndrome	Hemihypertrophy may occur with peculiar linear or swirled, macular or verrucous skin lesions.
4. Cutis Marmorata Telangiectatica	The skin has a reticulated vascular pattern.
D. Hemihypertrophy Associated with Dysmorphogenic Syndromes	
1. Russell–Silver Syndrome	Key features include prenatal growth deficiency, triangular facies, and clinodactyly of the fifth fingers. Hemihypertrophy has been described in some cases.
2. Beckwith–Wiedemann Syndrome	Important features of this disorder are postnatal somatic gigantism, macroglossia, omphalocele or umbilical hernia, transitory neonatal hypoglycemia, ear lobe grooves, and, in about 10%, hemihypertrophy. Wilms tumor and other tumors have been described.
3. Langer–Giedion Syndrome	Exostoses, asymmetry, sparse hair, hypoplastic alar cartilage, protuberant ears, brachyclinodactyly, and mild mental retardation may be present.
4. Hemihypertrophy, Macrodactyly, and Connective Tissue Nevi	A single case has been described.[1]

5. Proteus Syndrome | Accelerated growth, macrocephaly, macrodactyly, and thickening of the skin and subcutaneous tissue are other features.

II. Hemidystrophies
  A. Disturbances of Bone

1. Hypoplastic Bones | Short femora or tibiae are the most common.

2. Coxa Vara | Decreased angle of the head of the femur on the femoral shaft may give the impression of a shortened leg.

3. Dislocated Hip

4. Multiple Exostoses | Bowing of the extremity secondary to exostosis gives an asymmetric appearance.

5. Epiphyseal Trauma | Interference with bone growth secondary to injury to the epiphysis will result in a shortened limb.

6. Conradi–Hunermann Syndrome | Shortening of an extremity may result from punctate mineralization in epiphyses. Scoliosis is common; the facies may be flattened, hair sparse, skin coarse, and cataracts present.

7. Ollier Disease | Masses of hyaline cartilage occur asymmetrically, leading to decreased growth of affected bones.

8. Maffucci Syndrome | Multiple hemangiomata appear after birth along with enchondromata, resulting in asymmetric retarded growth of bones.

9. Postmeningococcal Skeletal Dystrophy | Epiphyseal and metaphyseal damage may follow sepsis and DIC, especially with meningococcemia, resulting in asymmetry.

  B. Linear Scleroderma | Bone growth may be retarded in areas of localized scleroderma.

  C. Neurologic Insults | Asymmetric development of parts of the body may follow various neurologic insults.

1. Cerebral Palsy
2. Poliomyelitis
3. Meningomyelocele

4. Sturge–Weber Syndrome | Atrophy of one limb may occur contralateral to the leptomeningeal angioma.

5. Spinal Dysraphism

D. Chromosomal Abnormality	Hemiatrophy has been observed in triploid and diploid mosaics. Other features include a very low birth weight, developmental retardation, and coloboma of the iris.
E. Congenital Torticollis	Asymmetry of the face will develop in children whose torticollis is not detected in early infancy.

REFERENCE

1. Temtamy SA, Rogers JG: Macrodactyly, hemihypertrophy, and connective tissue nevi: Report of a new syndrome and review of the literature. J Pediatr 89:924, 1976

SUGGESTED READING

Jaffe KM, Cohen MM Jr, Lemire RJ: Malformations of the limbs. In Kelly VC (ed): Practice of Pediatrics, Vol 10, Chap 54, pp 1–45. Hagerstown, Harper & Row, 1987

94

MUSCLE WEAKNESS

Evaluation of muscle weakness in children presents an interesting challenge. A few disorders account for most cases seen in the average pediatric practice. However, when the diagnosis is not obvious, the cause may be any of numerous rare and unusual conditions with long and confusing names. A full discussion of these disorders is beyond the scope of this chapter; for further details, neurologic texts such as those listed as Suggested Reading are recommended.

Diagnostic considerations include age of onset of the weakness; whether it occurred abruptly or was slowly progressive; whether there are associated systemic signs or symptoms; and, of course, whether there is a family history. It is also important to determine whether the weakness is static or progressive; whether it is focal or diffuse; and whether it is episodic or constant.

Results of the neurologic examination may indicate a specific anatomic site of the lesion. Upper motor neuron disease is suggested by an increase in deep tendon reflexes, clonus, presence of the Babinski sign, persistence of infantile reflexes, and frequently mental retardation. Anterior horn cell disease is likely to be associated with profound weakness, hyporeflexia, muscle atrophy and fasciculations, and the absence of sensory changes. Peripheral nerve disorders produce weakness, more pronounced distally, with sensory changes; deep tendon reflexes are usually absent or diminished. In myopathies, the weakness is usually proximal, and the deep tendon reflexes are reduced in proportion to the weakness; sensory changes are not part of the picture.

Weakness must be differentiated from other conditions such as ataxia, hypotonia, vertigo, and incoordination. In the following classification, disorders causing weakness are grouped according to mode of onset; however, there may be some overlap among categories.

I. Disorders with Acute Onset

A. Acute Infectious Myositis	This disorder is most commonly associated with influenzal infections. Calf and thigh pain are often severe. Muscle enzyme levels are elevated; myoglobinuria may be a finding. Bacterial myositis is relatively uncommon and is more likely to be unilateral.
B. Guillain–Barré Syndrome	Etiology is varied. Development of distal paresthesias, often with muscle pain, may be

sudden or gradual, followed by a progressive ascending muscle weakness, almost always symmetric. Deep tendon reflexes are lost. Cranial nerve involvement occurs in less than half of the cases. It often occurs 1 to 3 weeks after a nonspecific respiratory or gastrointestinal tract illness. Specific infectious agents incriminated include cytomegalovirus, Epstein–Barr virus, enterovirus, mycoplasma, and *Campylobacter jejuni* as well as after immunization.

C. Trauma

Weakness or paralysis may follow trauma to the head, spine, nerve roots, muscles, or peripheral nerves.

D. Hypokalemia

Loss of potassium from the gastrointestinal tract or kidneys, increased loss associated with drug therapy, or by iatrogenic induction may result in profound weakness. An ileus is often present.

E. Organophosphate Poisoning

Weakness is overshadowed by other symptoms including salivation, sweating, and tearing; coughing, choking, and dyspnea; vomiting, diarrhea, and abdominal cramps; anxiety, seizures, and confusion; and numerous other signs.

F. Atropine Poisoning

Mucous membranes are dry, and pupils are dilated; erythema of skin, fever, restlessness, and confusion are common.

G. Herpes Zoster

Weakness may occur in the distribution of the involved peripheral nerve.

H. Infectious Mononucleosis

Generalized or focal areas of weakness may occur.

I. Poliomyelitis

This disorder was formerly a common and important cause of flaccid weakness. There is usually a prodrome of fever, headache, vomiting, and diarrhea, followed by back pain, muscle tenderness, drowsiness, irritability, and stiff neck.

J. Diphtheria Toxin

Early signs include palatal paralysis, resulting in a nasal voice, difficulty in swallowing, and blurred vision, followed by other signs of cranial nerve involvement, loss of reflexes, and a neuropathy.

K. Botulism

Common presenting signs are diplopia, photophobia, and blurred vision, followed by difficulty in swallowing and weakness.

L. Tick Paralysis — The first symptoms may be some irritability and anorexia followed by an ascending weakness, often rapid in onset.

M. Epidural Abscess — Fever, back pain, and lower extremity weakness are typical; paralysis may occur rapidly if the problem goes untreated.

N. Transverse Myelitis — Back pain with the rapid onset of a flaccid paralysis is characteristic.

O. Myoglobinuria — Etiology is varied. Usually sudden onset of muscle pain with weakness occurs, followed by the passage of dark urine.

P. Polyarteritis Nodosa — Affected children generally have fever, abdominal pain, muscle pain and tenderness, arthritis, and nodular skin lesions, often purpuric.

Q. Anterior Spinal Artery Occlusion — The occlusion may be a result of trauma or local infection, a hypercoaguable state, or embolism. If occlusion occurs in the lumbar spine, weakness of the lower extremities, loss of deep tendon reflexes, and bladder difficulties occur.

R. Septic Arthritis/ Osteomyelitis — A pseudoparalysis may occur in the involved extremity.

S. Conversion Reaction — Hysterical weakness may be a reaction to rape, sexual abuse, or other stressful situations. The reflexes are normal and sensation is intact or altered in nonanatomical patterns.

T. Acute Central Cervical Cord Syndrome — This syndrome is produced by minor trauma to the cervical spine. It is characterized by more motor impairment of the upper than lower extremities; flaccid upper extremities with decreased or absent DTRs, while the lower extremities are spastic with increased reflexes.

II. Acute Onset—Episodic

A. Hypokalemic Periodic Paralysis — Periodic attacks of weakness may be hereditary or associated with chronic renal disease, hyperthyroidism, or aldosteronism; the ingestion of excessive amounts of licorice has also been implicated. In the familial form, attacks begin in adolescence. Quadriplegia and areflexia without pain may occur. Duration of weakness is a few hours to 2 days.

B. Hyperkalemic Periodic Paralysis — Attacks usually begin in the first decade; they may occur daily or several times a day but are less severe than in the hypokalemic form. Calf muscles may be enlarged. Weakness of facial muscles and myotonia are common.

C. Sodium-Responsive Periodic Paralysis

Onset is during the first decade. Attacks are severe, with quadriplegia and bulbar muscle involvement. Each episode may last 2 to 3 weeks, but oral or intravenous sodium chloride has been found effective.

D. Periodic Paralysis with Cardiac Dysrhythmias

Onset is during the first or second decade; attacks may occur at monthly intervals; they are of moderate severity; and they last 1 to 2 days.

E. Paroxysmal Paralytic Myoglobinuria

Onset is usually before 20 years of age. Recurrent attacks of muscle cramps with weakness and excretion of myoglobin in the urine are characteristic.

F. Acute Intermittent Porphyria

Attacks generally involve abdominal pain, disturbances of consciousness, apparent psychosis, seizures, and a rapidly progressing peripheral neuropathy. Urine is burgundy red. Onset is rare before puberty.

G. Aldosteronism

Muscle weakness may be episodic and can progress to paralysis. The lower extremities are more severely affected than the upper ones. Weakness is the result of potassium depletion. Other symptoms include polydipsia, polyuria, and hypertension.

H. Hyperthyroidism

There may be episodic muscle weakness associated with hypokalemia.

I. McArdle Disease (Glycogen Storage Disease, Type V)

Muscle weakness, stiffness, and painful cramps occur only after moderately severe exercise and they disappear with rest. Inheritance pattern is autosomal recessive.

J. Paramyotonia Congenita

Weakness is aggravated by cold and exercise. Findings on neurologic examination are normal except for percussion myotonia of the tongue or thenar eminence. Speech may be dysarthric after the ingestion of ice cream. Inheritance pattern is autosomal dominant.

III. Subacute Onset

A. Polymyositis

Onset can be sudden or chronic. There is a proximal muscle weakness of the pelvic and shoulder girdles. Muscles commonly ache and are tender to palpation. Muscle enzyme levels are increased; dysphagia and neck weakness are common.

B. Dermatomyositis — Symptoms are similar to those of polymyositis, but skin changes or discoloration of the upper eyelids, a facial butterfly erythema, or more commonly, erythematous papules over knees, elbows, and knuckles may also be findings.

C. Systemic Lupus Erythematosus — Muscle weakness is rarely an initial complaint. Arthritis, fever, rashes, and evidence of nephritis are common.

D. Heavy Metal Poisoning

   1. Lead — Signs of peripheral neuropathy such as footdrop may precede evidence of encephalopathy. Weakness may be symmetric.

   2. Mercury — Hypotonia is often severe. Affected children are very irritable, with photophobia, absent reflexes, weakness, erythema, tremors, and increased sweating and salivation.

   3. Arsenic — Following acute ingestion, gastrointestinal symptoms predominate. If the child survives, painful parasthesias followed by symmetric weakness occur within 1 to 6 weeks.

   4. Thallium — Acute ingestion results in profound weakness, first with paresthesias, followed later by hair loss.

   5. Gold and Zinc — Gold and zinc poisoning are rare causes of weakness.

E. Renal Disease — In chronic renal disorders with potassium loss, muscle weakness may be a symptom.

F. Steroid Myopathy — Excess production as in Cushing syndrome or more commonly from exogenous (iatrogenic) treatment may result in progressive muscle weakness, particularly proximally.

G. Hyperparathyroidism — Proximal muscle weakness and wasting, hypotonia and discomfort on movement with increased or decreased deep tendon reflexes, and muscle cramps have been described in hypercalcemia.

H. Hypopituitarism — Weakness and muscle atrophy may be part of the clinical picture.

I. Kocher–Debré–Sémélaigne Syndrome — Affected children appear to have well-developed musculature but are weak. The condition is secondary to hypothyroidism.

J. Hyperthyroid Myopathy

Rarely, proximal muscle weakness may be the initial symptom.

K. Neoplasia

Asymmetric weakness may be secondary to infiltrates of peripheral nerves or compression of nerves from tumors such as Hodgkin disease. In occult malignancies, myopathy may be a presenting sign.

L. Brain Stem Tumors

These tumors generally produce, among other symptoms, a progressive, symmetric spastic paraplegia or quadriplegia.

M. Spinal Cord Tumors

Spinal cord tumors may produce a flaccid weakness at the level of the lesion and a spastic weakness below. Extramedullary tumors may be associated with back pain, weakness, and in some cases, bladder or bowel dysfunction. Intramedullary tumors are painless and result in a symmetric weakness.

N. Brain Tumors

Cerebral hemisphere tumors produce a unilateral progressive spastic paraplegia.

O. Cat-Scratch Disease

If they occur, neurologic symptoms appear days to weeks after the initial adenitis. Fever, headache, weakness, and paralysis may be present. Encephalitis is more common, however.

P. Thiamine Deficiency

This is rare in childhood. Edema of the extremities, cardiomegaly, generalized hypotonia, and weakness may be present.

Q. Scleroderma

Very rarely, weakness may occur without obvious skin changes.

IV. Congenital or Onset in Early Infancy

A. Werdnig–Hoffman Disease

This disorder is also called infantile spinal muscular atrophy; it is the most common cause of severe hypotonia and progressive weakness during the first year of life. Diminished or absent reflexes, fasciculations of the tongue, and diaphragmatic breathing may be present. Inheritance pattern is autosomal recessive.

B. Cerebral Palsy

This disorder has a mixture of neurologic findings, the result of insults to the central nervous system causing spastic or flaccid weakness, poor coordination, lack of balance, and abnormal posturing.

C. Myasthenia Gravis — Onset in about one third of cases is at birth. Ptosis, difficulty in sucking, and respiratory difficulties may be present.

D. Benign Congenital Hypotonia — The etiology is poorly understood. Many cases probably represent primary muscle disease; there is a tendency to improve with age.

E. Congenital Laxity of Ligaments — If laxity is severe, the child may appear weak.

F. Down Syndrome

G. Prader–Willi Syndrome — Neonatal hypotonia may be severe. Hypogonadism, small penis, decreased reflexes, and retardation occur. Later, hyperphagia leads to obesity. Affected children are short in stature.

H. Myotonic Dystrophy — Weakness and muscular wasting may begin at any age. Infants have difficulty in swallowing and delay in achieving developmental milestones. Ptosis of eyelids and atrophy of facial muscles may occur early; cataracts, balding, and testicular atrophy occur later. The myopathy is associated with myotonia.

I. Tay–Sachs Disease — Affected infants appear normal until 4 to 6 months of age, when diminished muscle tone becomes evident. Loss of developmental milestones, progressive weakness, and decreased vision or blindness with a macular cherry-red spot are typical. Hyperacusis, myoclonic seizures, and generalized seizures occur. Affected infants are usually of Eastern European Jewish ancestry; inheritance pattern is autosomal recessive.

J. Pompe Disease (Glycogen Storage Disease, Type II) — The metabolic defect is a deficiency of acid maltase. Marked hypotonia and weakness are present from early infancy. The tongue becomes enlarged; cardiomegaly develops; and swallowing and respiratory difficulties become major problems. Death occurs in early infancy.

K. Arthrogryposis Multiplex Congenita — Multiple contractures of arms and legs are present at birth. There are various types, some with decreased anterior horn cells.

L. Lowe Syndrome — Marked hypotonia, cataracts, growth failure, severe retardation with proteinuria, aminoaciduria, and acidosis are findings. Inheritance pattern is sex-linked recessive.

M. Myopathies — Over the past two decades, a number of primary muscle disorders have been described. In all forms, symptoms may be similar, but characteristic findings on muscle biopsy allow differentiation.

1. Central Core Disease

Hypotonia and weakness are evident in infancy; motor milestones are delayed. Osteoarticular problems, including dislocated hips, kyphoscoliosis, and flat feet, are common.

2. Nemaline Myopathy

Weakness and hypotonia may be present at birth or appear much later. Affected children have a long, thin face and slender body build. There is gross motor weakness, but fine motor ability is undisturbed. Reflexes are variably affected. Inheritance pattern is autosomal dominant or recessive.

3. Myotubular Myopathy

Weakness and hypotonia may be present at birth or appear later. Most patients have facial weakness or extraocular movement problems. Deep tendon reflexes are normal or absent.

4. Mitochondrial Myopathies

This form probably represents a mixed bag of disorders. In some cases, a hypermetabolic state occurs, with weakness, hyporeflexia, profuse sweating, dyspnea, palpitations, polydipsia, polyuria, polyphagia, and unexplained rises in body temperature.

N. Canavan Disease

Symptoms appear in the first 6 months of life. Developmental failure, hypotonia, and moderate-to-severe head enlargement are early signs; spasticity and blindness occur later.

O. Gaucher Disease

The infantile form is characterized by a severe neurologic deficit with generalized hypotonia, opisthotonos, rigidity, dysphagia, laryngeal spasms, and mental and motor deterioration. Splenomegaly is followed by hepatomegaly.

P. Krabbe Disease (Globoid Leukodystrophy)

Psychomotor development is normal until 4 to 6 months of age, when progressive deterioration begins. Hypotonia is followed by progressive spasticity. Inheritance pattern is autosomal recessive.

Q. Generalized Gangliosidosis

Psychomotor retardation appears early in infancy. Hypotonia, facial and peripheral edema, frontal bossing, low-set ears, alveolar ridge hypertrophy, and hepatomegaly followed by splenomegaly are characteristic.

R. Dejerine–Sottas Disease (Progressive Hypertrophic Interstitial Neuropathy)
Delayed development is usually noted in early infancy. There is progressive weakness, especially in the lower extremities; sensory involvement results in ataxia. Nystagmus is common, as are muscle cramps. Palpation discloses peripheral nerve enlargement.

S. Congenital Hypomyelination Neuropathy
Symptoms are similar to those of Dejerine–Sottas disease but are more severe. Deep tendon reflexes are absent.

T. Hyperlysinemia
Mental and physical retardation occurs with hypotonia and laxity of ligaments.

U. Atonic Diplegia
Nonprogressive, generalized muscle weakness is characteristic. The cause is unknown. Leg weakness is usually more pronounced than arm weakness. Reflexes most frequently are hypoactive but may be normal.

V. Congenital Choreoathetosis and Congenital Ataxia
Affected infants may have marked hypotonia and weakness during the first year of life. Ataxia and posturing should be noticeable.

W. Glycogen Storage Disease, Type III
The onset of symptoms is in the first 6 months of life, with failure to thrive, hepatosplenomegaly, and liver failure with cirrhosis. Retarded muscular development and weakness with hypotonia may also be findings.

X. Congenital Hemiplegia
Congenital hemiplegia may be the result of acquired injuries to the brain, frequently causing porencephaly. A genetic form of porencephaly has been described.

Y. Lysinuric Protein Intolerance
This rare autosomal recessive disorder also features hepatosplenomegaly and osteoporosis.

V. Onset in Late Infancy or Early Childhood

A. Duchenne Type Muscular Dystrophy
Onset of symptoms is between 2 and 4 years of age. Affected children are often late in beginning to walk, with steady progression of weakness. Calf muscles appear enlarged. Reflexes are decreased or absent. Two thirds of the cases are hereditary (sex-linked recessive); one third are sporadic. Muscle enzyme levels are elevated.

B. Emotional Deprivation
Weakness and hypotonia may appear earlier in infancy also. Growth rate may be dimin-

ished. A change in environment brings about improvement.

C. Sulfatide Lipidosis (Metachromatic Leukodystrophy)

Onset of symptoms is by the end of the first year of life. Progressive weakness, hypotonia, and mental deterioration develop. Swallowing difficulties, optic atrophy, third or fourth cranial nerve palsies, nystagmus, and ataxia are prominent. There are three forms: infantile, juvenile, and adult. Inheritance pattern is autosomal dominant.

D. Subacute Necrotizing Encephalomyelitis

Onset of symptoms usually begins at less than 2 years of age. Feeding difficulties, vomiting, progressive hypotonia and weakness, asthma-like attacks, nystagmus, and normal or increased deep tendon reflexes are found.

E. Giant Axonal Neuropathy

Symptoms begin at 2 to 3 years of age, with clumsy gait and progressive weakness. Kinky hair is common; reflexes are absent.

F. Ataxia-Telangiectasia

Ataxia develops during the first 2 years of life. Progressive ataxia, choreoathetosis, oculocutaneous telangiectasia, and recurrent sinopulmonary infections are present. Hypotonia and weakness occur in later stages.

G. Chédiak–Higashi Syndrome

Features include defective pigmentation of hair and skin with pancytopenia, increased susceptibility to infections, and later, lymphatic malignancies. Mental retardation, seizures, and muscle weakness are common.

H. Refsum Disease

This disease is characterized by ichthyosis, hearing deficit, ataxia, and a polyneuritis with distal weakness.

I. Craniovertebral Anomalies

Spastic weakness with increased deep tendon reflexes is characteristic.

   1. Basilar Impression

The cervical spine invaginates into the base of the cranium. Abnormalities of the cervical vertebrae, such as the Klippel–Feil syndrome, may have this problem. Occipital headaches, lower cranial nerve palsies, nystagmus, and spastic paraplegia or quadriplegia may be seen.

   2. Occipitalization of Atlas; Atlantoaxial Dislocation;

There may be neck pain, ataxia, and posterior column deficits with numbness and pain in the arms and legs.

	Separated Odontoid Process of Axis
J. Familial Spastic Paraplegia	Progressive spasticity and weakness of the lower extremities without sensory changes begin in the first or second decade.
K. Late Infantile Acid Maltase Deficiency	Slow or regressing motor development, hip weakness, calf muscle hypertrophy, and toe walking from Achilles tendon contracture are found.
L. Infantile Neuroaxonal Dystrophy	Onset of symptoms is late in infancy, with progressive weakness, muscle atrophy, and hypotonia. Urinary retention, nystagmus, and blindness develop. Inheritance pattern is autosomal recessive.
M. Kugelberg–Welander Disease (Juvenile Spinal Muscular Atrophy)	Onset may be in childhood to adolescence. Proximal weakness and atrophy begin first in the legs. This slowly progressive disease is often mistaken for muscular dystrophy. Reflexes are diminished or absent.
N. Abetalipoproteinemia	Early in infancy, steatorrhea and abdominal distension develop; growth rate is retarded. By 7 to 8 years of age, ataxia and muscle weakness are present. Later visual acuity is lost, and retinitis pigmentosa and nystagmus develop. Ptosis and weak extraocular movements are present; deep tendon reflexes are absent, and loss of position and vibration sensation occurs. Inheritance pattern is autosomal recessive.
O. Tangier Disease	Hepatosplenomegaly and marked orangish yellow tonsillar enlargement with a variable peripheral neuropathy are present. Inheritance pattern is autosomal recessive.
P. Diaphyseal Dysplasia (Engelmann Disease)	Leg weakness and pain are characteristics of this hereditary bone disorder.
Q. Vitamin E Deficiency	Malabsorption of vitamin E leading to prolonged deficiency results in multiple neurologic signs. Hyporeflexia is the initial warning.

VI. Onset in Late Childhood or Adolescence

A. Myasthenia Gravis	Progressive fatigability is typical. Younger children have generalized muscle weakness

and partial or complete external ophthalmoplegia. Ptosis is common. Repetitive movements bring out weakness.

B. Diastematomyelia

Foot abnormalities, such as severe pes cavus, are common. Spastic weakness of lower legs, bladder dysfunction and muscular atrophy develop. There may be cutaneous abnormalities over the spine.

C. Charcot–Marie–Tooth Disease (Progressive Neuropathic [Peroneal] Muscular Atrophy)

Footdrop is often the first symptom; pes equinus deformity develops later. Reflexes are often absent; lower leg muscular atrophy is characteristic. Symptoms usually become apparent late in the second decade.

D. Limb–Girdle Muscular Dystrophy

Slowly progressive weakness begins at between 4 and 15 years of age. Pseudohypertrophy of calves and low back pain may be clues. Inheritance pattern is autosomal recessive.

E. Facioscapulohumeral Dystrophy

Onset of weakness is usually between 12 and 20 years, often with orbicularis oris, neck, and pectoral muscle weakness, and winging of the scapulae. Inheritance pattern is autosomal dominant.

F. Carnitine Deficiency

This disorder produces progressive muscle weakness and liver enzyme abnormalities. Myopathic facies and ptosis are present. Onset is usually before 10 years of age.

G. Amyotrophic Lateral Sclerosis

This disorder is rare in childhood. Muscle weakness and wasting, fasciculations, spasticity, and hyperactive reflexes are findings.

H. Uremia

Uremia is a rare cause of weakness in childhood. Peripheral neuropathy is characterized by dysesthesias, especially burning sensations, followed by slowly progressive weakness.

I. Diabetic Neuropathy

This is an unlikely cause of weakness in children.

J. Syringomyelia

Progressive inability to feel pain or temperature sensations develops, followed by weakness with decreased or absent deep tendon reflexes.

K. Glycogen Storage Disease, Type III

Features include hepatomegaly, hypoglycemia, and mild growth failure with late onset of weakness.

L. Muscle Phospho-fructokinase Deficiency — Motor development during the first decade is usually normal, but children have decreased exercise tolerance. They may complain of muscle stiffness and weakness and may have muscle cramps.

M. Late-Onset X-Linked Muscular Dystrophy (Becker) — The clinical picture resembles that in Duchenne type muscular dystrophy, but onset is later (in the second decade), and progression is slower. Pseudohypertrophy and Gowers sign are present. Severity of disease seems to be consistent in affected families.

SUGGESTED READINGS

Lagos JC: Differential Diagnosis in Pediatric Neurology. Boston, Little, Brown & Co, 1971

Swaiman KF, Wright FS: Pediatric Neuromuscular Diseases. St. Louis, CV Mosby, 1979

95

MUSCULAR HYPERTROPHY

Muscular hypertrophy is not a common sign or complaint in the pediatric age group. Although adolescents may develop hypertrophied muscles with exercise, in younger children this condition is unusual.

The causes of muscular hypertrophy have been divided into three categories: generalized, localized, and apparent. In the last group, loss of adipose or nearby muscle tissue creates the appearance of muscular hypertrophy.

I. Generalized Hypertrophy

A. Beckwith–Wiedemann Syndrome	In the neonatal period macroglossia and an omphalocele or umbilical hernia are quite noticeable. Hypoglycemia is common. The infants may be large at birth or grow rapidly thereafter. The viscera are large as well.
B. Adrenogenital Syndrome	21-Hydroxylase deficiency is the most common enzymatic defect. There is nearly always an excessive production of adrenal androgens. Girls show progressive virilization. The children grow rapidly and have increased muscle mass as well.
C. Virilizing Adrenal Tumors	In both boys and girls, the musculature is well developed, and linear growth is rapid. Girls become hirsute and virilized. The prepubertal boy has enlarged genitalia without testicular development.
D. Kocher Debré–Sémélaigne Syndrome	Muscular hypertrophy may occur in longstanding untreated hypothyroidism, either congenital, acquired, or induced. The hypertrophy is reversible upon treatment of the hypothyroidism.
E. Acromegaly	Excessive secretion of growth hormone after epiphyseal closure results in generalized enlargement, particularly of distal parts of the body. Initially there are generalized muscle hypertrophy and increased strength; however, muscle weakness occurs later.

F. Myotonia Congenita (Thomsen Disease)

Relaxation of voluntary muscle contraction is delayed. Newborns may have sucking and feeding difficulties and, later, slow motor development. The muscular difficulties are generally not noted until childhood or adolescence when difficulty in releasing grasped objects or initiating movements becomes obvious. Although the muscles appear large, they are mildly weak.

G. Paramyotonia Congenita

In this disorder the myotonia is aggravated by cold; it is associated with mild weakness; and it is not progressive. Inheritance pattern is autosomal dominant.

H. Myotonic Chondrodystrophy (Schwartz–Jampel)

This unusual disorder is characterized by short stature, kyphoscoliosis, pectus carinatum, a small mouth with a pinched facial expression, myotonia, and muscular hypertrophy. Inheritance pattern is autosomal recessive.

I. Generalized Muscle Enlargement, Severe Mental Retardation, and Central Nervous System Defects

This triad was described by DeLange in 1934. There is some question about whether this represents a single entity. The infants described had hypertonia and microcephaly with severe central nervous system defects including porencephaly.

II. Localized Hypertrophy (Calves)

A. Duchenne Type Muscular Dystrophy

This is the classic condition with calf pseudohypertrophy. The child may walk later than expected, but an abnormal gait is not noted until 3 or 4 years of age. The muscle weakness is progressive and initially most prominent in the hip girdle and later the shoulder girdle. The quadriceps, infraspinatus, and deltoid muscle groups may be enlarged as well.

B. X-Linked Muscular Dystrophy (Becker)

The clinical picture resembles that in the Duchenne type, but the signs develop later and progress slower with an onset often in the second decade.

C. Autosomal Recessive Pseudohypertrophic Muscular Dystrophy

Features of proximal muscle weakness and calf hypertrophy occur in both sexes. The onset is between 2 and 14 years of age.

D. Limb–Girdle Muscular Dystrophy

Muscle weakness develops in one or both groups of girdle muscles. Calf muscle hypertrophy occurs in a few cases.

E. Hyperkalemic Periodic Paralysis — Attacks of muscle weakness lasting 1 to 2 hours typically occur after exertion. The paralysis usually develops over a period of 30 to 40 minutes. The calf muscle may be enlarged. Inheritance pattern is autosomal dominant.

F. Late Infantile Acid Maltase Deficiency — In addition to calf muscle hypertrophy, hip weakness, slow or regressive motor development, atonic anal sphincter, and Achilles tendon contractures may be found.

G. Phosphoglucomutase Deficiency — The deficiency results in calf hypertrophy, mild generalized weakness, regression of motor development, and toe walking.

III. Apparent Hypertrophy

A. Lipodystrophy — Due to the loss of adipose tissue, the muscles in involved areas appear enlarged because of prominent muscle outline and veins.

1. Partial Lipodystrophy — Insidious loss of subcutaneous tissue from the face is first noted at about 5 years of age. The loss progresses to the neck, upper trunk, and arms but rarely to the lower extremities.

2. Total Lipodystrophy — In this form there is actually an increase in muscle mass. The abdomen is prominent, and the liver is enlarged. Diabetes resistance to insulin therapy generally develops.

B. Kugelberg–Welander Disease — In the juvenile form an abnormal gait develops between the ages of 2 and 17 years because of hip and thigh muscle weakness. Atrophy begins in the quadriceps and then involves the shoulder girdle. The calf muscles appear hypertrophied because of the severity of the quadriceps atrophy.

96

BOW LEGS AND KNOCK KNEES

Most infants have some degree of bowing of the legs as a result of intrauterine position. This physiologic phenomenon is responsible for the bowing seen in most infants. The bowing will often give way to knock knees as the infant begins standing and passes through the toddler stage. Pathologic conditions associated with bow legs have characteristic clinical or roentgenographic features that allow easy differentiation. Similarly, most children with knock knees are passing through a developmental phase, usually between 2 and 6 years of age, in which the condition is normal.

It should be noted that the Latin term *genu varum* is commonly but incorrectly used to refer to bow legs. *Genu varum* actually refers only to knock knees, and *genu valgum* to bow legs.[1] To avoid confusion, use of the straightforward descriptive terms is recommended.

I. Bow Legs

A. Physiologic Bowing	Most newborn infants have some degree of bowing, the result of intrauterine position with the legs crossed and flexed. The bowing will not begin to correct until some time after weight-bearing begins, usually at 6 to 12 months of age.
B. Rickets	Rickets, either vitamin D deficient or vitamin D resistant, is often blamed for the physiologic bowing. Roentgenographic examination should be performed if the bowing increases with age rather than improving, or if the separation of the medial femoral condyles is excessive (5 cm or more when the medial malleoli are touching and the patellae are facing forward).
C. Tibia Vara (Blount Disease)	This rather uncommon disorder results from a growth disturbance of the medial aspect of the proximal tibial epiphysis. It usually occurs in early walkers and is bilateral in 50% to 75% of cases. The bowing increases rather than de-

D. Asymmetric Growth Disturbance

creases with age. There is an adolescent form in which bowing does not develop until 8 to 13 years of age and is unilateral in most cases. Various types of injury to the distal femoral or proximal tibial epiphyses may result in subsequent bowing. Causes include trauma and osteomyelitis.

E. Familial Form

The bowing occurs in the lower third of the tibia so that the ankles seem to curve sharply inward.

F. Bowing with Internal Tibial Torsion

True internal tibial torsion is uncommon. Physiologic bowing often creates the erroneous impression of torsion.

G. Achondroplasia

H. Hypochondroplasia

In this mild short-limbed dwarfism with normal head size, the bowing is mild, and there is also ligamentous laxity.

I. Metaphyseal Dysostosis

Short stature and bow legs are apparent by 2 years of age. Roentgenographic changes in the metaphyses confirm the diagnosis.

J. Rheumatoid Arthritis

Some children with rheumatoid arthritis will develop bowing of the legs, although many more have knock knees.

K. Enchondromatosis (Ollier Disease)

This bone disorder of unknown cause is characterized by radiolucencies in the metaphyses and diaphyses of long bones, resulting in asymmetric limited growth.

L. Multiple Epiphyseal Dysplasia

Short stature and irregular mottled epiphyses on roentgenograms are findings in this rare disorder. The legs may be bowed or have a knock-kneed appearance. Inheritance pattern is autosomal dominant.

M. Cartilage–Hair Hypoplasia

This is a metaphyseal chondrodysplasia with features of short stature, fine sparse hair, and short limbs and hands. Mild bowing of the legs may be present.

N. Postmeningococcal Skeletal Dystrophy

Epiphyseal and metaphyseal damage may follow sepsis and DIC, especially with meningococcemia.

II. Knock Knees

A. Physiologic Knock Knees

Many children between 2 and 6 years of age pass through a knock-kneed phase. The natural history is one of improvement, usually by age 5; if it persists past age 8, the condition

	will not correct spontaneously. Obesity accentuates the problem.
B. Flatfoot	Pronation of the foot will result in a knock-kneed appearance.
C. Trauma	An injury to the distal femoral epiphysis or proximal tibial epiphysis may result in knock knees or bow legs. Causes include trauma, osteomyelitis, and rickets. A unilateral knock knee is almost always pathologic.
D. Adolescent Knock Knees	Adolescent children with knock knees are generally large in height, body build, and weight. The medial distal femoral condyles are higher than the lateral. The problem does not resolve spontaneously but rather tends to worsen with age.
E. Rheumatoid Arthritis	Children with juvenile rheumatoid arthritis are more likely to become knock-kneed than bow-legged.
F. Renal Rickets	Early signs may be growth failure and knock knees. Other symptoms include pallor, polydipsia, and polyuria.
G. Vitamin D–Resistant Rickets	The presenting symptom is usually a limb deformity, either bow legs or knock knees.
H. Chondroectodermal Dysplasia (Ellis–van Creveld Syndrome)	In this disorder inherited as an autosomal-recessive trait, features include sparse hair, defective nails and dentition, cardiac defects, dwarfism, and polydactyly.
I. Congenital Dislocation of the Patella	Permanent dislocation of the patella laterally will create a knock-kneed stance.
J. Diaphyseal Dysplasia (Camurati–Engelmann Disease)	The shafts of the femur and tibia become progressively thickened. The gait is often waddling, the limbs are thin, and leg pain is present even in infancy.
K. Diastrophic Dwarfism	This short-limbed dwarfism is characterized by severe club foot, limited flexion of some joints, a proximal thumb, and soft cystic masses in the auricles. Micrognathia and cleft palate may be present.
L. Morquio Syndrome	This is a mucopolysaccharidosis with features of short trunk, severe knock knees, short flat nose, wide mouth, and pectus carinatum.
M. Maroteaux–Lamy Syndrome (Mucopolysaccharidosis VI)	Coarse facies, growth deficiency, stiff joints, corneal opacities, and lumbar kyphosis are also common.

N. Multiple Epiphyseal Dysplasia Syndrome
: Slow growth is noted in early childhood. The gait is waddling, and joints are stiff. Roentgenograms reveal small, irregular epiphyses.

O. Spondyloepiphyseal Dysplasia
: Shortened trunk, kyphosis, short neck, and eventually, stiff joints are features. Inheritance is sex-linked recessive.

P. Homocystinuria
: In this aminoaciduria, affected children have a marfanoid appearance. Dislocated lenses, malar flush, mental deficiency, and arterial and venous thromboses are common.

REFERENCE

1. Houston CS, Swischuk LE: Varus and valgus—no wonder they are confused. N Engl J Med 302:471–472, 1980

SUGGESTED READING

Sharrad WJW: Pediatric Orthopaedics and Fractures. Oxford, Blackwell Scientific Publications, 1979

97

TOEING IN

In the evaluation of the relatively common pediatric problem of toeing in, examination should begin at the toes and move up to the hip. This chapter presents the most likely causes grouped by the anatomic location of the underlying problem.

I. Foot Problems

A. Metatarsus Adductus (Varus)

This deformity of the forefoot is most likely a result of forefoot compression *in utero*. The medial deviation of the forefoot should be apparent at birth. In most cases the deformity is mobile; that is, the forefoot can be abducted and is not fixed. The adduction may be compounded by the sleeping position; for example, the infant may lie prone with the feet turned in. Fixed deformities are best treated early on, long before the infant begins to walk with a toeing-in gait.

B. Talipes Equinovarus

In mild clubfoot, the forefoot adduction may be more severe than the eversion and equinus deformities.

C. Pronated Feet (Flatfeet)

The child with pes planus tends to stand with the feet in a valgus position, with the heel everted and the forefoot turned out. Because this position is not the most stable for walking or running, the child will toe in to shift the center of gravity toward the center of the foot.

II. Leg Problems

A. Internal Tibial Torsion

True internal tibial torsion is an uncommon problem, although it was invoked commonly in the past. Physiologic bowing of the legs in infancy gives the appearance of internal tibial torsion. The simplest clinical examination for tibial torsion is comparison of the relative positions of the medial and lateral malleoli while the child sits with legs extended and the patellae pointing straight ahead. Normally the me-

533

dial malleolus sits anterior to the lateral malleolus in the transmalleolar axis.

B. Knock Knees — Knock-kneed children toe in in order to shift the body's center of gravity medially.

C. Tibia Vara (Blount Disease) — Bilateral involvement produces genu varum, with resulting toeing in.

D. Bow Legs — Children with developmental bowing of the legs also tend to toe in when they walk.

III. Hip Problems

A. Femoral Anteversion — In this condition the head of the femur assumes a more anteriorly directed angle as it sits in the acetabulum. Toeing in is the result of an effort to create a more stable hip during walking. On examination, with the legs extended and the pelvis flat, there are excessive internal rotation (80° or more) and limited external rotation (30° or less) of the hips. In most cases the cause of femoral anteversion is unknown, but it can be associated with congenital hip dislocation, Legg–Calvé–Perthes disease, or congenital talipes equinovarus.

B. Paralytic Conditions — Toeing in may be seen in conditions such as cerebral palsy, as a consequence of poliomyelitis, or with myelomeningocele.

C. Spasticity of Internal Rotators of the Hip — This may be a consequence of cerebral palsy.

D. Maldirection of the Acetabulum — If the acetabulum is directed anteriorly, the child will toe in to swing the femoral head back into the hip joint for stability.

SUGGESTED READING

Tachdjian MO: Pediatric Orthopedics. Philadelphia, WB Saunders, 1972

98

TOEING OUT

Toeing out is a much less common problem than toeing in. In most cases, the toeing out is probably a result of intrauterine position.

The causes of toeing out are briefly outlined according to the anatomic location of the underlying problem.

I. Foot Problems

A. Talipes Calcaneovalgus	In this positional deformity, the foot is extremely dorsiflexed and everted, but it is flexible rather than rigid. With passive exercise in infancy, rapid correction is the rule.
B. Everted Flat Feet	Children with hypermobile, pronated feet may stand in a toeing-out position, but when walking they tend to toe in to improve the center of gravity.
C. Triceps Surae Muscle Contracture	Children with cerebral palsy may have toeing out at the foot because of spasticity affecting the triceps surae muscles (gastrocnemius and soleus). The foot is held in an equinus position.
D. Vertical Talus (Rocker-bottom Foot)	Children with congenital vertical talus have severe flatfoot. The forefoot is abducted and dorsiflexed.

II. Leg Problems

A. External Tibial Torsion	The condition may be present at birth or acquired. The medial malleolus lies much more anterior to the lateral malleolus than the normal 5° to 15°. External tibial torsion may be a consequence of femoral anteversion, in which external rotation of the hip is restricted, or of contracture of the iliotibial band, in which the internal rotation of the hip is limited.
B. Congenital Absence or Hypoplasia of the Fibula	In this uncommon congenital abnormality, shortening of the peroneal and triceps surae muscles results in bowing of the tibia and equinovalgus position of the foot. The lateral malleolus is absent.

III. Hip Problems

A. Femoral Retroversion	This condition is much rarer than femoral anteversion. The retroverted position of the femoral head results in limited internal rotation and excessive external rotation of the hip.
B. Flaccid Paralysis of the Internal Rotators of the Hip	
C. Physiologic Rotation in Newborns	Newborns whose intrauterine position was cross-legged have a relative external rotation contracture of the hips. When the legs are extended the toes will point out. Internal rotation at the hip is limited but improves rapidly with age.
D. Maldirection of the Acetabulum	The acetabulum may face posteriorly, resulting in outward turning of the leg.

SUGGESTED READING

Tachdjian MO: Pediatric Orthopedics. Philadelphia, WB Saunders, 1972

99

TOE WALKING

Toe walking is not a common primary complaint in childhood. This peculiarity of gait nevertheless may indicate an underlying disorder.

I. Physiologic Causes

A. Normal Variant

Toe walking may be seen intermittently in toddlers for the first 3 to 6 months after they begin ambulation. Joint mobility, reflexes, and development are normal.

B. Habit

Toe walking here tends to be intermittent. Dorsiflexion of the ankles is normal, as are patellar reflexes and muscle tone. The child can usually be persuaded to walk with the feet in the normal position.

C. Infantile Autism

Lack of interpersonal relationships, perseverations, and language delay are characteristic.

II. Disorders with a Shortened Achilles Tendon

A. Spastic Cerebral Palsy

This disorder is the commonest cause of toe walking. Depending on the type of cerebral palsy the abnormal gait may either be unilateral or bilateral. Associated signs include hyperactive reflexes, limited dorsiflexion of the ankle, tightness of extremity movement, and usually a delay in motor development.

B. Congenital Short Tendocalcaneus

In this uncommon cause of toe walking, the ankle is held in talipes equinus position. The knees must be fully extended to allow standing with the feet flat. Reflexes, muscle tone, and development are normal.

C. Late Infantile Acid Maltase Deficiency

Only a few patients have been described; they were asymptomatic during the first year of life but then developed a slowly progressive weakness. Symptoms may mimic those of Duchenne type muscular dystrophy. The gastrocnemius and deltoid muscles may be firm and rubbery; Gower's sign is present. Toe

	walking is secondary to Achilles tendon contracture.
D. Phosphoglucomutase Deficiency (Thomsen Disease)	The Achilles tendon is shortened, and calf muscles are bulky. One patient described had multiple episodes of supraventricular tachycardia in early infancy.
E. Spinocerebellar Degeneration	An abnormal gait develops in school-aged children, who eventually develop spasticity in their lower limbs and increasing ataxia, especially involving the upper extremities.

III. Disorders with a Shortened Extremity

A. Unilateral Hip Dislocation	Toe walking occurs on the affected side to compensate for the relative shortening of the leg. The range of motion of the affected hip is abnormal, particularly in abduction. Results of Trendelenberg test are positive.
B. Spinal Dysraphia	Lipoma of the cauda equina may be associated with enuresis, foot deformity, or leg shortening. Diastematomyelia should be considered if a cutaneous abnormality, such as a patch of hair, pigment, skin dimple, or sinus, is present over the spine. Talipes equinovarus or a shortened lower limb may be present with these deformities.

IV. Muscular Disorders

A. Duchenne Type Muscular Dystrophy	Toe walking may occur early. Since inheritance is sex-linked, only boys are affected. Pseudohypertrophy of the calves, the presence of Gower sign, and elevated creatinine phosphokinase levels are findings.
B. Viral Myositis	The acute onset of calf and thigh pain associated with influenzal infections may result in toe walking during the illness.
C. Myotonic Dystrophy	Weakness and muscle wasting may begin at any age. Ptosis of eyelids and atrophy of facial muscles may occur early. Myotonia is characteristic.
D. Emery–Dreifuss Muscular Dystrophy	Onset is in the first decade. Initial features are toe walking, partial flexion of the elbows, and inability to fully flex the neck and spine. A distinct pattern of contractures in the absence of major weakness is the earliest clue to diagnosis.

100

FLATFEET

Evaluation of flatfeet should begin with a determination of whether the condition is mobile or rigid. Most cases of flatfeet are a result of ligamentous laxity, producing a hypermobile flatfoot. The causes of rigid flatfeet are uncommon and are usually easily distinguishable.

I. Mobile Flatfeet

A. Newborn Fat Pad

Parents may mistake the presence of the normal pad of fat that occupies the medial arch of the foot in infancy for a flatfoot. The fat pad gradually disappears over the first 2 to 3 years of life. Absolutely no therapy is required, merely patient explanation to the concerned parent.

B. Ligamentous Laxity

The degree of normal joint extensibility shows great variation and may reflect a familial trait. Most children and adults with flatfeet have hypermobile joints as a result of ligamentous laxity. In a non-weight-bearing posture a medial arch appears to be present; on standing, however, the arch disappears, and the foot may tend to pronate (a combination of abduction and eversion) because the ligaments stretch. The condition is rarely symptomatic in children and requires no treatment. Other joints can be demonstrated to be hyperextensible as well, and examination of other family members usually reveals flatfeet or other evidence of the laxity.

C. Accessory Navicular Bone

Presence of this accessory bone, manifested by bony prominence at the arch, results in the loss of the principal support of the arch. Pain may be localized over the medial aspect of the foot, often because of a bursitis over the prominence, and along the posterior tibial tendon.

D. Talipes Calcaneovalgus

In this positional deformity found in infants, the foot is held dorsiflexed, giving a flatfoot appearance. The foot is flexible, however, and the position can be corrected easily.

II. Rigid Flatfeet

A. Vertical Talus (Rocker-bottom Foot)

Infants born with this rare anomaly have a severe rigid flatfoot with the appearance of a rocking-chair bottom. The heel is pointed downward, and the forefoot is held dorsiflexed. The vertical talus deformity may be seen in arthrogryposis or with meningomyelocele or the trisomy 18 syndrome.

B. Short Achilles Tendon

Owing to spasticity of the triceps surae group of muscles, dorsiflexion of the ankle past 90° is not possible. Hyperactive reflexes and ankle clonus may be present. Toe walking is common. This condition is most commonly found in children with cerebral palsy and, less frequently, in those with spinal epidural tumors.

C. Tarsal Coalition

Fusion of the tarsal bones occurs because of congenital bars, especially between the calcaneus and navicular. The principal feature on examination is lack of subtalar motion. Symptoms of foot pain with activity or walking do not usually occur until adolescence.

D. Low Insertion of the Soleus Muscle

Some children with tight heel cords may have an abnormally low insertion of the soleus muscle that can be palpated on examination.

SUGGESTED READING

Ehrlich MG: Foot disorders in infants and children. Current Probl Pediatr IV, No. 7, May 1974

101

RAYNAUD PHENOMENON AND ACROCYANOSIS

Intermittent episodes of color change in the extremities, usually associated with cold exposure or emotional stress, are called Raynaud phenomenon. Acrocyanosis refers to a persistent dusky discoloration of the hands and feet, which may be cold and sweaty as well; the pallor and discomfort characteristic of Raynaud phenomenon do not occur.

Recent findings with immunologic and arteriographic techniques indicate that the distinction between Raynaud disease and Raynaud phenomenon may not be as clear-cut as was once thought. Furthermore, other disorders produce color changes in the extremities. Differentiation of these conditions is important for the purposes of both prognosis and treatment.

I. Acrocyanosis

The duskiness may be transient after cold exposure or may persist throughout winter and, in some cases, summer as well. Slight hyperesthesias may occur. Trophic changes of the distal fingers and toes do not occur. The color change is always symmetric.

A. Transient Acrocyanosis	This type is commonly seen in newborn infants.
B. Recurrent Acrocyanosis	Adolescent girls are most frequently affected; there is often a family history of the condition.
C. Ehlers–Danlos Syndrome	Affected children may have acrocyanosis in addition to the characteristic loose jointedness, skin stretchability and fragility, and easy bruising.
D. Infection Related Causes	Cold-induced acrocyanosis has been described following infectious mononucleosis and mycoplasma infections.
E. Sympathomimetic Drugs	

II. Chilblain (Perniosis)

This disorder is characterized by a relatively persistent bluish or vivid red discoloration of the extremities; it is seen in damp cold climates and affects particularly young girls; it is not commonly described in the United States. Warmer or dryer weather may bring about improvement. The discoloration tends to blanch on pressure. There may be a doughy swelling, nodules, and severe pruritus or burning. Subepidermal bullae may form in severe forms.

III. **Raynaud Phenomenon**

Episodic attacks of color changes of the fingers or other acral areas, generally consisting of pallor followed by cyanosis and redness on warming, may be precipitated by cold exposure and occasionally emotional stress.

A. Primary Raynaud Disease

Criteria for diagnosis include (1) episodes of Raynaud phenomenon brought on by cold or emotion; (2) bilateral involvement; (3) absence of extensive gangrene; (4) exclusion of any secondary causes; and (5) a history of symptoms for 2 or more years.[1] It is most commonly seen in women; the hands and less often the feet are affected. In 25% of the cases, digital trophic changes may develop gradually. The primary disease was formerly thought to account for most cases of Raynaud phenomenon, but with more sophisticated diagnostic procedures uncovering the secondary form, a significantly lower percentage has the primary form.[2]

B. Secondary Raynaud Phenomenon

Numerous disorders have been implicated: a vasculitis associated with immune complex disorders, vasospasm, or poorly understood mechanisms of arterial obstruction. Involvement may not be symmetric.

1. Connective Tissue Disorders

   a. Scleroderma (Progressive Systemic Sclerosis)

Raynaud phenomenon occurs in most cases; in almost half, the color change precedes other symptoms. Pain is common. The presence of digital ulcerations suggests this diagnosis.

   b. Systemic Lupus Erythematosus

Arthralgias or arthritis, rashes, hair loss, and other systemic signs are clues.

   c. Rheumatoid Arthritis

Joint findings usually predominate.

   d. Morphea (Localized Scleroderma)

Raynaud phenomenon may occur, especially in linear scleroderma of the extremities.

e. Dermato-myositis	Muscle weakness, tenderness, and cutaneous changes are present.	
f. Periarteritis	Fever, malaise, and various rashes secondary to the vasculitis are found.	
g. Mixed Connective Tissue Disease	Symptoms of various connective tissue disorders may be present.	
h. Sjögren Syndrome	Arthritis, dryness of eyes and mouth, and recurrent parotid swelling are clues.	

2. Blood Disorders

a. Cold Agglutinins	These may occasionally be a cause in childhood, especially with viral infections and mycoplasmal pneumonia. Intracapillary agglutination of red cells occurs in the acral areas of the body which are cooler. The process tends to be transient in infections but can be chronic when associated with malignancies. A hemolytic anemia may be present.
b. Cryoglobulinemia	A wide variety of disorders may be associated with monoclonal or polyclonal immunoglobulin proliferation, producing cold sensitivity, Raynaud phenomenon, and peripheral vascular occlusion precipitated by cold. Chronic infections, connective tissue diseases, and malignancies have been implicated. A low erythrocyte sedimentation rate and rouleaux formation on blood smear suggest this possibility or cold agglutinins as the cause.
c. Cryofibrinogenemia	A cold-precipitable protein is present in the plasma but not in serum. Various causes include acute bronchiolitis in infants, pneumococcal pneumonia and meningitis, connective tissue disorders, and malignancies. Cold intolerance or thrombotic episodes in severe underlying disease may be presenting signs.

3. Thoracic Outlet Syndromes — Cervical ribs or pressure by the scalenus anticus muscle or even the clavicle may produce color changes in one extremity or a few digits secondary to traction or compression of the subclavian vessels or brachial plexus. Aggravation of symptoms by neck or shoulder motion may be used as a test.

4. Intoxications — Poisoning by lead, arsenic, or ergot may produce the phenomenon.

5. Occupational Trauma	This is obviously rare in children; it is seen in pianists, typists, pneumatic hammer operators, and so forth.
6. Chronic Occlusive Arterial Disease	Children are not affected; the disorders may include arteriosclerosis obliterans or thromboangiitis obliterans. Involvement is asymmetric in both, often with gangrene.
7. Miscellaneous Causes	
a. Pheochromocytoma	Raynaud phenomenon may be seen; usual symptoms include nausea, vomiting, sweating, headaches, polyuria and polydipsia, hypertension, and weight loss.
b. Primary Pulmonary Hypertension	Raynaud phenomenon rarely may be part of an altered arterial reactivity.
c. Reflex Sympathetic Dystrophy	This uncommon phenomenon follows injury or surgery; vasospasm occurs later. Usually only one extremity is affected; the pain may be severe and burning.
d. Oral Contraceptives	

REFERENCES

1. Harper FE, Maricq HR, Leroy EC: Raynaud's phenomenon. In Demis DJ (ed): Clinical Dermatology, Vol 2, Unit 7:36. Hagerstown, Harper & Row
2. Porter JM, Bardana EJ, Baur GM, et al: The clinical significance of Raynaud's syndrome. Surgery 80:756–764, 1976

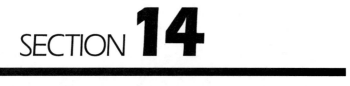

SECTION **14**

NERVOUS SYSTEM

102

SEIZURES

$\mathcal{S}$eizures are common in childhood; various studies have estimated that 4% to 8% of all children will have a seizure prior to reaching adulthood. Seizures may be generalized or focal; some involve motor activity, whereas others are characterized by changes in sensation, in behavior, or in autonomic function. In seizure disorders termed epilepsy, episodes are recurrent. Seizures may occur only during the acute phase of an illness.

Seizures are often classified by type: major motor, myoclonic, absence, akinetic, and so forth. In this chapter, common causes of seizures are given for each childhood age group in approximate order of frequency. A category of seizure mimics is also included; many of these disorders may be mistaken for seizures by parents and relatives.

I. Newborn and Neonatal Period

A. Metabolic Derangements

1. Hypocalcemia — Seizures may be focal or tonic-clonic. In many series, hypocalcemia is the most common cause of neonatal seizures; those occurring after 3 or 4 days of life have been related to the high phosphate content of milk. Hypocalcemia may also be secondary to maternal hyperparathyroidism, idiopathic neonatal hypoparathyroidism, or DiGeorge syndrome.

2. Hypoglycemia — Low blood sugar may be caused by many factors including perinatal stress, hyperviscosity, and maternal diabetes.

3. Hypomagnesemia — Tetany, convulsions, and hypocalcemia are characteristic.

4. Hyponatremia — This condition may follow the administration of excessive intravenous fluid without adequate sodium to the mother or disorders causing inappropriate release of antidiuretic hormone.

5. Hypernatremia — Diarrhea with excessive water loss or poisonings in which salt is substituted for sugar in the feeding formula may be a cause.

6. Disorders of Amino Acid Metabolism	The early onset of lethargy, vomiting, and seizures indicates the possibility of one of these disorders; many are associated with elevated blood ammonia levels. Phenylketonuria, maple syrup urine disease, and argininosuccinic aciduria are but a few.
7. Galactosemia	The presence of jaundice, diarrhea, and vomiting requires a urine test for reducing substances.
B. Intracranial Birth Injury	Ischemic insults and hypoxic episodes are more likely to be responsible for these injuries than traumatic injuries.
1. Intracranial Hemorrhage	
a. Subdural Hemorrhage	A tense fontanel, retinal hemorrhages, and progressive enlargement of the head suggest a subdural hemorrhage.
b. Subarachnoid Hemorrhage	Spells of apnea and poor color are additional signs.
c. Intracerebral Hemorrhage	This type is more common in full-term infants born after prolonged, difficult labor.
d. Intraventricular Hemorrhage	Premature infants born by spontaneous deliveries are most commonly affected.
2. Perinatal Anoxia	Anoxia may lead to intracerebral capillary bleeding, brain edema, and seizures.
C. Central Nervous System Infection	
1. Bacterial Meningitis	In the neonatal period almost any unusual change in the infant may be a sign of central nervous system infection or sepsis. An infant who has a seizure should have a lumbar puncture performed.
2. Viral Infection	Various congenital and acquired viruses may be responsible. Herpes simplex, rubella, cytomegalovirus or Coxsackie virus infections, and others are included.
3. Other Infections	
a. Syphilis	
b. Neonatal Tetanus	

  c. Toxoplas-
    mosis
D. Congenital Cere-
   bral Malformation

1. Cerebral Agenesis or Dysgenesis	Chromosomal abnormalities, teratogenic drugs taken by the mother, or fetal radiation exposure may be a cause.
2. Holoprosencephaly	Hypotelorism and microcephaly with midline facial defects may be present.
3. Porencephaly	This is a cystic area of absent cerebral tissue.
4. Hydrocephalus	This problem is often associated with a myelomeningocele.

E. Drugs and Chemicals

1. Withdrawal	Tremulousness, irritability, tachypnea, vomiting, diarrhea, sweating, and a shrill cry, especially in a premature infant or one who is small for gestational age, suggest this possibility.
2. Toxic Reactions	Seizures may follow intravenous injections of drugs such as penicillin or even absorption of hexachlorophene from the skin. Inadvertent injection of caudal anesthetic into the infant's scalp during the delivery process is another uncommon cause.

F. Developmental Abnormalities

1. Incontinentia Pigmenti	Seizures are common in this disorder, which is lethal to males *in utero*. Cutaneous changes include vesicles and verrucous lesions, often in a linear distribution, and later, pigmented swirls.
2. Sturge–Weber Syndrome	A port-wine stain of the face, involving the area supplied by the ophthalmic branch of the trigeminal nerve, may be associated with ipsilateral cerebral angiomatosis leading to seizures.
3. Tuberous Sclerosis	The earliest sign is the presence of hypopigmented macules on the skin.
4. Linear Sebaceous Nevus	Any linear macular or papular lesion on the skin, especially on the head, may indicate an underlying central nervous system abnormality.

G. Miscellaneous
   Disorders

1. Postmaturity	Postmature infants have an increased incidence of seizures for various reasons, including hypoglycemia.
2. Pre-eclamptic Toxemia	Maternal toxemia may be a cause.
3. Kernicterus	Jaundice, irritability, a shrill cry, and opisthotonos are features.
4. Hyperviscosity	Sludging in cerebral vessels and hypoglycemia may be responsible for seizures.
5. Pyridoxine Dependency or Deficiency	Seizures from this rare cause are treatable by pyridoxine. An intravenous test dose of vitamin B_6 may be given to an infant with seizures from no apparent cause.
6. Cardiac Dysrhythmias	
H. Unknown Cause	In 25% to 33% of infants with seizures, no cause can be found.

II. Infancy

A. Febrile Seizures	Febrile seizures are by far the most common cause of seizures in children 9 months to 5 years of age. It is important to distinguish febrile seizures from seizures associated with fever. The criteria for febrile seizures include: (1) the seizure must occur with fever; (2) the seizure must be generalized, not focal; (3) the child must not have had previous nonfebrile seizures and must not have had abnormal neurologic findings or a history of central nervous system injury in the past; (4) the seizure is of short duration, less than 20 minutes; and (5) there must be no evidence of intracranial infection or other cause. The onset is generally between 6 months and 3 years of age.
B. Intracranial Birth Injury	Seizures may begin after the neonatal period in infants who have sustained perinatal intracranial injuries.
1. Perinatal Hypoxia or Anoxia	
2. Intracranial Hemorrhage	
C. Congenital Cerebral Malformations	The onset of seizures may occur in infancy. Look for signs of physical abnormalities or developmental delays (see I-D).

D. Infections
   1. Bacterial Infec-   Meningitis and cerebral abscesses are exam-
      tions   ples.
   2. Viral Infections Aseptic meningitis or encephalitis may cause
                         seizures. Some congenital infections may not
                         produce seizures until later.
   3. Other Infec-
      tions
      a. Roseola   The exact mechanism of seizures in roseola is
                         not known; some are febrile seizures.
      b. Shigella   The seizure may be toxin-related.
      c. Tubercu-
         lous Men-
         ingitis
      d. Parasitic   Toxoplasmosis and, rarely, other parasites
                         may be responsible. Cysticercosis, caused by
                         the larval form of the pork tapeworm *Taenia
                         solium,* is most commonly seen in immigrants
                         from Mexico and Latin America. Seizures and
                         signs of increased intracranial pressure are the
                         most common manifestations in children.
E. Toxic Reactions   Exposure to various toxins may result in an
                         encephalopathy with seizures.
   1. Heavy Metals   Seizures may be a sign in lead, mercury, or
                         thallium poisoning.
   2. Drugs   Amphetamines, camphor, hexachloraphene,
                         and scabicides have been implicated.
   3. Ingestion of   Organophosphates and hydrocarbons are ex-
      Other Toxic   amples.
      Substances
   4. Immunizations Seizures may represent a toxic reaction to per-
                         tussis toxoid.
F. Metabolic Causes
   1. Hypoglycemia Blood glucose levels should always be deter-
                         mined in children with seizures. Ketotic hypo-
                         glycemia is a poorly understood disorder that
                         occurs not uncommonly in infants and young
                         children, who may develop hypoglycemia
                         after long fasts, especially if they are ill.
   2. Hyponatremia Excessive water intake or the syndrome of
                         inappropriate antidiuretic hormone secretion
                         from various causes may cause hyponatremia.
                         In water intoxication young infants are offered
                         dilute formula or breast milk supplemented
                         with water. All have increased vasopressin.

3. Hypernatremia	This disorder may occur in hypertonic dehydration during a gastroenteritis, in diabetes insipidus, or from accidental solute overload. The seizures occur most commonly after rehydration.

G. Trauma
  1. After Concussions — Post-traumatic seizures are common.
  2. Subdural Hematoma
  3. Child Abuse — There may be external evidence of trauma. With shaking injuries, no external signs of trauma may be visible, but retinal hemorrhages are common.
  4. Anoxic Episodes — Seizures may follow anoxic insults.

H. Inborn Errors of Metabolism — Seizures may develop in the neonatal period or later in infancy.
  1. Aminoacidopathies
  2. Organic Acidopathies
  3. Degenerative Diseases — Metachromatic leukodystrophy, Tay–Sachs disease, gangliosidoses and other storage diseases, Menkes' syndrome and Lowe syndrome, all have other striking findings on examination.
  4. Biotin-Responsive Multiple Carboxylase Deficiency — Other features include ataxia, periorificial dermatitis and alopecia.

I. Neurocutaneous Disorders — Careful skin examination may reveal clues to underlying central nervous system disorders.
  1. Tuberous Sclerosis
  2. Incontinentia Pigmenti
  3. Sturge–Weber Syndrome
  4. Linear Sebaceous Nevus
  5. Neurofibromatosis

J. Miscellaneous Causes

1. Intracranial Hemorrhage	Hemorrhage may occur in arteriovenous malformations, in severe thrombocytopenia, or rarely in coagulation disturbances.
2. Post Infectious	A seizure focus may be the result of preceding bacterial meningitis or viral encephalitis.
3. Tumors	
4. Convulsive Syncope	Pain or sudden fright may trigger cardiac asystole, which if greater than 10 seconds, may result in an anoxic seizure.
5. Cardiac Dysrhythmias	
K. Unknown Causes	In a significant number of seizures the cause is of unknown etiology; some perhaps reflect a genetic predisposition.

III. Childhood

A. Unknown Causes	Idiopathic seizures are the most common cause in childhood.
B. Infections	
1. Meningitis	Bacterial and rarely tuberculous infections may be associated with seizures.
2. Encephalitis	
3. Encephalopathy	Infectious diseases, such as shigellosis and legionnaires' disease, may produce an encephalopathy with seizures.
4. Cerebral Abscess	
5. Parasitic Infestations	These are seen particularly in countries other than the United States.
6. Tetanus	
C. Genetic Predisposition	In as many as 4% to 8% of epileptics hereditary factors appear to be operative. Petit mal seizures are a common example.
D. Trauma	
1. Head Injury	Post-traumatic seizures may occur at the time of the injury or months to years later.
2. Anoxic Injury	
3. Burn Encephalopathy	Seizures may occur within a few days of the burn.
4. Subdural Hematoma	
5. Epidural Hematoma	
6. Previous Insult	Seizures may occur months to years following infection, trauma, or anoxia.

E. Toxic Reactions—
   Poisonings

   1. Drugs

   2. Heavy Metals

   3. Chemicals

F. Vascular Causes

   1. Hypertensive
      Encephalop-
      athy

   2. Subarachnoid
      Hemorrhage

   3. Cerebral Em-
      bolization

   4. Vascular
      Thrombosis

   5. Sickle-Cell
      Disease

   6. Vasculitis

G. Other Causes

   1. Reye Syn-
      drome

   2. Tumors

   3. Metabolic Dis-
      orders

   4. Subacute
      Sclerosing
      Panencephalitis

   5. Convulsive
      Syncope

   6. Dysrhythmias

A host of drugs, chemicals, and metals may be responsible.

Toxic reactions to acetylsalicylic acid, amphetamines, antihistamines, atropine, aminophylline, penicillin, narcotics and their congeners, steroids, or tricyclic antidepressants may occur.

Lead, mercury, or thallium poisoning may cause seizures.

Organophosphates, hydrocarbons, LSD, and phencyclidine are examples.

Seizures may be a presenting sign of acute glomerulonephritis.

Hemorrhage may result from a cerebral aneurysm. The neck is usually stiff.

Emboli are more common in cyanotic congenital heart disease but may also occur in subacute bacterial endocarditis.

This disorder may occur in severe dehydration.

The vasculitis associated with systemic lupus erythematosus may cause seizures.

The toxic encephalopathy follows a viral illness, often influenza or varicella. Vomiting and, later, seizures may precede the central nervous system depression.

Central nervous system tumors are still an uncommon cause of seizures in this age group.

The causes listed for other age groups are less likely in childhood, but hyponatremia and hypoglycemia may be found.

Some years after rubeola infection, personality changes are noted; focal seizures and myoclonic jerks occur later.

Pain or sudden fright may trigger cardiac asystole, which if greater than 10 seconds may result in an anoxic seizure.

Syncope followed by hypoxic seizures may be seen in various cardiac dysrhythmias, including the congenital long QT syndrome.

7. Rett Syndrome | In this syndrome slowly progressive neurologic deterioration is seen exclusively in girls. Onset is between 4 and 18 months with behavioral changes. Seizures usually begin between 2 and 4 years of age. Choreoathetosis, ataxia, and hypotonia are other features.

IV. Adolescence

A. Unknown Causes | In most seizures in this age group, the cause is unknown.

B. Trauma | Various acute and posttraumatic causes account for a significant percentage of seizures in this age group.

C. Infection | Meningitis and encephalitis and abscesses are examples.

D. Genetic Predisposition

E. Drug Abuse

F. Tumors | Tumors may account for as many as 2% of seizures in this age group.

G. Vascular Malformations

H. Other Causes | Causes listed in the preceding section, Childhood, may be responsible in this age group also.

V. Seizure Mimics

A. Breath-Holding | Episodes occur most commonly between 6 and 36 months of age; they are triggered by a sudden fright or anger, whereas seizures are not. The child cries, holds his breath, and becomes cyanotic; a loss of consciousness and a few clonic twitches may follow. In pallid breath holding the child suddenly turns pale rather than blue and faints.

B. Syncope | Simple fainting spells are short-lived and not followed by a postictal period; there is no amnesia for the event as with a seizure.

C. Migraine | Headache, visual complaints, nausea, and vomiting, along with a family history of migraine, suggest this disorder.

D. Hyperventilation | This phenomenon usually occurs in adolescents rather than young children. The extremities may become numb, with the fingers and toes in spasm; headache and shortness of breath are common.

E. Drugs

Phenothiazines are notorious for producing the extrapyramidal tract symptoms of the oculogyric crisis, commonly mistaken for a seizure. The child is, however, awake.

F. Myoclonic Jerks

One or more sudden body muscle contractions, especially when falling asleep, may occur normally.

G. Tics

Movements are repetitive and stereotyped and involve the same muscle groups.

H. Pavor Nocturnus

Night terrors sometimes are confused with seizures.

I. Hysteria

Preceding events allow easy distinction from seizures.

J. Malingering

A feigned seizure can usually be readily distinguished from a genuine one.

K. Spasmus Nutans

There are often three components: head nodding, head tilt, and nystagmus; it occurs in young infants and disappears during sleep.

L. Cardiac Dysrhythmias

Cardiac dysrhythmias or severe aortic stenosis may be accompanied by fainting episodes.

M. Masturbation

In young children masturbatory activity may simulate seizures. The children often rock back and forth, become flushed, and perspire; they resist interference during this activity.

N. Labyrinthitis

Attacks of vertigo may simulate epilepsy. In benign paroxysmal vertigo the attacks are sudden; the child is pale and frightened and attempts to hold onto anything close.

O. Shuddering Attacks

This benign disorder is characterized by rapid tremors involving the head and arms similar to shivering, but of longer duration. There are no EEG abnormalities.

SUGGESTED READINGS

Holmes GL, Russman BS: Shuddering attacks. Am J Dis Child 140:72–73, 1986

Snyder CH: Conditions that simulate epilepsy in children. Clin Pediatr 11:487–491, 1972

Swaiman KF, Wright FS: The Practice of Pediatric Neurology, 2nd ed. St. Louis, CV Mosby, 1982

103

COMA

Coma—the loss of consciousness and of responsiveness to environmental stimuli—is a distressing symptom that calls for immediate evaluation to determine the cause as well as prompt institution of measures to prevent permanent brain injury or death. Because the patient is unconscious, information about preceding events may not be available. Coma of sudden onset is most likely to be associated with trauma, poisonings, seizure disorders or intracranial hemorrhage.

In this chapter the possible causes of coma are arranged according to the mnemonic AEIOU–TIPS:

Alcohol ingestion and acidosis	Trauma
Epilepsy and encephalopathy	Insulin overdose and inflamma-
Infection	tory disorders
Opiates	Poisoning and psychogenic causes
Uremia	Shock

A group of relatively uncommon causes of coma is also included.

I. Alcohol Ingestion

Young children may accidentally ingest alcohol in amounts sufficient to cause stupor or coma; ingestion by older children and adolescents may be intentional. Important considerations in management include (1) hypoglycemia as the primary cause of or an added insult in the comatose state resulting from alcohol ingestion; (2) the additive effects of alcohol and other drugs; (3) aspiration of stomach contents with resulting hypoxia and serious lung disease; and (4) methanol rather than ethanol ingestion.

II. Acidosis and Metabolic Problems

Conditions that produce coma as a result of acidosis or metabolic problems are usually gradual rather than sudden in onset. The preceding clinical course supplies diagnostic clues.

A. Diabetes Mellitus	Polyuria, polydipsia, weight loss, dehydration, and a fruity odor to the breath are signs.
B. Dehydration	Hyper- or hypotonic dehydration may result in seizures and coma.
C. Hypercapnia	Respiratory failure occurring in primary lung disease or with neurologic disturbances may cause the comatose state or add complications.

D. Hepatic Failure	Any severe, acute, or chronic liver disease may result in coma. Plasma ammonia nitrogen levels are usually elevated. Progressive stages are usually evident: mild depression, alterations in speech, and insomnia; drowsiness, inappropriate behavior, and loss of sphincter control; somnolence and confusion; and finally coma. Various precipitating factors include nitrogen overload, fluid and electrolyte abnormalities, infection and other stresses, and drugs.
1. Reye Syndrome	This is an important, relatively common cause of coma that usually follows a viral infection (influenza or varicella). After a period of apparent recovery from the infection the child begins vomiting. Confusion and delirium frequently precede the increasing obtundation.
2. Fulminant Hepatitis	
3. Wilson Disease	
4. Alpha$_1$-antitrypsin Deficiency	
5. Cystic Fibrosis	
6. Biliary Atresia	
7. Toxin Ingestion	Acetaminophen in particular has been implicated.
E. Hypoglycemia	See the Insulin Overdose and Hypoglycemia category.
F. Hypoxia	Insufficient oxygen delivery to the brain may be a cause. Near drowning, carbon monoxide poisoning, congestive heart failure, and lung disorders must be considered.
G. Water Intoxication	Inappropriate antidiuretic hormone release may occur in a variety of disorders. Iatrogenic intravenous overload occasionally occurs. Rarely, the problem is of psychogenic origin.
H. Electrolyte Disturbances 1. Hypernatremia	

2. Hypona-
   tremia

3. Calcium   Either hypocalcemia or hypercalcemia may
                    occur.

4. Magnesium   Hypermagnesemia or hypomagnesemia may
                    be a cause.

I. Uremia   The severity of coma is poorly correlated with
                    serum urea nitrogen levels.

J. Alkalosis   Metabolic or respiratory alkalosis may cause
                    alterations in consciousness.

K. Inborn Errors of   In most of these disorders, onset of symptoms
   Metabolism   is early in life, with vomiting, seizures, and
                       acidosis. Although all are uncommon, some
                       are more prevalent than others.

   1. Maple Syrup
      Urine Dis-
      ease

   2. Methylma-
      lonic Acidu-
      ria

   3. Ketotic Hy-
      perglycine-
      mia

   4. Isovaleric
      Acidemia

   5. Argininosuc-   The subacute form presents a Reye syndrome-
      cinic Lyase   like picture. Hepatomegaly is marked.
      Deficiency

   6. Propionic
      Acidemia

L. Endocrine Dis-   Coma is a rare presentation of these disorders.
   orders
   1. Addison
      Disease
   2. Cushing
      Syndrome
   3. Congenital   In the salt-losing form, dehydration and hypo-
      Adrenal Hy-   natremia may be presenting signs.
      perplasia
      (Adrenogen-
      ital Syn-
      drome)
   4. Pheochromo-   Hypertensive encephalopathy may occur.
      cytoma

    M. Hepatic Porphy-
       rias
      1. Acute Inter-
         mittent
         Porphyria
      2. Variegate
         Porphyria

III. Epilepsy

The postictal patient or the patient in status epilepticus may be coma-
tose.

IV. Encephalopathy

Various metabolic and infectious insults may result in an encephalopathy presenting as coma. In many cases the insult may not be identi-
fiable.

V. Infection

A. Meningitis	A lumbar puncture should be performed on every comatose patient, although there may be a great dilemma when signs of increased intracranial pressure are present.
1. Bacterial Infection	
2. Viral Infection	
3. Fungal Infection	
4. Protozoal Infestation	
5. Mycobacterial Infection	
B. Encephalitis	A wide variety of viruses and rickettsial organisms may be responsible. Cat-scratch disease has also been implicated.
C. Severe Systemic Infection	Stupor or coma may occur in severe infections such as pneumonia or pyelonephritis.
D. Postinfectious or Parainfectious Encephalomyelitis	An encephalomyelopathy may follow a viral illness, as a result of either direct invasion by the virus or an altered immunologic state. Immunization material, particularly pertussis toxoid, may produce such a response.
E. Brain Abscess	Fever and headache precede the coma.

F. Subdural or
   Epidural Empy-
   ema

VI. Opiates
An overdose of narcotics, either illegal drugs or opiate congeners present in medications such as propoxyphene hydrochloride (Darvon) or diphenoxylate hydrochloride with atropine (Lomotil), may be responsible for coma. A trial dose of a narcotic antagonist may be diagnostic.

VII. Uremia
Preceding coma, other neurologic signs such as tremors, myoclonus, asterixis, convulsions, and a change in mental status are findings. The severity of the coma does not correlate well with the elevation of the blood urea nitrogen.

VIII. Trauma and Other Physical Causes

A. Blunt Trauma	Concussions produce alterations of consciousness lasting less than 24 hours. A contusion of the brain produces greater periods of unresponsiveness and indicates bruising.
B. Subdural Hematoma	The bleeding may be of sudden onset or present for some time.
C. Epidural Hematoma	The classic picture is one of immediate loss of consciousness following the trauma and then a lucid period followed by a gradual onset of obtundation.
D. Heat Stroke	The body core temperature is generally greater than 106°F.
E. Marked Hypothermia	Excessive body cooling may result in coma.
F. Electric Shock	A period of cardiac asystole usually produces the coma.
G. Decompression Sickness	The formation of gaseous microemboli, usually nitrogen, in the "bends" may affect the brain.
H. Blood Loss	Blood loss may be a consequence of major trauma or may occur with minor trauma in association with clotting disorders.

IX. Insulin Overdose and Hypoglycemia
Various disorders may produce hypoglycemia and consequent coma. Insulin overdose must always be considered as the cause in a known diabetic. However, infants and children are prone to develop hypo-

glycemia during fasting, especially with infections and in the new-born period. Determination of blood sugar is mandatory in the coma-tose child.

X. Inflammatory Disorders
Coma may occur with cerebral involvement in systemic lupus erythe-matosus and polyarteritis nodosa.

XI. Poisoning
Ingestion of a drug or toxin must always be considered as the cause of coma, especially if the onset of the illness producing the unre-sponsive state is acute. Phenothiazines, hydrocarbons, organophos-phates, phencyclidines, salicylates, barbiturates and other sedatives, and antihistamines are the most common offenders. Lead poisoning with encephalopathy is usually characterized by a subacute course with vomiting, headache, and increasing lethargy.

XII. Psychogenic Causes
Hysterical unresponsiveness is generally short-lived. The history of-ten provides diagnostic clues.

XIII. Shock
A shock-like state may be associated with many of the causes in this chapter.

XIV. Miscellaneous Causes
A. Vascular Disor-ders

1. Subarachnoid Hemorrhage	Trauma or rupture of an aneurysm may cause the bleeding. Although a stiff neck is present in most adults, this finding is not consistent in children.
2. Venous Thrombosis	Venous thrombosis may follow severe dehy-dration or a pyogenic infection of paranasal sinuses, middle ear, or mastoid. The presence of periorbital edema or scalp edema with di-lated veins on the scalp and face is a clue.
3. Arterial Thrombosis	This cause is unusual in children. However, children with homocystinuria are prone to develop arterial thromboses; they have a mar-fanoid appearance with dislocated lenses and mental retardation.
4. Intracerebral and Intraven-tricular Hem-orrhages	In newborns, these lesions may follow birth asphyxia or trauma; in older children the cause is usually a disturbance of the clotting mechanisms.

5. Cerebral Emboli	Subacute bacterial endocarditis is the prototype; splinter hemorrhages, splenomegaly, and microscopic hematuria are suggestive findings.
6. Acute Infantile Hemiplegia	An acute seizure, followed by coma and hemiparesis, is characteristic.
B. Cardiac Disorders	Any disorder resulting in diminished blood supply to the brain may lead to the sudden onset of loss of consciousness.
1. Ventricular Fibrillation	
2. Stokes–Adams Attacks	Heart block leads to unconsciousness.
3. Aortic Stenosis	Severe aortic stenosis may lead to attacks of unconsciousness secondary to diminished cardiac output.
C. Hypertension	Hypertensive encephalopathy may follow acute glomerulonephritis or may be associated with pheochromocytomas, the Riley–Day syndrome, or drug ingestion.
D. Neoplasia	
1. Brain Tumors	The most common cause of a loss of consciousness is increased intracranial pressure. Other symptoms precede coma, except when a sudden hemorrhage into the tumor results in sudden increase in intracranial pressure or obstruction of cerebrospinal fluid outflow.
2. Metastatic Tumors	Wilms and Ewing tumors may metastasize to the brain.
3. Meningeal Infiltration	This lesion may be seen in acute leukemia.

SUGGESTED READING

Swaiman KF, Wright FS: The Practice of Pediatric Neurology, 2nd ed. St. Louis, CV Mosby, 1982

104

FLOPPY INFANT SYNDROME AND HYPOTONIA

Generalized weakness or hypotonia in the newborn or young infant, the floppy infant syndrome, may be congenital or acquired. Affected infants are much like rag dolls; if suspended over the palm of the hand, they literally droop around it. Signs of hypotonia include a weak cry, poor sucking reflex, and decreased body movement, as well as respiratory difficulty. Hypotonia should always be considered in the differential diagnosis of neonatal respiratory distress.

Many disorders that may cause hypotonia, especially with onset at later than 6 months of age, are listed in Chapter 94, Muscle Weakness, and are not repeated here. This chapter covers only those disorders that produce hypotonia in the first 6 months of life. Texts for further review are listed at the end of this chapter.

I. Trauma
- A. Birth or Intrauterine Anoxia
- B. Intracerebral Hemorrhage
- C. Spinal Cord Injury

II. Infection
A. Sepsis	Acquired infections may produce profound weakness.
B. Congenital Infections—The STORCH Complex	Syphilis, toxoplasmosis, rubella, cytomegalovirus, and herpes simplex have been implicated. Poliomyelitis acquired *in utero* has also been described.

III. Inborn Errors of Metabolism
A. Hypothyroidism	
B. Congenital Joint Laxity and Ehlers–Danlos Syndrome	There is a wide variety in the expression of these disorders, but extreme hyperextensibility of joints may give the impression of hypotonia.

C. Pompe Disease (Glycogen Storage Disease, Type II)

A deficiency of acid maltase is the basic defect.

D. Osteogenesis Imperfecta (Autosomal Recessive Form)

Short-limbed growth deficiency, large fontanels with multiple wormian bones of skull, and multiple fractures of bones are features.

E. Marfan Syndrome

Arachnodactyly and joint hyperextensibility are evident early in life. Hypotonia may be marked in some cases.

F. Cerebrohepatorenal Syndrome (Zellweger Syndrome)

Large fontanels, high forehead, hepatomegaly, and redundant skin folds of the neck are characteristic. In some affected infants, the appearance resembles that in Down syndrome. The cause of the high serum iron levels and excessive iron storage is unclear.

G. Oculocerebrorenal Syndrome (Lowe Syndrome)

H. Williams Syndrome

This syndrome was previously called idiopathic hypercalcemia and supravalvular aortic stenosis with failure to thrive. Anteverted nose and a long philtrum are characteristic.

I. Pseudodeficiency Rickets

The course is similar to that in early-onset severe rickets, with growth failure, large fontanels, hypotonia, hypocalcemia, and in some cases, seizures. Inheritance pattern is autosomal recessive.

J. Generalized Gangliosidosis

Coarse features may suggest Hurler syndrome, but signs are evident at birth. Storage of ganglioside GM_1 occurs in liver, spleen, and brain. Inheritance pattern is autosomal recessive.

K. Fucosidosis

Progressive developmental retardation with hypotonia begins early but is not evident at birth. Affected children later become hypertonic and develop cardiomegaly.

L. Mannosidosis

Affected infants may be hypotonic at birth. Hepatosplenomegaly, macroglossia, repeated infections, and lens opacities are other findings.

M. Infantile Thiamine Deficiency

Onset of symptoms is in the first 3 months of life if maternal intake of thiamine has been poor and exogenous sources are deficient. Anorexia, vomiting, lethargy, pallor, ptosis, edema of the extremities, and cardiac failure are characteristic.

N. Hypercalcemia
O. Hypokalemia
P. Adenylate Deaminase Deficiency

It is not clear whether this muscle enzyme deficiency is primary or secondary.

Q. Copper Deficiency

Affected infants are pale, hypopigmented with hepatosplenomegaly.

R. Biotin Deficiency

Usually develops at age 3 to 6 months. Periorificial dermatitis, alopecia, conjunctivitis, irritability, and ataxia may also be present.

S. Hyperuricemia and Growth Retardation

This is an X-linked recessive disorder.

IV. Amino Acid and Organic Acid Disorders

A. Argininosuccinicaciduria

Severe mental retardation occurs. Seizures, ataxia and hypotonia may be noted; the hair tends to be fragile with nodes along the shaft.

B. Hyperlysinemia

Severe mental retardation with muscular hypotonia and ligament laxity is characteristic.

C. Pipecolatemia

Mental retardation, hepatomegaly, and hypotonia have been described.

D. Nonketotic Hyperglycinemia

Poor feeding, apneic episodes, and seizures occur in the neonatal period. Severe mental and developmental retardation develops in survivors.

E. Maple Syrup Urine Disease

Poor feeding, lethargy, and seizures begin early. Affected infants may be hypertonic or hypotonic.

F. Multiple Carboxylase Deficiency

Episodes of ketoacidosis, hyperglycemia, and hyperammonemia are brought on by ingestion of large amounts of protein. Vomiting, lethargy, and hypotonia are common.

V. Toxins and Drugs

A. Bilirubin

Hyperbilirubinemia may result in kernicterus. Early signs include hypotonia, lethargy, poor appetite, and decreased activity. The hypotonia is replaced by spasticity and opisthotonos in a few days to weeks.

B. Magnesium — Hypermagnesemia in newborns may result from magnesium given to their mothers during labor. Severely affected infants may be flaccid and cyanotic and require respiratory assistance.

C. Phenobarbital — Maternal therapy rarely results in neonatal depression with flaccidity.

D. Botulism — Botulism must be considered in infants with sudden onset of hypotonia, lethargy, constipation, and poor feeding.

E. Fetal Warfarin Syndrome — Maternal therapy with warfarin during pregnancy may cause hypotonia, developmental delay, seizures, a hypoplastic nose, and stippling of the epiphyses on x-ray films.

F. Fetal Aminopterin Syndrome — Maternal exposure during pregnancy may result in a markedly abnormal phenotype, occasionally with hypotonia.

G. Aluminum Toxicity — Infants receiving aluminum containing phosphate binders may develop an osteodystrophy. Poor muscle tone, a ricket-like picture, and bulging fontanel may be found.

VI. Neuromuscular Disorders

A. Werdnig–Hoffman Disease

B. Neonatal Myasthenia — This condition, which may be transient or persistent, is characterized by ptosis, weak cry, difficulty in swallowing, and generalized weakness.

C. Congenital Myopathies — The many types are distinguishable by special stains of muscle biopsy material.
   1. Central Core Disease
   2. Nemaline Myopathy
   3. Congenital Fiber Type Disproportion
   4. Myotubular Myopathy

D. Myotonic Dystrophy — Neonatal problems include difficulty in swallowing and in sucking, facial diplegia, ptosis, arthrogryposis, respiratory difficulty, and talipes equinovarus. Maternal hydramnios may have been noted.

E. Benign Congenital Hypotonia

F. Congenital Muscular Dystrophy   There is marked hypotonia with swallowing and sucking difficulties, ptosis, thin extremities, and joint contractures that are often present at birth.

G. Atonic Paraplegia   Atonic cerebral palsy may be a cause.

H. Congenital Ataxia and Congenital Choreoathetosis

I. Infantile Neuroaxonal Dystrophy

J. Congenital Hypomyelination Neuropathy   Affected infants are hypotonic and inactive and have palpably enlarged nerves.

K. Polymyositis   This disorder is rare in infants.

L. Dejerine–Sottas Disease   Onset in infancy is rare. Weakness, hypotonia, delayed motor milestones, and areflexia are typical. Nerve biopsy is pathognomonic.

VII. Syndromes with Hypotonia

A. Down Syndrome

B. Prader–Willi Syndrome

C. Achondroplasia

D. Familial Dysautonomia   Additional findings include feeding difficulties, absent lacrimation and corneal reflexes, decreased or absent deep tendon reflexes, and absent fungiform papillae of tongue.

E. Trisomy 13 Syndrome   This chromosomal defect may cause hypotonia as well as numerous other abnormalities. Cleft lip or palate, microcephaly, cardiac defects, polydactyly, microphthalmia, and seizures are commonly found.

F. Cri du Chat Syndrome   Most affected infants are hypotonic. A cat-like cry, hypertelorism, growth failure, downward slanting of the palpebral fissures, and microcephaly are prominent figures.

G. Short-Arm Deletion of Chromosome 4 (4p⁻ Syndrome) — Typical features include ocular hypertelorism, a broad or beaked nose, microcephaly, cranial asymmetry, low-set ears, and hypotonia.

H. Long-Arm Deletion of Chromosome 18 (18q⁻ Syndrome) — Midface flattening, microcephaly, hypotonia, long fingers, and ear abnormalities are usually present.

I. XXXXY Syndrome — Common findings include hypogenitalism, limited elbow pronation, low nasal bridge, and hypertelorism, as well as hypotonia in one third of the cases.

J. Marinesco–Sjögren Syndrome — This syndrome is characterized by cerebellar ataxia, cataracts, and weakness. Hypotonia may or may not be present.

K. Cohen Syndrome — Hypotonia and weakness occur early; obesity is noted later. Protruding maxillary incisors are part of the picture.

L. Stickler Syndrome — Flat facies, cleft palate, myopia, hypotonia, hyperextensible joints, and an arthropathy are characteristic.

M. Langer–Giedion Syndrome — Redundant or loose skin is noted in the neonatal period. The nose appears bulbous. Multiple bony exostoses occur.

N. Thanatophoric Dwarfism — Short-limbed dwarfism with feeble fetal activity, polyhydramnios, and hypotonia are characteristic. Affected infants die shortly after birth.

O. Coffin–Siris Syndrome — Growth failure, sparse hair, hypotonia, and absent fifth finger and toenails are among the more prominent features.

P. Rieger Syndrome — A myotonic dystrophy of variable degree with iris dysplasia and dental abnormalities are features of this disorder inherited as an autosomal-dominant trait.

Q. Multiple Endocrine Adenomatosis Syndrome — Infants with the mucosal neuroma syndrome may be hypotonic at birth. Lingual neuromas may be present at birth or appear in the first few years.

VIII. Miscellaneous Causes

A. Kwashiorkor

B. Dietary Chloride Deficiency — Cases due to errors in formula production as well as breast milk chloride deficiency have been described. Key features also include failure to thrive and anorexia.

SUGGESTED READING

Dubowitz V: The floppy infant syndrome. In Muscle Disorders of Childhood, pp 223–231. Philadelphia, WB Saunders, 1978

Smith DW: Recognizable Patterns of Human Malformation, 3rd ed. Philadelphia, WB Saunders, 1982

Swaiman KF, Wright FS: Pediatric Neuromuscular Diseases, 2nd ed. St. Louis, CV Mosby, 1982

105

ATAXIA

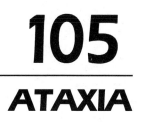

The ataxic gait is characterized by unsteadiness, staggering, and wide-based, lurching movements in any direction. When truncal muscles are primarily involved, ataxia is not as obvious. Because infants normally have poor balance and poorly controlled movements, the incoordination usually cannot be demonstrated until the end of the first year of life. In infants, muscular hypotonia associated with the ataxia may be the only finding.

The causes of ataxia may be grouped by mode of onset. Ataxia of short duration suggests toxic, infectious, or neoplastic causes. Slowly progressive ataxia may occur with posterior fossa tumors, but it may also be a sign in any of a large number of hereditary degenerative disorders. Nonprogressive, chronic ataxia is associated with congenital lesions.

The four most common causes of ataxia are diphenylhydantoin intoxication, acute cerebellar ataxia, infectious polyneuritis, and posterior fossa tumors.

I. Infections

A. Acute Cerebellar Ataxia
Profound truncal ataxia of sudden onset is typical; it is often preceded by a nonspecific illness occurring 2 to 3 weeks before. Tremors, hypotonia, scanning speech, photophobia, headache, and nystagmus may also be present; the deep tendon reflexes remain intact. Children 1 to 5 years of age seem most susceptible. An association with this disorder has been reported in various infections including echovirus, Coxsackie virus, poliomyelitis, herpes simplex, varicella, Epstein–Barr virus, *M. pneumoniae,* and legionellosis.

B. Ataxia During Acute Infections
Ataxia has been noted during the following infections.
1. Mumps
2. Pertussis
3. Poliomyelitis
4. Infectious Mononucleosis

5. Diphtheria
6. Coxsackie virus and Echovirus Infections
7. Rubeola
8. Varicella
9. Typhoid   Other bacterial enteritides may also cause ataxia.
10. *M. pneumoniae*
11. Lyme Disease
12. Scarlet Fever
13. Leptospirosis
14. Legionnaires' Disease

C. Meningitis   Ataxia is not uncommon during recovery from bacterial meningitis; occasionally it may occur preceding the diagnosis of meningitis.

D. Acute Febrile Polyneuritis (Guillain–Barré Syndrome)   Ataxia may occur during the course of this ascending polyneuropathy. The absence of deep tendon reflexes should make this disorder readily separable from acute cerebellar ataxia. The onset occurs 1 to 3 weeks after a nonspecific respiratory or gastrointestinal tract illness. Specific infections incriminated include cytomegalovirus, Epstein–Barr virus, enterovirus, *Mycoplasma pneumoniae*, and Campylobacter jejuni as well as immunizations.

E. Cerebellar Abscess   This usually occurs in children with chronic middle ear infections. Bacteremia in children with cyanotic congenital heart disease is responsible for a minority.

F. Fisher Syndrome   This rare disorder is characterized by the acute onset of ophthalmoplegia, ataxia, and hyporeflexia. An antecedent URI may occur. Most cases recover spontaneously without sequelae.

G. Acute Labyrinthitis   Acute onset of vertigo, nausea, and vomiting is typical. Ataxia may be found. Results of tests of labyrinthine function are abnormal.

H. Cerebellar Abscess

I. Acute Viral Cerebellitis

J. Lyme Disease — Aseptic meningitis, encephalitis, chorea, cerebellar ataxia, cranial neuritis, and a host of other neurologic as well as systemic problems may occur.

K. Tuberculosis — Central nervous system infection may result in increased intracranial pressure and cerebellar dysfunction.

L. Congenital Syphilis — Onset of CNS dysfunction occurs in late preschoolers or adolescents. Memory loss, personality changes, and academic failure are other signs. Stigmata of congenital syphilis are present.

M. Parasitic Disease — Cerebellar echinococcosis is a rare cause.

N. HIV Infection — Ataxia is one part of the progressive encephalopathy described in children with AIDS.

O. Kuru — This chronic slow virus infection may produce cerebellar disease in children. It is primarily found in New Guinea.

II. Ingestions

Ataxia may occur with intoxication by various drugs and metals, whether deliberate, accidental, or iatrogenic. Some of the more common ones are listed.

A. Alcohol

B. Anticonvulsants — Diphenylhydantoin, phenobarbital, primidone, carbamazepine, and clonazepam have been implicated.

C. Lead, Thallium, Organic Mercurials

D. Antihistamines

E. Tranquilizers (Diazepam)

F. Sedatives

G. Gamma Benzene Hexachloride (Lindane)

H. DDT (Chlorophenothane)

I. 5-Fluorouracil

J. Phencyclidine

III. Neoplasms

A. Posterior Fossa Tumors — This possibility must always be considered in any child with the gradual onset of ataxia, especially if headache, vomiting, and papilledema are present. Neck stiffness and head tilt may be other signs. A medulloblastoma may produce ataxia of a relatively abrupt onset.

B. Neuroblastoma/ Ganglioneuroblastoma — Acute cerebellar ataxia may be a presenting symptom of an occult neuroblastoma. Opsoclonus (irregular, jerking eye movements) and myoclonic jerks of the body may also be present. The ataxia may persist after treatment.

C. Brain Stem Tumors — In addition to the ataxia, evidence of cranial nerve deficits is also found.

D. Cerebral Hemisphere Tumors — A small percentage of children with cerebral tumors may have ataxia; in these cases, the tumor is often misdiagnosed as a posterior fossa mass.

E. Spinal Cord Tumors — Extramedullary tumors may produce ataxia along with weakness, spasticity, and sensory changes.

IV. Hereditary Disorders

A. Friedreich's Ataxia — Early signs include loss of vibratory and position senses. Distal muscle weakness becomes evident generally between 7 and 13 years of age. Deep tendon reflexes are absent. Pes cavus and kyphoscoliosis are common. Death by 20 years of age is the rule. Inheritance pattern is autosomal recessive.

B. Ataxia–Telangiectasia — Progressive cerebellar ataxia usually begins between 1 and 3 years of age. Telangiectatic lesions, most commonly affecting the conjunctivae and skin of the ear, appear later. Frequent sinopulmonary infections are typical. Deep tendon reflexes are decreased, and dysarthria is often present. Inheritance pattern is autosomal recessive.

C. Spinocerebellar Degeneration — An abnormal gait develops in school-age children, who eventually develop spasticity in their lower limbs and increasing ataxia, especially involving the upper extremities. Affected children walk on their toes and have a broad-based gait and pes cavus.

D. Roussy–Lévy Disease

This disorder may represent a mild and incomplete form of Friedreich's ataxia; peroneal muscular atrophy also occurs.

E. Abetalipoproteinemia

The first sign is steatorrhea during the first year of life; progressive ataxia and muscle weakness develop later. Acanthocytes are found on peripheral blood smears.

F. Pelizaeus–Merzbacher Disease (Familial Centrolobar Sclerosis)

This sex-linked disorder is characterized by the gradual development of spasticity, ataxia, intention tremor, choreoathetosis, and intellectual deterioration. Nystagmus may be a finding in the first year of life.

G. Marinesco–Sjögren Syndrome

In this rare syndrome inherited as an autosomal recessive trait, short stature, cataracts, and mental retardation are found.

H. Dentate Cerebellar Ataxia (Ramsay Hunt Syndrome)

Initial symptoms include generalized convulsions, myoclonic jerks, tremors, and ataxia. Coordinated movements become difficult to perform. Onset of this disorder inherited as an autosomal recessive trait is between 7 and 16 years of age.

I. Acute Intermittent Cerebellar Ataxia

In a number of families, the sudden onset of ataxia, intention tremors, and gait disturbances has been described.

J. Familial Calcification of Basal Ganglia

This disorder is characterized by convulsions, involuntary movements, and intellectual impairment.

K. Ataxia, Retinitis Pigmentosa, Vestibular Abnormalities, and Intellectual Deterioration

L. Cerebellar Ataxia with Deafness, Anosmia, Absent Caloric Responses, Nonreactive Pupils, and Hyporeflexia

M. Familial Ataxia with Macular Degeneration

N. Familial Intention Tremor, Ataxia, and Lipofuscinosis

O. Hereditary Cerebellar Ataxia, Intellectual Retardation, Choreoathetosis, and Eunuchoidism

P. Hereditary Cerebellar Ataxia with Myotonia and Cataracts

Q. Olivopontocerebellar Atrophy (Dejerine–Thomas Atrophy)

Onset of progressive ataxia, parkinsonian rigidity, resting tremors, and speech impairment is usually in adulthood. Both autosomal-dominant and autosomal-recessive types have been described.

R. Periodic Attacks of Vertigo, Diplopia, and Ataxia

Inheritance pattern is autosomal dominant.

S. Posterior and Lateral Column Difficulties, Nystagmus, and Muscle Atrophy

T. Progressive Cerebellar Ataxia and Epilepsy

U. Dejerine–Sottas Disease (Progressive Hypertrophic Interstitial Neuropathy)

The peripheral nerves are thickened and easily palpable. Pupillary irregularity, nystagmus, intention tremor, scanning speech, and scoliosis are features.

V. Biemond Posterior Column Ataxia

One family with ataxia secondary to progressive degeneration of the posterior columns of the spinal cord has been described.

W. Benign Familial Chorea of Early Onset

The gait is ataxic in this disorder inherited as an autosomal-dominant trait.

V. Trauma

A. Concussion	Acute cerebellar or, less commonly, frontal lobe edema may result in ataxia of short duration.
B. Posterior Fossa Subdural or Epidural Hematoma	
C. Heat Stroke	Prolonged hyperthermia may cause cerebellar degeneration.

VI. Congenital Disorders

A. Ataxic Cerebral palsy	Various causes have been described including cerebellar malformations, perinatal brain damage, and acquired infections. An underlying cause should be sought.
B. Agenesis or Hypoplasia of the Cerebellum	Symptoms are usually noted during the first year of life; clumsiness and developmental delay may be seen.
C. Dandy–Walker Syndrome	Obstructive hydrocephalus is due to congenital atresia of the foramina of Luschka and of Magendie. The cerebellum atrophies as the fourth ventricle becomes enlarged. Hydrocephalus dominates the clinical picture.
D. Hydrocephalus	Progressive hydrocephalus may be associated with ataxic diplegia.
E. Arnold–Chiari Malformation	Displacement of the brain stem and cerebellar tonsils may be associated with ataxia.
F. Encephalocele	
G. Cerebellar Dysplasia with Microgyria, Macrogyria, or Agyria	
H. Basilar Impression (Platybasia)	Margins of the foramen magnum invaginate resulting in posterior displacement of the odontoid and compression of the spinal cord or brain stem. Other features include stiff neck, nystagmus, and cortical tract signs.
I. Craniovertebral Anomalies	Occipitalization of the atlas, separated odontoid process of the axis, and chronic atlantoaxial dislocation may all produce symptoms similar to those of platybasia, including spastic weakness, neck pain, ataxia, and numbness and pain in the extremities.

VII. Metabolic Disorders

A. Niemann–Pick Disease (Type C)
Neurologic symptoms predominate in this form of the disease, which usually appears between 2 and 4 years of age with myoclonic or akinetic seizures and ataxia. A cherry-red macular spot is present.

B. Metachromatic Leukodystrophy
In the infantile type, ataxia begins between 1 and 2 years of age, followed by bulbar signs, hypotonia, and then spasticity. In the juvenile form, a previously normal child develops a gait disturbance, spasticity, and a progressively downhill course.

C. Hypoglycemia
The cerebellum may be damaged by frequent and severe episodes of hypoglycemia during the first year of life.

D. Argininosuccinic Aciduria
Affected infants present with seizures, intermittent ataxia, hypotonia, hepatomegaly, and unusual kinky hair.

E. Juvenile Gaucher Disease
Progressive hepatosplenomegaly, intellectual deterioration, cerebellar ataxia, and spasticity are characteristic.

F. Refsum Disease
Prominent features include ataxia, ichthyosis, and retinitis pigmentosa.

G. Hartnup Disease
Intermittent attacks of ataxia may be accompanied by a pellagra-like rash, mental changes, and double vision.

H. Pyruvate Decarboxylase Deficiency
Attacks of intermittent ataxia are precipitated by fever or stress.

I. Maple Syrup Urine Disease
The intermittent variant occurs in infants and children who are otherwise normal but have attacks of acute ataxia, irritability, and, sometimes, coma.

J. Vitamin E Deficiency
In chronic deficiency, as might occur in chronic intra- or extrahepatic cholestatic disorders, a mild ataxia is a late finding. Hyporeflexia is the initial sign appearing between 1 and 4 years of age.

K. Biotin Responsive Multiple Carboxylase Deficiency
Other features include seizures, hearing loss, developmental delay, periorificial dermatitis, alopecia, and eventually death.

L. Galactosemia
Tremors and ataxia may be seen in some infants. The urine should be checked for reducing substances.

M. Pyruvate Decarboxylase Deficiency — A progressive neurologic disease with variable symptoms, usually ataxia, weakness of ocular mobility and peripheral nerve disease. Acute episodes of weakness or ataxia may occur.

N. Cerebrotendinous Xanthomatosis — Ectopic xanthomas occur in the brain and lung as well as along the tendons. Other findings include spinal cord damage, mental impairment, and corneal opacities. Onset is as early as 10 years of age with progression throughout life.

VIII. Hysterical Ataxia

This cause can usually be differentiated by observation and a careful neurologic examination.

IX. Vascular Disorders

A. Cerebellar Embolism

B. Cerebellar Thrombosis

C. Von Hippel–Lindau Disease (Cerebelloretinal Angiomatosis) — Retinal angiomas enlarge during childhood and may cause visual problems later. Cerebellar angiomas produce signs of cerebellar dysfunction as they enlarge, but usually not until the third decade. Inheritance pattern is autosomal dominant.

D. Posterior Cerebellar Artery Disease

E. Basilar Artery Migraine — Transient blindness, scotomata, formed hallucinations, vertigo, ataxia, loss of consciousness, and drop attacks may be part of this syndrome.

X. Miscellaneous Causes

A. Multiple Sclerosis — This disorder is rare in children, but acute intermittent attacks of optic neuritis, ataxia, or regional parasthesias are strongly suggestive findings.

B. Benign Paroxysmal Vertigo of Childhood — Attacks of ataxia and vertigo are self-limited, lasting minutes. The etiology is unknown.

C. Tick Paralysis — Ataxia is an early sign, but impressive muscular weakness rapidly follows.

D. Hypothyroidism	Ataxia has been described in hypothyroid adults.
E. Seizures	Children may develop sudden ataxia as a result of frequent transitory impairment of consciousness associated with repetitive minor motor seizures.
F. Systemic Lupus Erythematosus	Ataxia has been described in severe cases.
G. Rett Syndrome	A slowly progressive neurologic deterioration seen exclusively in girls. Onset is between 4 and 18 months with behavioral changes. Seizures occur later along with choreoathetosis, ataxia, and hypotonia.

SUGGESTED READING

Swaiman KF, Wright FS: The Practice of Pediatric Neurology, 2nd ed. St. Louis, CV Mosby, 1982

106

CHOREA

Chorea is a movement disorder characterized by explosive, involuntary, and purposeless jerking movements. The movements may involve the trunk and face as well as the extremities.

This movement disorder is relatively uncommon in children. In this chapter, the possible causes have been divided into three categories: cerebral palsy, in which choreiform movements are fairly common; disorders that usually appear after infancy but are infrequent; and a potpourri of much less common causes.

I. Cerebral Palsy
Choreiform movements are usually not detected until later in infancy when attempts at purposeful movements are made. Hypotonia is often present and more prominent early on than chorea.

II. Disorders to Consider First
The disorders in this group are the more common causes of chorea, although overall they are uncommon diseases.

A. Sydenham Chorea	This is the most common cause of acquired chorea, despite an apparently decreasing incidence in developed countries. Although the etiology is still unclear, this disorder seems to follow a streptococcal infection by weeks or months. Evidence of preceding streptococcal infection often is lacking at the time of onset of chorea. The abnormal movements most often begin insidiously and increase in severity over a few weeks. The entire episode rarely lasts more than 3 months. Early signs are often attributed to an emotional disorder. Affected children cannot control their movements and become hyperkinetic, emotionally labile, and often hypotonic. These problems cause interference with normal activities.
B. Bilirubin Encephalopathy (Kernicterus)	Children who survive eventually develop choreoathetosis, often not evident until a few years later. The neonatal history is of great importance. Other features include deafness,

mental retardation, and paralysis of upward gaze.

C. Systemic Lupus Erythematosus
Chorea is rarely a presenting symptom; however, more cases with chorea are being reported.

D. Familial Paroxysmal Choreoathetosis
This unusual disorder is characterized by the sudden onset of choreoathetosis lasting seconds to 4 hours without changes in consciousness. In most cases the movements last less than 1 minute. The episodes may be precipitated by exercise, fatigue, or the ingestion of coffee, tea, or alcohol. It is thought to be a form of reflex epilepsy and responds to anticonvulsants.

E. Benign Familial Chorea of Early Onset
In this disorder transmitted as an autosomal dominant trait, the early onset of chorea may interfere with motor development. The gait is ataxic. No abnormal results of laboratory tests have been found, and there is no mental deterioration.

F. Ataxia–Telangiectasia
Although truncal ataxia is the predominant feature, in some cases there is severe choreoathetosis.

G. Huntington Chorea
In this disorder inherited as an autosomal-dominant trait, the average age of onset is 35 years. In childhood onset, seizures may be an initial manifestation. The chorea is progressive and relentless with mental deterioration, hypotonia, and death after 5 to 18 years. Psychosis is also a prominent feature.

H. Wilson Disease (Hepatolenticular Degeneration)
Hepatic symptoms are often prominent in children. Neurologic symptoms include abnormal posturing, muscle hypertonia, dystonia, chorea, athetotic movements, and tremors. Inheritance pattern is autosomal recessive.

I. Encephalitis
Choreiform movements have been described in encephalitis associated with rubeola, mumps, and varicella and in St. Louis encephalitis.

J. Lesch–Nyhan Syndrome
Chorea, dystonia, tremor, and athetosis are findings in this sex-linked disorder. Self-mutilation often occurs; affected boys must be restrained from injuring themselves. Serum uric acid levels are elevated.

K. Drugs   Choreiform movements may be seen in chil-
                            dren taking amphetamines, methylphenidate,
                            and phenothiazines and upon recovery from
                            diphenylhydantoin intoxication. Phenytoin,
                            without toxic levels, may cause choreoatheto-
                            sis in young children with a pre-existing CNS
                            insult.

III. Even Less Common Causes

The disorders in this group are either rare or are rarely associated with
chorea. The list has been modified from the text by Swaiman and
Wright.[1]

A. Congenital Disor-
   ders
   1. Progressive   Choreiform movements are a consequence of
      Atrophy of   atrophy of the pallidal system of the corpus
      Globus Palli-   striatum.
      dus
B. Degenerative
   Disorders
   1. Canavan Dis-   Symptoms begin between 2 and 4 months of
      ease (Spongy   age. Additional features include optic atrophy,
      Degeneration   hypotonia, and developmental failure. The
      of Central Ner-   head circumference usually increases by 6
      vous System)   months of age. Seizures and spasticity follow.
                           Choreoathetotic movements are occasionally
                           noted.
C. Genetic Disorders
   1. Dystonia   Spasmodic dystonic movements, opisthotonos,
      Musculorum   and writhing, twisting movements are charac-
      Deformans   teristic.
   2. Friedreich's   Affected children usually do not begin walk-
      Ataxia   ing when expected. Ataxia, abnormal speech,
                           and incoordination of hand movements occur
                           later.
   3. Phenylketo-   Some children may have twisting movements
      nuria   suggestive of chorea.
   4. Incontinentia   Linear vesiculopustular lesions followed by
      Pigmenti   the appearance of verrucose lesions and later
                           pigmented swirling suggest this disorder.
   5. Hallervorden–   Choreoathetosis occurs in some cases. More
      Spatz Disease   prominent features are progressive rigidity
                           and dementia. The inheritance pattern is auto-
                           somal recessive.

6. Pelizaeus–Merzbacher Disease (Familial Centrolobar Sclerosis)
   In this sex-linked disorder, the development of spasticity, ataxia, intention tremor, choreoathetosis, and intellectual deterioration is gradual.

7. Abetalipoproteinemia
   Steatorrhea begins during the first year of life. Progressive ataxia and muscle weakness develop later.

8. Fabry Disease (Angiokeratoma Corporis Diffusum)
   Presenting signs of this sex-linked disorder may include weight loss, fever, joint and abdominal pain, and burning pains in the extremities. Punctate angiomas appear on the lower abdomen and scrotum in late childhood.

9. Familial Microcephaly, Retardation, and Chorea

10. Chorea with Curvilinear Bodies
    Two cases have been described with onset at 6 and 7 years of age. Severe chorea, seizures, and intellectual deterioration were found.

11. Porphyria
    Acute intermittent porphyria usually begins at puberty with episodes of abdominal pain, vomiting, and diarrhea. Neurologic symptoms include seizures, peripheral neuropathy, and personality changes.

D. Infections
   1. Diphtheria
   2. Pertussis
   3. Typhoid Fever
   4. Neurosyphilis
   5. Legionellosis
   6. Lyme Disease

E. Endocrine Disorders
   1. Addison Disease

   2. Hypoparathyroidism
      Tetany is the prominent finding.

   3. Thyrotoxicosis
      Short, rapid, uncoordinated jerks may be present.

F. Metabolic Derangements
   1. Hypocalcemia
   2. Hypoglycemia

3. Hypomagne-
semia
4. Hypernatremia
5. Thiamine Defi-
ciency
6. Vitamin B_{12}
Deficiency in
Infants

G. Neoplasms — Chorea has been described in association with cerebellar tumors.

H. Toxins
1. Carbon Mon-
oxide — Chorea may occasionally be seen in patients surviving acute or chronic poisoning.
2. Isoniazid
3. Lithium
4. Mercury
5. Oral Contra-
ceptives
6. Reserpine
7. Scopolamine
8. Phencyclidine

I. Vascular Disor-
ders
1. Henoch–
Schönlein Pur-
pura
2. Sturge–Weber
Syndrome — Chorea rarely occurs as a result of cerebral angiomatosis.
3. Cerebral In-
farction

J. Trauma — Burns in children may cause an encephalopathy with choreiform movements.

K. Miscellaneous
Causes
1. Pregnancy — Chorea gravidarum may be a recrudescence of rheumatic chorea.

2. Polycythemia
3. Hyperkinetic
Syndrome — Choreiform movements are sometimes seen, but this is not true chorea.
4. Nevus Unius
Lateralis — Central nervous system and bony abnormalities have been described in association with this skin disorder.
5. Rett Syndrome — A slowly progressive neurologic deterioration seen exclusively in girls. The onset is between 4 and 18 months with behavioral changes.

Seizures occur later accompanied by choreo-athetosis, ataxia, and hypotonia.

REFERENCE

1. Swaiman KF, Wright FS: The Practice of Pediatric Neurology, 2nd ed. St. Louis, CV Mosby, 1982

SUGGESTED READINGS

Herd JK, Medhi M, Uzendoski DM et al: Chorea associated with systemic lupus erythematosus: Report of two cases and review of literature. Pediatrics 61:308–315, 1978

Kinast M, Erenberg G, Rothner AD: Paroxysmal choreoathetosis: Report of five cases and review of literature. Pediatrics 65:74–77, 1980

107

DELIRIUM

Delirium is a frightening alteration in consciousness characterized by hallucinations, disorientation, and delusions. Normal thought processes are impaired, judgment is altered, and rational behavior is lost. The cause may be a metabolic derangement, an acute infection, or in a distressing number of cases, drug abuse.

I. Infections

A. Acute Systemic Infections	Children may become delirious during acute infections, both bacterial and viral. Bacterial sepsis, pneumococcal pneumonia, measles, and other viral disorders with exanthems and high fever are relatively common causes.
B. Central Nervous System Infections	Children with meningitis, encephalitis, brain abscesses, and other central nervous system infections often act delirious.
C. Malaria	
D. Syphilis	Neurosyphilis is relatively uncommon in children.
E. Rocky Mountain Spotted Fever	Delirium with hallucinations may precede the appearance of the rash. At onset of the illness, symptoms include fever, headache, muscle aches, and shaking chills.
F. Rabies	

II. Drugs and Toxins

A. Alcohol	Acute intoxication and, less commonly in older children, withdrawal from alcohol may cause delirious behavior.
B. Amphetamines	Tremor, dry mouth, tachycardia, hyperactivity, and occasionally, hypertension are signs.
C. Hallucinogenic Drugs	LSD, mescaline, and psilocybin produce vivid hallucinations. Tremors, dilated pupils, abdominal pain, and nausea may be present.
D. Phencyclidine ("Angel Dust")	Affected children have tachycardia, hyperreflexia, visual hallucinations, and hypertension. Ataxia and nystagmus with small or normal-sized pupils suggest this ingestion.

E. Opiates
F. Marihuana;
   Hashish
G. Antihistamines
H. Phenothiazines
 I. Atropine; Sco-
   polamine
J. Caffeine
K. Aminophylline
L. Barbiturate With-
   drawal
M. Salicylates
N. Camphor
O. Lead; Mercury;
   Arsenic
P. Glucocorticoids
Q. Organic Solvents

III. Metabolic Derangements

A. Hypoglycemia

B. Diabetic Ketoaci-
   dosis

C. Hyponatremia — Hyponatremia may occur in various disorders with inappropriate antidiuretic hormone secretion. Lethargy and seizures may be other signs.

D. Uremia — Fatigue, irritability, and difficulty in concentrating occur early; delirium generally appears later.

E. Acidosis

IV. Psychoses

Delirium and hallucinations are less commonly reported in children with affective disorders than in adults.

V. Central Nervous System Disorders

A. Head Injury — Delirious behavior may follow significant head injury.

B. Migraine — Visual hallucinations are relatively common, but less so than scotomata, transitory blindness, blurred vision, and hemianopsia. An acute confusional state can be seen as a form of complicated migraine.

C. Increased Intra-
cranial Pressure

Headache and vomiting in the presence of papilledema suggest this problem.

D. Epilepsy

Olfactory and visual hallucinations may be
part of a preconvulsive aura or occur in the
postictal state.

E. Brain Tumor

F. Cerebral Throm-
bosis or Embo-
lism

G. Cerebral Degen-
erative Disease

VI. Diminished Cerebral Oxygenation

A. Acute Blood Loss

B. Severe Anemia

C. Congestive Heart
Failure

D. Hypoxia

Any cause of hypoxemia may alter cerebral
function producing hallucinations, disorientation, and other symptoms of delirium.

VII. Miscellaneous Causes

A. Fatigue

B. Dehydration

C. Heat Stroke

D. Hepatic Failure

Common initial symptoms are alterations in
consciousness, including disorientation, restlessness, slurred speech, and delirium. Tremors and decerebrate and decorticate rigidity
may follow.

E. Reye Syndrome

Delirious behavior often rapidly follows vomiting and precedes stupor and coma.

F. Insect and Spider
Bites

Potent toxins may be released by various bit-
ing insects and spiders.

G. Burn Encepha-
lopathy

H. Chorea

I. Systemic Lupus
Erythematosus

Cerebral vasculitis may be associated with
psychotic behavior. It may be difficult to separate effects of steroid therapy from those due
to the disease.

J. Pellagra

In severe vitamin deficiency delirium, tremors,
spasticity, polyneuritis, and optic atrophy may
overshadow the skin changes.

K. Hartnup Disease   This rare inherited disorder is characterized by a pellagra-like skin rash, cerebellar ataxia, and psychological disturbances. Attacks of these symptoms may be intermittent.

L. Porphyria   Attacks of psychotic behavior usually do not begin until late adolescence or early adulthood.

108

VERTIGO (DIZZINESS)

Vertigo is a subjective symptom in which the affected person feels as though he or his environment were moving, usually spinning. This complaint is not a common one in children, probably because of the difficulty young children have in expressing this sensation.

Studies in vertigo in childhood are distinctly uncommon, but in a thorough evaluation of this symptom in 42 children by Eviatar and Eviatar,[1] a seizure focus was the cause in 25; psychosomatic vertigo, migraine, and vestibular neuronitis each accounted for 5 cases.

The evaluation of this symptom is a complex procedure and requires specialized expertise.

I. Central Causes

A. Vertiginous Seizures	These seizures may be characterized by sudden attacks of vertigo alone, or sometimes with headache, nausea, vomiting, falling, and loss of consciousness, or combinations of these symptoms. The electroencephalogram may show a temporal lobe abnormal focus, or the tracing may be diffusely abnormal.
B. Infection	Vertigo may accompany or follow meningitis, meningoencephalitis, or a brain abscess. The symptom of vertigo is generally less noticeable than other signs and symptoms of infection.
C. Trauma	Vertigo may be associated with temporal bone fractures, brain contusions, and occasionally cervical spine injuries. Fractures of the temporal bone usually cause hearing loss, tinnitus, and nystagmus; the vertigo appears a few days to weeks after the trauma.
D. Migraine	Vertigo may be an aura prior to the onset of migraine and sometimes persists during the other symptoms. Dizziness or true vertigo may occur with or without a headache. Basilar artery migraine often presents with dizziness.
E. Demyelinating Disease	Dizziness or vertigo occurs at some time during the onset or course of multiple sclerosis in most cases.

591

F. Tumors	Cerebellopontine angle tumors, such as acoustic neuromas, or increased intracranial pressure may cause vertigo.
G. Vertebrobasilar Artery Ischemia	The most common symptom of this problem is dizziness. The attacks are recurrent and spontaneous and last 5 to 15 minutes. Other symptoms such as diplopia, difficulty in speaking, weakness, headache, and impaired consciousness may occur.
H. Vestibulocerebellar Ataxia	Postural vertigo may occur in this rare form of hereditary ataxia. Nystagmus is usually present. The vertigo may precede the onset of ataxia.

II. Peripheral Causes

A. Vestibular Neuronitis	Most patients have symptoms of a recent viral illness, usually an infection of the upper respiratory tract. The vertigo usually begins abruptly, often with nausea, but without hearing loss or central nervous system disturbance.
B. Benign Paroxysmal Vertigo	This disorder occurs primarily in young children between 1 and 4 years of age, with recurrent, sudden, short-lived attacks of vertigo. The attacks disappear over a variable period of time. This disorder may represent a migraine equivalent, especially if there is a positive family history. Classic migraine may follow in later life.
C. Paroxysmal Torticollis of Infancy	This may be a variant of benign paroxysmal vertigo. Attacks are characterized by the head tilting to one side, with resistance to straightening. Vomiting, pallor, and agitation occur in some cases. The average duration is 2 to 3 days.
D. Middle Ear Disease	
1. Acute Otitis Media	Vertigo or dizziness may be a secondary complaint.
2. Chronic Serous Otitis Media	The tympanic membrane is immobile and retracted.
3. Chronic Suppurative Otitis	Labyrinthitis occurs from spread of middle ear infection to the inner ear. Hearing is lost, and there is a history of chronic ear drainage.

E. External Auditory Canal	Children with complete obstruction of the canal and pressure on the tympanic membrane may have dizziness and decreased hearing.
F. Postural Vertigo	Most cases are due to inner-ear disorders, but rarely it may be idiopathic in children. Vertigo is precipitated by changes in head position.
G. Labyrinthitis	Common viral infections such as mumps, influenza, measles, and the common cold may cause transient hearing loss and vertigo.
H. Herpes Zoster Oticus (Ramsay Hunt Syndrome)	Vesicles are found in the external auditory canal. Ear pain is usually severe.
I. Vascular Accidents	
1. Hemorrhage	Inner-ear bleeding with destruction of the vestibular labyrinth and cochlea may occur in leukemia and other blood dyscrasias.
2. Embolus	
3. Thrombus	The arterial blood supply to the inner ear may be blocked; this may occur in collagen–vascular diseases such as periarteritis nodosa.
J. Meniere Disease	This disorder is characterized by recurrent attacks of vertigo associated with hearing loss and often a sensation of fullness in the ear. As the attacks continue deafness may occur. It is rare before puberty and probably has many causes.
K. Perilymphatic Fistula	A rupture in the oval or round window allows fluid to leak into the middle ear. The injury may be caused by direct ear trauma or severe pressure changes. Hearing loss and tinnitus are present.

III. Psychogenic Vertigo

Vertigo or dizziness may be a chronic or recurrent complaint in psychological disturbances. There may be other complaints or unusual behavior. Chronic headaches are common.

IV. Miscellaneous Causes

| A. Hypertension | Dizziness may be a complaint in children with hypertension. |
| B. Hyperventilation | Dizziness commonly occurs during episodes of hyperventilation, along with headache, chest |

pain, anxiety, paresthesias of fingers and toes, and carpopedal spasm.

C. Hypoglycemia

D. Drugs

Vestibular damage may be caused by various drugs, resulting in balance problems. Common offenders include the aminoglycosides. Larger doses of aspirin and long-term therapy with large doses of phenytoin may also result in disturbances of vestibular function.

E. Pellagra

F. Cardiac Dys-
rhythmias

Dizzy spells may be caused by a number of rhythm disturbances.

G. Syncope Associ-
ated

Dizziness rather than syncope may be present with any of the disorders reported in Chapter 61.

REFERENCE

1. Eviatar L, Eviatar A: Vertigo in children: Differential diagnosis and treatment. Pediatrics 59:833–837, 1977

SUGGESTED READINGS

Cody DTR, Kern EB, Pearson BW: Diseases of the Ears, Nose and Throat. Chicago, Year Book Medical Publishers, 1981

Fried MP: The evaluation of dizziness in children. The Laryngoscope 90:1548–1560, 1980

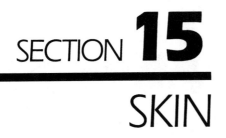

SECTION **15**

SKIN

109

ALOPECIA (HAIR LOSS)

Alopecia—derived from the Greek word for "fox mange"—refers to hair loss. In the evaluation of alopecia in children, it is important to determine whether the hair loss is congenital or acquired; whether it is diffuse or patchy; and whether there is associated scarring or preceding scalp disease.

The classification of conditions causing alopecia in this chapter has been modified from an approach used by Weston.[1] The first category represents the most common causes of alopecia found in children, which accounts for most cases seen by the primary-care physician. In the remaining categories, possible causes are grouped by characteristic patterns of hair loss.

The congenital diffuse alopecias contain several primary hair defects that can often be distinguished on microscopic examination of the hair shaft (a primary presenting complaint is that the child's hair does not seem to grow); a relatively long list of malformation syndromes associated with hair abnormalities is also included in this category. Acquired diffuse hair loss usually results from an underlying systemic disorder; since most of these disorders are correctable, early diagnosis is of particular benefit.

I. Most Common Causes of Hair Loss

A. Alopecia Areata	This condition is characterized by the complete or almost complete loss of hair in circumscribed areas. The scalp is smooth and not inflamed. Total loss of scalp or body hair may occur, and hair loss often begins suddenly.
B. Trichotillomania	Irregular areas of hair loss are the result of self-inflicted pulling; broken-off hairs are readily apparent in the areas of alopecia. The scalp is usually not abnormal.
C. Traction Alopecia	Various types of prolonged or recurrent pull or tension on the hair may lead to areas of alopecia. "Corn-row" and ponytail hair styles and the use of hot combs are relatively common causes.
D. Tinea Capitis	This disorder must always be considered as the cause of any alopecia. Broken hairs are usually present in the affected area. The scalp is often scaly, and the hair in the involved

areas is dull. It is usually seen only in prepubertal children.

II. Congenital, Circumscribed Areas of Hair Loss

A. Sebaceous Nevus or Epidermal Nevus	There is no hair growth in the area of the yellowish tan plaque-like lesion of a sebaceous nevus whose surface resembles pigskin. The epidermal nevi tend to be verrucous rather than flat.
B. Aplasia Cutis Congenita	At birth affected areas appear as punched-out, ulcer-like lesions. They generally heal in a scar devoid of hair.
C. Conradi–Hunerman Syndrome	Affected children have mild to moderate growth deficiency, low nasal bridge, flat facies, asymmetric short limbs, scoliosis, stippled epiphyses, and occasionally areas of alopecia.
D. Incontinentia Pigmenti	Patchy alopecia, especially of the posterior scalp, may be found in 20% of the cases. The skin lesions are the main diagnostic clues. There may be a progression of lesions from linear bullae and vesicles, to verrucous looking lesions, to hyperpigmented streaks and swirls. Eye, teeth, and central nervous system abnormalities may occur.
E. Myotonic Dystrophy	Frontal baldness usually develops during childhood. Muscle myotonia, weakness, and an immobile facies are early clues.
F. Goltz Syndrome	Areas of hair loss, focal dermal hypoplasia (areas of atrophic skin with outpouchings of subcutaneous tissue), syndactyly of fingers and toes, strabismus, and dystrophic nails may be found.

III. Acquired, Circumscribed Areas of Hair Loss with Scarring

A. Following Infection

1. Kerion	Hypersensitivity reaction to tinea capitis may, if untreated, lead to scarring with hair loss.
2. Pyoderma	Scalp infections if deep enough may destroy hair follicles.

3. Recurrent Herpes Simplex

4. Varicella

5. Dissecting Cellulitis; Folliculitis Decalvans	Destruction of hair follicles secondary to the inflammatory process leads to scarring.
6. Tuberculosis; Sarcoid; Leprosy	Localized areas of inflammation may result in alopecia.

B. Following Inflammation

1. Lupus Erythematosus	Both systemic and discoid lupus may cause patches of alopecia. In the systemic form scarring may not always be present.
2. Morphea	Areas of localized scleroderma in the scalp result in atrophy of hair follicles.
3. Keratosis Follicularis	This disorder, transmitted as an autosomal trait, is characterized by the development of papules on the face, chest, back, and extremities. The lesions may coalesce to form scaly, greasy masses. Scalp involvement leads to hair loss. The buccal mucosa and nails are also involved.
4. Lichen Planus	Small, flat-topped, polygonal papules first appear on the extremities and may become generalized. Scalp involvement may lead to scarring.
5. Porokeratosis of Mibelli	A plaque-like lesion surrounded by a keratotic ridge.

C. Following Trauma

1. Physical Trauma	Chronic traction, neurotic excoriations, or clumps of hair pulled out with force result in hair follicle disruption with scarring.
2. Chemical or Thermal Burns	Caustics, acids or alkalis, and phenol as well as burns may cause permanent hair loss.
3. Radiation Injuries	

IV. Congenital, Diffuse Alopecia

A. Hair Shaft Defects

1. Trichorrhexis Nodosa

a. Familial Form	An increase in hair fragility is the only finding. On microscopic examination the hair resembles two brooms that have been pushed together end to end. Excessive combing, permanent treatments, and the like provide the

	trauma. The condition is more common in blacks, especially adolescents.
b. Arginino-succinic Aciduria	The hair is stubby and fragile in affected infants, who are severely mentally retarded.
2. Pili Torti (Twisted Hair)	
a. Classic Form	The hair appears normal at birth but by 2 or 3 years of age it looks brittle and spangled. The condition occasionally is associated with deafness.
b. Menkes' Syndrome	In this severe X-linked neurodegenerative disorder, kinky short hair is characteristic.
3. Monilethrix (Beaded Hair)	This rare disorder transmitted as an autosomal dominant trait is characterized by breaking off of scalp hair.
4. Trichorrhexis Invaginata	On microscopic examination the hairs look like bamboo shoots. The disorder is associated with ichthyosis (Netherton syndrome).
B. Congenital Hypothyroidism	
C. Anhidrotic Ectodermal Dysplasia	The skin seems thin and wrinkled giving an aged appearance. A saddle nose, thick lips, and dental abnormalities accompany the hypotrichosis.
D. Hidrotic Ectodermal Dysplasia	Hypoplasia of hair with painfully thickened nails is typical.
E. Progeria	This is a fascinating, rare disorder producing premature aging.
F. Atrichia Congenita	Familial cases of sparse to absent hair have been reported.
G. Marinesco–Sjögren Syndrome	Main features are cerebellar ataxia, growth deficiency, cataracts, and weakness. Sparse hair has also been reported.
H. Rothmund–Thomson Syndrome	Striking, irregular hyperpigmentation and depigmentation of the skin with telangiectactic lesions are characteristic. Alopecia, photosensitivity, and cataracts are common.
I. Cartilage–Hair Hypoplasia	Fine, sparse hair with short stature, short limbs, short hands, and irregularly scalloped metaphyses on roentgenograms are findings.
J. Ellis–van Creveld Syndrome (Chondroectodermal Dysplasia)	A combination of hair and dental abnormalities occurs with shortened extremities; trunk size is normal. Polydactyly and congenital heart disease are also prominent features.

K. Trichorhinopha-langeal Syndrome (Langer–Giedion Syndrome)

Sparse hair, a pear-shaped nose, and short metacarpals are the main physical findings.

L. Cockayne Syndrome

Growth deficiency becomes evident after 1 year of age. Mental retardation, an unsteady gait, tremors, deafness, sunken eyes, skin photosensitivity, joint movement limitations, and sparse hair create a striking picture.

M. Hallermann–Streiff Syndrome (Oculomandib-ulofacial Syndrome)

This syndrome is characterized by small stature, prominent forehead, congenital cataracts, a small, thin nose with "pinched" facies, hypoplastic teeth and sparse hair.

N. Oculodentodigital Dysplasia

Microphthalmos, a thin nose with hypoplastic alae, enamel hypoplasia, fixed and flexed fifth fingers, and sparse, dry, slow-growing hair are important features.

O. Crouston Syndrome

Physical findings include thick, dyskeratotic palms and soles; hyperpigmentation over knuckles, elbows, axillae, and pubic area; nail dysplasia; and hair abnormalities ranging from hypoplasia to alopecia.

P. Laurence–Moon–Biedl Syndrome

Hypotrichosis is seen occasionally in affected children; prominent findings include short stature, obesity, polydactyly, mental retardation, and hypogonadism.

Q. Homocystinuria

The hair of children with this aminoaciduria may be sparse and light. A marfanoid slender build, subluxated lenses, malar flush, and venous thromboses are prominent features.

R. Werner Syndrome

This is a syndrome of premature aging that begins in adolescence.

S. Oral–Facial–Digital Syndrome, Type I

Abnormalities include cleft soft palate, asymmetric shortening of digits, and webbing of buccal mucosa and alveolar ridges. Alopecia is a rare finding.

T. Seckel Syndrome

This syndrome, originally called the "bird-headed dwarf" syndrome, may occasionally have sparse hair.

U. Dyskeratosis Congenita

Dystrophy of nails with chronic paronychiae develops first, followed by the appearance of mucous membrane blisters and reticular brown pigmentation of the skin.

V. Acquired Diffuse Hair Loss

A. Telogen Effluvium — Various stressful circumstances may cause the abrupt, premature cessation of growth in certain normal hair bulbs. These hairs then enter an involutional phase, followed by the resting or telogen phase during which they may be shed. The period between the causative stress and the hair loss is 2 to 4 months. Rarely, more than 50% of the hair is lost. Various stressful situations that have been implicated are listed below.

    1. Febrile Illnesses — High fevers associated with various illnesses, particularly pneumonia, influenza, and typhoid fever, may be followed by hair loss.

    2. Physiologic Hair Loss in Newborns

    3. Parturition

    4. Psychogenic Factors

    5. Crash Diets

    6. Traction

    7. Surgery and Anesthesia

B. Endocrine Disorders

    1. Androgenetic Alopecia — Physiologic male pattern baldness may occur in adolescents.

    2. Hypothyroidism — Diffuse thinning of scalp hair may occur with some patchy areas of alopecia.

    3. Hypopituitarism — Scalp, eyebrow, and sexual hair is sparse. The skin is thin and prematurely wrinkled.

    4. Hypoparathyroidism — Hair is thin and coarse and sheds easily; the loss may be complete or patchy. Muscle cramps, tetany, and convulsions are more impressive features.

    5. Diabetes Mellitus

C. Chemicals and Drugs

    1. Heavy Metals — Thallium, arsenic, and lead ingestion may cause hair loss. Arsenic may be inhaled via smoke from the burning of outdoor grade lumber treated with preservatives.

2. Antithyroid Drugs

3. Heparin; Coumarin

4. Antimetabolites

5. Trimethadione

6. Carbamazepine (Tegretol)

D. Nutritional Disorders

1. Hypervitaminosis A	Chronic ingestion may lead to hair loss, peeling of the skin, bone pain, and soft-tissue calcifications.
2. Acrodermatitis Enteropathica	Zinc deficiency in affected children is associated with alopecia, irritability, diarrhea, and perioral and perianal as well as distal extremity rashes.
3. Marasmus and Kwashiorkor	The nutritional deficiency must be severe for hair loss to result.
4. Celiac Disease	
5. Iron Deficiency	Thinning of hair may occur with chronic, severe iron-deficiency anemia.
6. Rickets	

E. Miscellaneous Causes

1. Seborrhea	Chronic involvement of the scalp with thick scales may lead to thinning of the hair.
2. Psoriasis	Heaped-up layers of silvery scale may lead to hair loss in involved areas.
3. Biotin Responsive Multiple Carboxylase Deficiency	Biotinidase deficiency results in seizures, ataxia, hearing loss, developmental delay, periorificial dermatitis, alopecia, and eventually death.

REFERENCE

1. Weston WL: Practical Pediatric Dermatology, pp 269–284. Boston, Little, Brown & Co, 1979

SUGGESTED READING

Price VH: Disorders of the hair in children. Pediatr Clin North Am 25:305–320, 1978

110

HYPERTRICHOSIS AND HIRSUTISM

Hirsutism is the term usually used to denote an increase in body hair; however, it refers specifically to the excess growth of hair, in an adult male distribution pattern, that may be seen in women and children. Hypertrichosis is the correct term to describe a generalized or localized increase in body hair.

Hirsutism results from an excess production of androgens from either adrenal or ovarian sources or from a constitutional increase in sensitivity of hair follicles, or possibly from both. In this chapter the causes of increased hair growth are divided into disorders with hypertrichosis and those with hirsutism.

I. Hypertrichosis
  A. Generalized Hypertrichosis
    1. Genetic Trait — Certain races and certain families may have more hair.
    2. Drug-Induced Hypertrichosis — Diphenylhydantoin, diazoxide, streptomycin, and hexachlorobenzene are among the drugs that have been implicated.
    3. Central Nervous System Disorders — Hypertrichosis has been reported following encephalitis and concussions, and in multiple sclerosis.
    4. Starvation and Anorexia Nervosa
    5. Hypothyroidism — Hair is increased, especially on the back and limbs.
    6. Dermatomyositis — Generally, increased hair is seen on the legs and temples.
    7. Epidermolysis Bullosa
    8. Dysmorphogenic Syndromes — Hypertrichosis has been described in Hurler, Bloom, Seckel, de Lange, Rubinstein–Taybi, leprechaunism, Marshall–Smith, and trisomy 18 syndromes and in generalized gangliosi-

604

dosis. It may also occur in children with idiopathic gingival fibromatosis who have never received treatment with anticonvulsants.

9. Acrodynia — Increased hair is an unusual feature in chronic mercury poisoning; it occurs primarily on the limbs.

10. Congenital Hypertrichosis — Excessively long lanugo hair is present at birth and increases during childhood. The hair is soft and silky.

11. Lipodystrophy — Children with congenital or generalized lipodystrophy tend to have increased body hair.

12. Porphyria — Children with congenital erythropoietic porphyria develop increased body hair, but other signs and symptoms such as red urine, marked photosensitivity with bullae formation and scarring, and, eventually, red to pink teeth are more prominent. Affected persons were the so-called werewolves of old.

B. Localized Hypertrichosis

1. Trauma — Increased hair growth may occur at sites of trauma or chemical irritation.

2. Nevi and Hamartomas — Localized hair growth may occur in various nevi or over spinal cord defects or other lesions.

II. Hirsutism

A. Idiopathic Hirsutism — In most cases no cause for the hirsutism can be found. There may be a family history. Support for the idiopathic appellation includes a history of normal menses, no deepening of the voice, and lack of frontal hairline recession. As more sensitive assay techniques for androgens are developed most patients will be shown to have an underlying abnormality of androgen metabolism.

B. Iatrogenic Hirsutism — Among the exogenous causes are progestational agents, anabolic steroids, and testosterone. Systemic steroids and adrenocorticotropic hormones cause an increase in lanugo hair. Phenytoin, diazoxide, and minoxidil are also drugs that should be considered.

C. Physiologic Hirsutism — Hirsutism without virilization may occur in precocious puberty, at puberty, and during pregnancy.

D. Adrenal Disorders

1. Congenital Adrenal Hyperplasia (Adrenogenital Syndrome)

Classic adrenogenital syndrome as well as compensated forms involving 11- and 21-hydroxylation and 3-β-hydroxysteroid dehydrogenase activity demonstrate hirsutism and other signs of virilization. In the latter intermittent elevations of cortisol precursors may be missed.

2. Virilizing Tumors

Clitoral enlargement in girls and phallic enlargement in prepubertal boys are important clinical signs.

3. Cushing Syndrome

Other signs are more prominent including moon facies, truncal obesity, short stature, and hypertension.

E. Ovarian Disorders

1. Virilizing Ovarian Tumors

Arrhenoblastoma and granulosa–theca cell tumors are uncommon causes.

2. Stein–Leventhal Syndrome

Features include amenorrhea or dysfunctional uterine bleeding with infertility, with or without obesity, in association with polycystic ovaries. Other non-neoplastic causes of ovarian androgen production may present a spectrum of severity of clinical findings less obvious than the above.

3. Pure Gonadal Dysgenesis

F. Pituitary Disorders

Acromegaly associated with an eosinophilic pituitary tumor may be accomplished by diabetes and hirsutism.

G. Miscellaneous Causes

1. Achard–Thiers Syndrome

Obesity and facial hirsutism develop by 15 to 30 years of age. Hypertension and diabetes occur later.

2. Male Pseudohermaphroditism

SUGGESTED READINGS

Emans SJ, Grace E, Fleischnick E et al: Detection of late-onset 21-hydroxylase deficiency congenital adrenal hyperplasia in adolescents. Pediatrics 72:690–695, 1983

Kustin J, Rebar RW: Hirsutism in young adolescent girls. Pediatr Ann 15:522–528, 1986

111

PURPURA (PETECHIAE AND ECCHYMOSES)

Purpura is the name given to the discoloration of the skin or of mucous membranes caused by extravasation of red blood cells; the areas of discoloration do not blanch upon pressure. Petechiae are purpuric lesions that are 2 mm or less in diameter; ecchymoses are larger purpuric lesions.

Purpuric lesions are generally the result of a defect in the circulating blood or the blood vessels. Although in this chapter the causes of purpuric lesions are divided into categories of thrombocytopenic, nonthrombocytopenic, vascular, and coagulation disorders, more than one defect may be involved: For instance, infections may cause purpura with or without thrombocytopenia, and thrombocytopenia and vascular damage may occur together.

Petechiae and random ecchymoses are characteristic of thrombocytopenias and thrombocytopathies (platelet dysfunction). Coagulation disturbances cause hemostasis problems in large vessels and usually produce ecchymoses rather than petechiae. Vascular disorders may produce either type of lesion. Causes of purpura in the neonatal period have been treated as a separate grouping.

I. Neonatal Purpura

A. Infection	Infections of various types are the most common cause of neonatal purpura. Thrombocytopenia or disseminated intravascular coagulation may or may not be associated.
1. Bacterial Infection	Group B streptococci, *E. coli*, *Listeria*, and other organisms have been implicated.
2. Viral Infection	Infections may be congenital or acquired. Important congenital infections include cytomegalovirus infection, rubella, and herpes simplex; the last may be acquired, usually during passage through the birth canal.
3. Parasitic Infestation	Toxoplasmosis may be associated with purpura.
4. Other Infections	Purpura may be a finding in syphilis.

B. Immunologic Disorders

1. Isoimmune Neonatal Thrombocytopenia — Maternal IgG antibody against fetal platelets crosses the placenta. The maternal platelet count is within normal limits.

2. Maternal Auto-antibody Disease — Maternal disorders associated with autoantibody formation may cause thrombocytopenia in the offspring. Examples are maternal idiopathic thrombocytopenic purpura and systemic lupus erythematosus.

3. Erythroblastosis Fetalis — In severe disease the platelet count may be depressed.

C. Disseminated Intravascular Coagulation — Triggering mechanisms include infection, shock, severe hyaline membrane disease (or any cause of severe hypoxia and acidosis), and necrotizing enterocolitis, among others.

D. Purpura with Congenital Defects

1. Thrombocytopenia with Absent Radii (TAR) Syndrome

2. Wiskott–Aldrich Syndrome — Thrombocytopenia and eczema usually develop later, as do the recurrent infections.

3. Trisomy 13 and 18 Syndromes

E. Other Blood Clotting Defects

1. Hemorrhagic Disease of the Newborn — Occurrence is rare now that vitamin K is given at birth. The bleeding typically occurs on the second or third day of life and most commonly is from the gastrointestinal tract, not the skin.

2. Congenital Deficiencies of the Coagulation Factors — Bleeding associated with these deficiencies generally does not take place in the first few weeks of life but has been reported in severe deficiencies, particularly those involving factors VIII and IX. Less commonly, bleeding has been reported with von Willebrand disease and deficiencies of factors V, VII, X, XI, and XIII.

F. Miscellaneous
   Causes
   1. Congenital
      Leukemia
   2. Giant Heman-   Purpuric lesions are a consequence of platelet
      gioma   trapping.
   3. Renal Vein
      Thrombosis
   4. Maternal Drug   Maternal warfarin therapy and chronic mater-
      Ingestion   nal anticonvulsants such as barbiturates and
                        phenytoins may be associated with low levels
                        of vitamin K in the newborn.
   5. Congenital
      Thyrotoxicosis

II. Purpura Secondary to Platelet Disorders

A. Disorders with
   Thrombocyto-
   penia
   1. Idiopathic   This condition may be chronic or develop
      Thrombocyto-   abruptly. A viral illness often precedes the
      penic Purpura   appearance of the petechiae. The bone mar-
      (ITP)   row contains an abundance of megakaryo-
                        cytes.
   2. Infection   Various infections may cause purpura with or
                        without thrombocytopenia, including menin-
                        gococcemia, other bacterial septicemias, and
                        some viral infections.
   3. Drugs   Sulfonamides, iodides, digitoxin, quinine, and
                        quinidine may cause thrombocytopenia.
   4. Autoimmune   Examples include systemic lupus erythema-
      Disorders   tosus, acquired hemolytic anemia, and hyper-
                        thyroidism.
   5. Neoplastic   Leukemias, lymphomas, and other tumors
      Disorders   may replace the bone marrow, with a result-
                        ing decrease in platelet production.
   6. Disseminated   In addition to thrombocytopenia, children
      Intravascular   with DIC have hypofibrinogenemia, reduced
      Coagulopathy   factors II, V, and VIII, and fibrin-split prod-
      (DIC)   ucts in the serum. DIC has many precipitating
                        causes including infections (bacterial, viral,
                        rickettsial, and protozoal), malignancies, head
                        injury, shock, and transfusion reactions.
   7. Hemolytic–   Hemolytic anemia, acute renal failure, and
      Uremic Syn-   thrombocytopenia are the classic findings; it
      drome   usually follows a gastroenteritis. This syn-

drome occurs chiefly in young children, although its signs may mimic those of thrombotic thrombocytopenic purpura in young adults.

8. Aplastic Anemia

The condition may be idiopathic or drug-induced. The bone marrow may also be suppressed by radiation and chemicals.

9. Disorders Producing Hypersplenism

Splenic enlargement may result in platelet trapping as seen in thalassemia major and Gaucher disease. Liver disorders causing portal hypertension may also induce thrombocytopenia.

10. Inherited Disorders with Decreased Platelet Production

   a. Fanconi Syndrome

   Pancytopenia usually does not appear until 5 years of age or later. Various abnormalities may be found in affected children including short stature, hyperpigmentation, thumb abnormalities, strabismus, renal problems, and microcephaly. Inheritance pattern is autosomal recessive.

   b. Thrombocytopenia with Absent Radii (TAR) Syndrome

   In this disorder inherited as an autosomal recessive trait, the thrombocytopenia is of most concern during the first year of life.

11. Inherited Disorders with Increased Platelet Destruction

   a. Wiskott–Aldrich Syndrome

   This is a sex-linked disorder characterized by recurrent infections, an eczematoid rash, and thrombocytopenia.

   b. May–Hegglin Anomaly

   Giant platelets and inclusions in leukocytes are findings in this inherited blood defect. One third of patients have decreased platelets.

   c. Bernard–Soulier Disease

   This rare blood disorder is characterized by giant platelets, often decreased in number. Bleeding may be severe.

12. Miscellaneous Disorders
    a. Iron-Deficiency Anemia — In severe cases iron deficiency may be associated with thrombocytopenia.
    b. Osteopetrosis — Replacement of marrow by bone eventually leads to severe anemia and thrombocytopenia.
    c. Giant Hemangioma — Platelets may be trapped in the hemangioma.
    d. Cyanotic Congenital Heart Disease
    e. Acquired Immune Deficiency Syndrome — Petechiae may be the presenting sign in infants. In older children the thrombocytopenia is overshadowed by opportunistic infections.

B. Normal Platelet Counts with Abnormal Platelet Function
   1. Drug-Induced Thrombocytopathies
      a. Aspirin — Small doses of aspirin may cause prolonged platelet effects.
      b. Other Drugs — Antihistamines, phenothiazines, sulfonamides, antidepressants, and local anesthetics are among the offenders.
   2. Uremia
   3. Inherited Thrombocytopathies
      a. Glanzmann Thrombasthenia — This disorder inherited as an autosomal recessive trait is characterized by mucosal and cutaneous bleeding from early life. The bleeding time is prolonged; clot retraction is absent or deficient.
      b. Adenosine Diphosphate (ADP) Storage Pool Disease — Mild purpura may occur in this rare disorder inherited as an autosomal-dominant trait.

c. Adenosine Diphosphate (ADP) Release Disease | A mild bleeding tendency is present.

III. Purpura Secondary to Vascular Disorders (Nonthrombocytopenic)

A. Trauma | Trauma is the most common cause of purpura overall. The following should be considered.

1. Child Abuse | Unexplained or poorly explained bruising in a young child suggests abuse.

2. Factitious Lesions | Bruises unusual in shape and position in teenagers may be factitious.

3. Autoerythrocyte Sensitization | This disorder was originally thought to represent an unusual autosensitivity to the erythrocytes, resulting in purpuric areas. More recently, a psychogenic origin has been suggested; the lesions may be self-induced.

4. Cupping and Coin Rubbing | In some cultures lesions caused by attempts to "bring out" the cause of illness may be the result of vacuum-induced purpura from cupping or rubbing the skin with coins.

B. Raised Intravascular Pressure | Coughing, vomiting, or choking may cause petechiae on the head and neck.

C. Henoch–Schönlein Purpura | The lesions tend to be located on the lower extremities, almost never on the trunk. Abdominal pain, arthritis, or nephritis occurs in about one half of the cases. The etiology is still unknown.

D. Infection | Petechiae may appear during sepsis without thrombocytopenia. Viral infections, particularly with Coxsackie viruses A9 and B3 and echoviruses 9 and 4, may be associated with purpuric lesions. Petechiae of the head and neck may be found in streptococcal pharyngitis. Rocky Mountain spotted fever and atypical measles may also produce a vasculitis.

E. Septic Emboli | Purpuric lesions may be a presenting sign in subacute bacterial endocarditis.

F. Drug-Induced Lesions | Ingestion of sulfonamides, penicillins, iodides, mercury, bismuth, and other substances may produce purpuric lesions. A vasculitis secondary to drug reactions has been described with a wide variety of drugs including penicillins, sulfonamides, hydantoin, and allopurinol. Palpable purpura should suggest vasculitis. Hemorrhagic vesicles and bullae may also appear.

G. Corticosteroids — Easy bruising may be seen in patients on prolonged steroid therapy or, rarely, with Cushing syndrome.

H. Scurvy — This disorder is unusual in children in the United States. Perifollicular petechiae with swollen gums and painful limbs are suggestive findings.

I. Inherited Vascular Disorders

1. Ehlers–Danlos Syndrome — Various types have been described. Easy bruisability, skin hyperelasticity, and joint laxity may be seen.

2. Hereditary Hemorrhagic Telangiectasia — Telangiectatic lesions usually do not appear until late childhood. Epistaxis and gastrointestinal bleeding are more likely than cutaneous bleeding.

3. Marfan Syndrome — Bleeding problems are more likely to involve the large vessels, such as the aorta, with dissecting aneurysm.

4. Osteogenesis Imperfecta — Capillary fragility may lead to increased bleeding tendency.

J. Progressive Pigmentary Dermatosis (Schamberg Disease) — This disorder is characterized by the insidious onset and slow progression of grouped petechiae over the extremities, usually the lower. The lesions contain fresh and old petechiae, giving rise to various colors. Adolescents may be affected.

K. Dysproteinemias — Abnormal plasma proteins, such as seen in hyperglobulinemias, cryoglobulinemias, or macroglobulinemias, may be associated with purpura.

L. *Maculae Cerulae* — Faint, grayish purpuric lesions of the lower abdomen and back may be caused by pubic lice, simulating purpuric lesions.

M. Vasculitis — A host of disorders may be associated with vasculitis, creating palpable purpura especially in dependent areas. Lupus, Wegener's granulomatosis, other connective tissue disorders and diseases associated with immune complexes, complement and immunoglobulin deposition should be sought.

IV. Coagulation Disturbances

Clotting factor disorders are more likely to cause deep muscular or joint bleeding than superficial skin bleeding, although purpura may occur in any of these disorders (all are not listed).

A. Von Willebrand Disease	In this relatively common disorder transmitted as an autosomal-dominant trait, there is a deficiency of a circulating plasma protein related to factor VIII. The most common presenting sign is excessive bleeding after dental extraction, tonsillectomy, or other surgical procedure.
B. Factor VIII, IX, XI, or XII Deficiency	These disorders are characterized by a prolonged partial thromboplastin time (PTT) and a normal prothrombin time (PT).
C. Factor V, X, II (Prothrombin), or I (Fibrinogen) Deficiency	Both PTT and PT are prolonged.
D. Factor VII Deficiency	The PT is prolonged; the PTT is normal.
E. Factor XIII Deficiency	Bleeding from the umbilical stump as the cord separates is the most common sign.
F. Late Hemorrhagic Disease	Vitamin K deficiency states may occur in various disorders including diarrhea, cystic fibrosis, biliary atresia, alpha-1-antitrypsin deficiency, hepatitis, abetalipoproteinemia, celiac disease, and chronic warfarin exposure. Breast-fed infants occasionally develop late hemorrhagic disease.
G. Protein C Deficiency	Protein C is an important physiologic anticoagulant. Congenital deficiency is an autosomal dominant disorder and leads to recurrent episodes of superficial thrombophlebitis, deep vein thrombosis, and pulmonary embolism.

SUGGESTED READINGS

Corrigan JJ Jr: Disseminated intravascular coagulopathy. Pediatr In Rev 1:37–46, 1979

Lane PA, Hathaway WE: Vitamin K in infancy. J Pediatr 106:351–359, 1985

Miller DR, Pearson HA, Baehner RL et al (eds): Smith's Blood Diseases of Infancy and Childhood, 4th ed. St. Louis, CV Mosby, 1978

Oski FA, Naiman JL: Hematologic Problems in the Newborn, 2nd ed. Philadelphia, WB Saunders, 1972

Sills RH, Marlar RA, Montgomery RR et al: Severe homozygous protein C deficiency. J Pediatr 105:409–413, 1984

112

PRURITUS

Pruritus—which comes from the Latin *prurire*, "to itch"—is a most annoying symptom. It is a subjective complaint of an uncomfortable skin sensation that leads to the response of scratching. Scratching often results in relief of this sensation, but the relief is only temporary.

Pruritus may or may not be associated with skin lesions that may provide diagnostic clues. It is important to remember, however, that repeated scratching of the skin will cause excoriations, and if the scratching persists, lichenification or thickening of the skin will result.

Exogenous causes of pruritus such as contactants, parasitic infestations, and environmental factors (drying, high humidity, and excessive bathing) are the most common; the atopic person is especially susceptible. Psychogenic causes of pruritus are less common in children than in adults. Endogenous causes account for very few of the cases except perhaps for drug reactions, although, because of their lethality, neoplasia cannot be ignored as a possible cause.

When a thorough investigation fails to reveal an underlying cause for the pruritus, it may be said to be idiopathic.

I. Exogenous Causes

A. Contactants	Various substances, either irritants or allergens, may produce pruritus upon contact with the skin; only a few examples are listed. In most cases, a rash occurs with the pruritus; typically it is localized and well-defined with sharp borders.
1. Irritants	Harsh soaps, bubble bath, saliva, citrus juices (especially on perioral skin), urine and feces (diaper dermatitis), chemicals (creosote), wool (especially in atopic children), and caterpillar contact may cause skin irritation.
2. Allergens	Poison ivy (plant dermatitis), jewelry (nickel), topical medications (especially anesthetics and antihistamines), clothing dyes, and cosmetics may cause allergic reactions.

615

B. Parasitic Infestations and Insect Bites

1. Scabies — The recent pandemic of scabies requires consideration of this infestation in the differential diagnosis of any pruritic rash of recent onset, especially if the characteristic distribution (hands, wrists, axillae, gluteal cleft, and genitalia) and papular, papulovesicular, or nodular lesions, as well as involvement of other family members, are found.

2. Papular Urticaria — Bites of insects, especially fleas and mosquitoes, may be followed by localized pruritus. In some cases, periods of intense pruritus are associated with many papules having a central punctum on an erythematous base.

3. Pediculosis — Body lice may be difficult to see, but their egg sacs (nits) are stationary, attached to hairs.

4. Cercarial Infestations — Swimmers' itch may develop following bathing in certain freshwater lakes.

5. Other Mites; Chiggers; Hookworm (Creeping Eruption)

C. Foreign Bodies — Fiberglass is probably the best recognized and the most common, particularly if clothing is washed with materials containing fiberglass. Cactus spines and hair may also cause pruritus.

D. Environmental Factors

1. Drying of Skin — Low humidity, especially in temperate climates, may be a factor, most commonly in the winter months when the heat is turned on.

2. Excessive Bathing — Removal of natural oils allows drying of the stratum corneum and resultant pruritus.

3. High Humidity — Retention of moisture in the skin may produce pruritus, which may be associated with miliaria rubra (prickly heat).

II. Endogenous Causes

A. Drug Reactions — A large number of drugs may produce pruritus, often without primary skin lesions. Occasionally exposure to sunlight precipitates the itch. Among the more common offenders are aminophylline, aspirin, barbiturates, opiates, erythromycin, gold, griseofulvin, isoniazid, phenothiazines, and vitamin A.

B. Internal Malignancies and Lymphomas

This is the most worrisome group of disorders that may cause pruritus, although overall they make up a tiny percentage. The pruritus may precede other manifestations of neoplasia by months or even years; curiously, it may be localized as well as generalized.

C. Blood Dyscrasias

Polycythemia vera is a well-recognized cause of pruritus in adults but is rare in children. Iron deficiency has even been suggested as a cause.

D. Renal Disease

Retention of products usually excreted by the kidney may cause pruritus. The association of pruritus with uremia is well known. Uric acid and other products, as yet undetermined, may play a role.

E. Hepatic Disorders

Pruritus may occur with or without jaundice. Cholestatic conditions such as familial cholestasis or biliary atresia and cholestasis secondary to drugs may produce itching. In acute hepatitis pruritus often precedes jaundice and may be associated with urticaria. Repeated scratching will produce excoriations and eczema.

F. Endocrine and Metabolic Causes
  1. Hypothyroidism

The associated dry skin may be the cause of the pruritus.

  2. Hyperthyroidism

This condition rarely may be associated with itching.

  3. Hypoparathyroidism

  4. Diabetes Mellitus

Pruritus most commonly occurs on the lower extremities.

  5. Carcinoid Tumors

Pruritus may rarely accompany flushing attacks.

  6. Hypercalcemia

Immobilization as well as other causes of hypercalcemia may result in various symptoms including pruritus.

G. Autoimmune Disorders
  1. Systemic Lupus Erythematosus

2. Juvenile Rheu- matoid Arthri- tis	The characteristic rash is occasionally pruritic.
H. Parasitic Diseases	Trichinosis and hookworm infestations may be associated with itching.
I. Pregnancy	
J. Congenital Ecto- dermal Defects	Both the anhidrotic and hidrotic forms of ecto-dermal dysplasia may be associated with pruritus.

III. Psychogenic Pruritus
Before a psychological origin is considered, a thorough search must be made for organic causes.

IV. Pruritus Associated with Skin Disorders
Pruritus may be a problem in many skin disorders. Only a few important conditions are listed.

A. Atopic Dermatitis	This apparently hereditary condition of the skin is common. It was aptly described years ago as an "itch that rashes," since if the child could be prevented from scratching, no rash would appear. Several exogenous factors as well as stress may produce pruritus in the atopic child.
B. Infections	Pruritus may accompany fungal, candidal, bacterial, or viral skin infections.
C. Pityriasis Rosea	Pruritus may occur in 5% to 10% of affected persons.
D. Psoriasis	
E. Urticaria Pigmen- tosa	Occasionally pruritus without pigmented skin lesions may be present or precede the more typical lesions. Dermatographia in these cases may be intense.
F. Urticaria	Urticarial skin lesions are pruritic (see Chap. 113, Urticaria).
G. Erythropoietic Protoporphyria	Burning pruritus may occur within a few minutes following exposure to sunlight, erythema, urticarial wheals, or vesicles develop. A laboratory hallmark of this disorder is a high free erythrocyte protoporphyrin.
H. Neurodermatitis	Repeated scratching of the skin may lead to the itch–scratch–itch cycle. Various stimuli trigger the phenomenon.

V. Idiopathic Pruritus

113

URTICARIA

Hives are easily recognizable, even by most laymen, because they are such a common sign. It has been estimated that as many as 15% of the population may experience urticarial lesions at some time during their lives. The recognition of hives is one matter; finding the underlying cause is another. Most of the literature on this subject divides hives into two categories: acute and chronic. Acute hives last less than 6 weeks; chronic hives are present or recur for more than 6 weeks. In roughly three fourths of patients, particularly those with chronic hives, no definite etiology can be established.

Urticaria is characterized by the presence of wheals that come and go and are usually pruritic. The wheals vary in size, ranging from a few millimeters to many centimeters. There may or may not be other signs and symptoms. Careful investigation may reveal characteristic features. Information about the duration of episodes and the pattern of occurrence is important. The hives may occur only in certain places, such as home or school. There may be an association with certain activities, such as food ingestion or exercise.

The pathogenic mechanisms are many and often poorly understood. Immunologic and nonimmunologic mechanisms may be involved.

I. Drugs

Drug reactions are among the most commonly recognized causes of acute urticaria. Almost any drug is a potential offender, especially penicillins, sulfas, sedatives, tranquilizers, analgesics, laxatives, hormones, and diuretics. Drugs such as penicillin may be present in trace amounts in foods, especially cow's milk. There may be no clear history of exposure. Aspirin may be responsible for the exacerbation of chronic urticaria in as many as 20% to 40% of patients; the effects of aspirin may last for a few weeks rather than just a few days as is commonly thought.

II. Foods

Foods are another common cause, especially of acute urticaria. The causative factor may be food protein or added preservative. Commonly incriminated foods are nuts, fish, eggs, lobster, strawberries, yeasts, salicylates, citric acid, azo dyes, and benzoic acid. A food diary, as well as elimination and readdition diets, may be helpful in identifying the offending substance. Often more than one food may be the cause.

III. Inhalants

Reactions are seen primarily in atopic persons with a history of allergic rhinitis and asthma in a seasonal occurrence pattern. Pollens, mold spores, animal danders, aerosols, and plant products may be responsible. Identification may be aided by skin tests.

IV. Infections and Infestations

Transient urticaria may be associated with a variety of infections, sometimes as a prodromal feature. Included in this group are streptococcal infection, viral hepatitis, infectious mononucleosis, Coxsackie virus and adenovirus infections, and parasitic infestations (trichinosis, giardiasis or roundworms). Chronic focal bacterial infection (such as sinus, dental, genitourinary, or gastrointestinal), dermatophytosis, or candidiasis is probably an uncommon cause of chronic urticaria despite popularity in the old literature. Giardiasis, malaria, and infestations with *entamoeba histolytica* are uncommon causes of chronic urticaria.

V. Insect and Arthropod Bites and Stings

These usually cause acute, transient episodes of urticaria. Bees, wasps, fleas, mites (especially *Sarcoptes scabei*), bedbugs, mosquitoes, scorpions, spiders, and jellyfish are included.

VI. Penetrants and Contactants

A wide variety of types of materials may be the cause of urticaria. Possibilities include foods, textiles, animal dander and saliva, plants, medicaments, chemicals, and cosmetics.

VII. Systemic Diseases

This group of disorders is an uncommon cause of urticaria in children. In adults lymphomas, visceral carcinomas, and hyperthyroidism are more prominent as causes. In children juvenile rheumatoid arthritis, systemic lupus erythematosus, acute rheumatic fever, and Henoch–Schönlein purpura must be considered. Urticaria may be an early manifestation of these disorders or be associated with other signs and symptoms. *Urticaria pigmentosa* is usually associated with pigmented macules or nodules; stroking these lesions causes them to become edematous. Hives, bullae, or erythema may occur in areas of skin free of the pigmented lesions.

VIII. Psychogenic Urticaria

Unfortunately, chronic urticaria is often labeled as psychogenic in origin, usually because other causes cannot be found. Chronic pruritic lesions can cause psychological disturbances in almost anyone. Recent evidence indicates that psychological stress may exacerbate urticaria but rarely is the sole cause.

IX. Genetic Disorders

These conditions are rare causes of urticaria. People with hereditary angioneurotic edema do not really develop hives. Others in this group include familial cold urticaria, familial localized heat urticaria, vibratory angioedema, the heredofamilial syndrome of urticaria with deafness and amyloidosis (Muckle–Wells syndrome), and erythropoietic protoporphyria.

X. Physical Factors

A few of the conditions in this category deserve singling out.

A. Dermatographia	Some reviewers estimate that dermatographia accounts for 8% to 9% of all cases of urticaria. Wheal and erythema follow minor stroking or pressure.
B. Cholinergic Factors	From 5% to 7% of all cases of urticaria may be induced by heat, emotion, stress, or exercise. Wheals 1 to 3 mm across are surrounded by large erythematous flares.
C. Cold	Urticaria may be associated with cryoglobulin formation and immune complex disease, especially collagen–vascular diseases, although these are rare in children. An acquired form is characterized by the appearance of wheals in a cold-exposed area after rewarming.
D. Pressure	This form occurs primarily in adolescents. Deep, painful swelling appears 4 to 6 hours following prolonged pressure.
E. Solar	In this uncommon form, pruritus, erythema, and wheals appear within a few minutes of sun exposure. The lesions are localized to exposed skin.

XI. Urticarial Vasculitis

Urticarial lesions tend to remain in the same areas, generally the extremities, for 24 to 72 hours. Malaise, arthralgias, fever, elevated sedimentation rates, and decreased serum complement levels are generally found. The clinical picture may suggest serum sickness.

SUGGESTED READINGS

Harris A, Twarog FJ, Geha RS: Chronic urticaria in childhood: Natural course and etiology. Ann Allergy 51:161–165, 1983

Maize JC: Urticaria. In Demis DJ (ed): Clinical Dermatology, Vol 2, Unit 7–9. Hagerstown, Harper & Row

Monroe EW, Jones HE: Urticaria. Arch Dermatol 113:80–90, 1977

Weston WL: Practical Pediatric Dermatology. Boston, Little, Brown & Co, 1979

Index

Numbers followed by a *t* indicate a table.

ISBN 0-397-50863-8

90000

9 780397 508631